Qualitative Methods for Health Research

INTRODUCING QUALITATIVE METHODS provides a series of volumes which introduce qualitative research to the student and beginning researcher. The approach is interdisciplinary and international. A distinctive feature of these volumes is the helpful student exercises.

One stream of the series provides texts on the key methodologies used in qualitative research. The other stream contains books on qualitative research for different disciplines or occupations. Both streams cover the basic literature in a clear and accessible style, but also cover the 'cutting edge' issues in the area.

For a list of all titles in the series, visit www.sagepub.co.uk/iqm

Qualitative Methods for Health Research

Second Edition

Judith Green and Nicki Thorogood

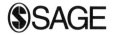

Los Angeles • London • New Delhi • Singapore • Washington DC

First edition 2004
Rprinted 2005
Second edition 2009

SAGE Publications Ltd
1 Oliver's Yard
55 City Road
London EC1Y 1SP

SAGE Publications Inc.
2455 Teller Road
Thousand Oaks, California 91320

SAGE Publications India Pvt Ltd
B 1/I 1 Mohan Cooperative Industrial Area
Mathura Road
New Delhi 110 044

SAGE Publications Asia-Pacific Pte Ltd
33 Pekin Street #02-01
Far East Square
Singapore 048763

Library of Congress Control Number: 2009921347

British Library Cataloguing in Publication data

A catalogue record for this book is available from
the British Library

ISBN 978-1-84787-073-5
ISBN 978-1-84787-074-2 (pbk)

Typeset by C&M Digitals (P) Ltd, Chennai, India
Printed in Great Britain by CPI Antony Rowe, Chippenham, Wiltshire
Printed on paper from sustainable resources

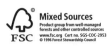

Mixed Sources
Product group from well-managed
forests and other controlled sources
www.fsc.org Cert no. SGS-COC-2953
© 1996 Forest Stewardship Council
FSC

Contents

List of Boxes

List of Case Studies

Preface

The craft skills needed for qualitative research may change rather slowly, but the world in which we use those skills has moved on, even over the five years since the first edition of this textbook. Most obviously, there have been developments in technologies available for computer aided analysis, and an increasing availability of qualitative health research on bibliographic databases, which has made systematic reviews of qualitative research more feasible and useful. These developments are reflected in updated sections of this book, but there have also been changes to the contexts in which qualitative health research gets commissioned and conducted which we have also tried to address. First, the popularity of qualitative methods with policy makers, health research commissioners and health care programme planners has generated more work opportunities for researchers who do not necessarily have a social science background. Second, many health providers are now obliged to 'do research' as part of their professional development, or to contribute to their organisation's commitment to a research based culture. We have explicitly addressed some of these research settings in Chapter 9, given that the traditional orientations of qualitative research can sit uneasily in more applied projects. We have also taken on board comments from many readers that some of the social science terminology and concepts they come across when reading qualitative outputs may be unfamiliar, and that it would be useful to have them explained in an introductory text. These terms include 'phenomenology' and 'reflexivity', which are now explained in more detail. Recognising that few read a textbook sequentially, cover to cover, we have also now included a glossary to aid readers dipping into chapters, who may miss the first explanation of a term.

In general, though, this edition has the same aims and structure as the first. Our aim was to produce a text that predominantly met the needs of our postgraduate students, who have considerable professional experience but little prior knowledge of the social sciences. They come from almost all countries in the world, and want an introduction to qualitative methods that is sensitive to the practicalities of doing sound research on health topics in a wide variety of settings. Although the principles of research design and conduct may be the same wherever it is happening, and whatever the topic studied, clearly the practice is not. First, the context of health research may be rather different from that of general social research. It is increasingly undertaken within multi-disciplinary teams, in which the legitimacy of using qualitative methodologies is still challenged. It is undertaken in institutional contexts (medical schools, health authorities, hospitals) in which the assumed model of research may be clinical, rather than social. Although none of this has any impact on the principles of 'doing good research', it does demand a particular range of skills from the researcher, including the ability to explain those principles to a wide range of collaborators and potential users, and an understanding of why the most common conflicts over issues such as research design may occur. Second, most of the social research texts on the market assume a Western setting, and it may be difficult for a reader to grasp the principles if their initial reaction is 'But that wouldn't work in my country!' The first incentive for producing this text was, then, to provide an introduction to qualitative methods that used examples of health research from a number of different settings, so that we can demonstrate how key methodological issues may have different implications in different contexts. We have been aided in this task by colleagues from the London School of Hygiene and Tropical Medicine who work across the world, and we have used examples from their research liberally to illustrate key points.

Having taught methodology courses to students from a range of low-, middle- and high-income countries, we have realized that there is a huge amount to learn from reflecting on the differences and similarities between what is possible and productive in diverse contexts. Being forced to reflect on, for instance, different assumptions made about research interviews can aid an awareness of the cultural specificity of the interview format in any setting – something we can easily forget if all our interviewees share similar cultural backgrounds to ourselves. Thinking through how the methodological aims may be shaped by practical constraints can be a very useful way of clarifying exactly what our aims are in using particular designs, or particular methods of collecting data. Confronting examples from work in different settings helps all of us challenge our assumptions about what we are trying to do in conducting qualitative research of and for health.

A second incentive for writing this book was to bridge a gap that is sometimes apparent between policy-orientated field guides that aim to provide 'toolboxes' for novice researchers and theoretical introductions to social research that may appear to have little relevance to researchers working in applied areas. A key argument of this book is that good-quality applied qualitative work *has* to be theoretically informed: doing policy-orientated studies is no excuse for poor design, or inadequate attention to methodology. But it is not always obvious how this is to be done, particularly if faced with the constraints of short-term funding or inadequate training in social science methods. We hope this book will help more practically minded researchers to see the value of attending to theoretical issues, both for producing more useful findings and for unpacking some of the debates they will inevitably have about the validity, generalizability and implications of their findings.

Following from this, a third aim of this book is to explore the contribution of qualitative methods to understanding health and health behaviour. Although there is now largely an acceptance of the value of qualitative methods in public health research, many of our students and colleagues still report having to 'justify' their use to collaborators who are sceptical or simply poorly informed. Qualitative researchers still face questions about the validity and generalizability of their methods, and lack of understanding of what qualitative research

aims to do. Throughout this book we have suggested how this kind of scepticism can be met – not to convince our readers, who are presumably already
convinced, but to help in potential discussions with colleagues from other
research traditions. The second edition therefore also includes, in Chapter 1, an
explicit discussion of some of the main criticisms to which qualitative
researchers occasionally have to respond.

   This book is intended primarily, then, for public health, primary care,
health promotion and nursing practitioners and managers, in high-, middle-
or low-income countries, with little previous experience of social science theory, who need to commission, use or conduct qualitative research. The aims
are to introduce readers to some of the debates in qualitative methodology, to
demonstrate the uses of qualitative designs and methods of data generation
in a wide range of health research projects, and to suggest ways of improving
their own research practice. We also hope it will be a useful text for social
research students, in introducing some of the particular methodological possibilities and challenges of researching health.

   The structure of the book is straightforward. The chapters in Part 1 deal
with methodological principles, research designs and ethics. They introduce
some of the key terms used in methodology, and some of the underlying principles of qualitative approaches. Those in Part 2 discuss four common strategies for producing or collecting qualitative data: in-depth interviews, group
interviews, observation and documentary research. These chapters provide
overviews of these methods of generating data and suggestions for improving
research practice. The final chapter in this section is an introduction to some
common ways of analysing qualitative data. Part 3 highlights the practical
issues raised by 'doing' qualitative health research, with chapters on working
in applied and multi-disciplinary settings and on writing and reading qualitative work. Throughout the book we have drawn on examples of social research
on health from a number of settings. Some of these are extended case studies,
which are summaries of published research. It would be helpful to look at the
sources of these wherever possible, as a good way of learning about methods
is to read how others have approached questions of design and conduct. Even
better as a learning tool is *doing* research, and there are suggestions for exercises to develop your own skills at the end of each chapter.

   Finally, we would like to acknowledge the input of our past and current
colleagues and students from the London School of Hygiene and Tropical
Medicine, whose experiences, both published and unpublished, have been
drawn on widely in writing this book and revising it for the second edition.
We are particularly grateful to: the students who have taken Qualitative
Methodologies and the staff and students who have participated in the
Qualitative Analysis workshop over the last few years, whose lively discussions and comments have contributed to many of the ideas here (often in
ways they may not approve of!); Simon Lewin and Gillian Hundt, whose
research experiences have been drawn on in a number of chapters; Geraldine
Barrett, for her contributions to Chapter 8; and Simon Carter, for contributions to Chapter 10. Thanks also to Alvaro Alonso-Garbayo, Jacqueline

Fitzgerald and Catherine Montgomery, whose experiences and suggestions have contributed to the second edition, and to Avril Porter, whose help with the manuscript has been invaluable.

Judith Green and Nicki Thorogood

Part 1

Principles and Approaches in Qualitative Health Research

Qualitative Methodology and Health Research

1

CHAPTER SUMMARY

This chapter introduces the theoretical perspectives that have generated qualitative research both of and for health, and argues that an understanding of these is vital for both conducting good quality research and for researching in a multidisciplinary environment. Some broad orientations common to much qualitative research are then outlined, and the criticisms these can attract from other approaches discussed. The contribution of qualitative research to areas such as public health, health promotion and health services research is identified as that of providing contextual, in-depth understanding of the perspectives of participants.

Introduction

'Health' and 'illness' have long been topics of interest for social science disciplines such as sociology, social anthropology and history.

- *Sociology* is the study of human society. It has traditionally focused on developed countries, with the sociology of health and illness addressing such issues as concepts of health and illness, inequalities in health, experiences of health and health care systems (Annandale 1998).

- *Social anthropology*, the study of people in the context of culture and society, has traditionally studied cultures 'other' than that of the researcher. Medical anthropologists have focused on how a society's beliefs and practices relating to health and illness (including healing systems and folk practices) are embedded in other aspects of its culture (Helman 1984).
- *History of medicine* has contributed to understanding the history of medicine and medical knowledge, understanding the role of health and illness in social history, and to policy studies in the health arena (James 1994).

Maintaining health and dealing with ill health are universal challenges, and there is now a large research literature within these disciplines on how these have been accomplished over time and across different human societies. Health professionals have a long history of integrating insights from social science research into their understanding of human health (see, for instance, Henderson 1935; Kleinman 1973; Helman 1984). More recently, the *methods* of social research have become an accepted part of health research in areas such as public health, primary care, health promotion and nursing. Disciplines such as sociology, social anthropology and history have their own methodological traditions, but have in common perhaps a focus on human behaviour in context, whether social, cultural or historical. Health care practitioners, managers and policy-makers have increasingly turned to the qualitative methods of social inquiry used within the social sciences to enhance understanding of health, health behaviour and health services, and to improve the management and provision of health services. As the problems of public health are increasingly those of human behaviour, rather than the development of new technical interventions, those trained primarily in health sciences, such as medicine or nursing, are turning to social research to help understand how to improve health and health care. This book is intended for both qualitative social scientists interested in applying their disciplines to health research, and for health professionals interested in using qualitative research approaches.

We focus on the particular contribution of qualitative research methods to health research. What we mean by 'health research' includes two broad strands of work. First are critical studies *of* health from various social science perspectives, which address questions such as: What are health and illness? How are they managed, and in whose interests? Second are studies *for* health, from within the disciplines of public health, health promotion or health services research, in which the contributions of social science are defined in terms of the health agenda. The distinction between these two sorts of investigation is perhaps a useful one for thinking about the aims of the study. (Is it basic research, aiming to expand our knowledge of society, or applied research, aiming to address an existing health care problem?) How the two kinds of investigation are written up may also differ, in order to meet the expectations of different intended audiences (see Chapter 10). However, the distinction does not imply different criteria for methodological rigour. Doing applied research *for* health is not an excuse for inadequate research design, a superficial approach to data collection or under-theorized analysis. Producing useful findings involves, as a necessary condition, producing sound findings. Indeed, if the research has been funded to produce policy-relevant findings, there is perhaps even more reason for rigorous design and analysis. The principles of qualitative research are, therefore, exactly the same, whether the study is primarily academic (such as a PhD thesis in Anthropology) or more 'applied', such as a funded evaluation of a health care project. Similarly, the same principles of good design and conduct apply whether the research setting is a health service organization in a high-income country, or a rural village in a low-income country. Clearly the practicalities of carrying out the study will differ, but we hope to show how the same elements of research planning are involved. Whatever the setting, the researcher has to consider the local cultural and social context, and this is an essential part of adapting methodological techniques to a particular research project. Throughout this book we have used examples from a variety of settings, and we hope this range will illustrate the universal applicability of methodological principles.

What is qualitative research?

Health research, then, includes any study addressing understandings of human health, health behaviour or health services, whatever the disciplinary starting point. What is meant by 'qualitative' research is perhaps more contentious. Some have seen the division between 'quantitative' and 'qualitative' approaches as a false one, and it is perhaps impossible (and unhelpful) to characterize qualitative research in a way that is completely separate from quantitative research. Although qualitative research tends to use language data (written or oral), and quantitative research numerical data, for instance, this is not always the case. Many qualitative studies use simple frequency counts, whereas language data can be used in quantitative studies. Although qualitative research tends to have smaller sample sizes, it certainly does not follow that any study with a small sample is a qualitative study.

There are some methods of data collection that are particularly associated with qualitative research. These are discussed in the chapters in Part 2 of this book. However, these methods of data collection can also be used in quantitative studies, so it is not merely the way in which data are collected (such as through an interview, or by observation) that characterizes a study as qualitative. It might be more useful to characterize qualitative research not by the kind of data produced or the methods used to produce them, but by the overall aims of the study. The most basic way of characterizing qualitative studies is to describe their aims as seeking answers to questions about the 'what', 'how' or 'why' of a phenomenon, rather than questions about 'how many' or 'how much'. Box 1.1 shows some examples of qualitative research studies reported in social science and biomedical journals, together with their main methods of data collection and the stated aims of the study.

Note that many of the studies in Box 1.1 have 'examine' or 'explore' as an aim. These are studies which were conducted to understand more about a phenomenon, rather than 'measure' it, and to investigate health, illness or health services from the perspective of the communities and individuals affected, or the professionals who provide health services for them. Understanding questions such as these as legitimate aims for research is the consequence of having a particular theoretical perspective on the role of knowledge, how we acquire it from research activities, and what 'counts' as valid knowledge about the world. Although theoretical assumptions in research articles are not often made explicit, they nonetheless frame the kinds of questions researchers decide to ask, how they go about answering them, and how debates about the soundness of their findings are conducted. Therefore, a consideration of the theoretical approaches and broad orientations that are typical of qualitative approaches is fundamental to understanding the contribution of qualitative research to the study of health.

Box 1.1	**Some examples of qualitative health research questions**	
Title of paper	**Methods of data collection**	**Aims**
Using qualitative methods to understand the determinants of patients' willingness to pay for cataract surgery: a study in Tanzania (Geneau et al. 2008)	Semi-structured interviews, informal discussions	'to understand better cataract patients' willingness to pay for surgery'
Cancer patients' information needs and help-seeking behaviour (Leydon et al. 2000)	In-depth interviews	'to explore why cancer patients do not want or seek information about their condition other than that supplied by physicians'
Doctor in the house (Hardey 1999)	Household interviews	'[to examine] the internet as a source of knowledge about health in relation to the broader sociological debates about deprofessionalization and consumerism'

| Leprosy among the Limba (Opala and Boillot 1996) | In-depth interviews | 'examines Limba concepts of leprosy within the wider context of Limba world view' |
| Parents' perspectives on the MMR immunization (Evans et al. 2001) | Focus group interviews | 'to investigate what influences parents' decisions on whether to accept or refuse ... [measles, mumps and rubella] immunization' |

Theoretical approaches

'Theory' is central to research, even the most applied research. By this we do not mean that researchers have to start with grand theoretical concerns, or that research should be testing or building theory. Some studies are designed to do this, but many other health research projects are properly designed to address empirical questions, without any explicit theoretical aims. In Box 1.1, for instance, the study of parents' perspectives on MMR immunization (Evans et al. 2001) is designed to examine how parents make decisions in this particular context, not to generate theory about decision making in general, although of course it may do this as well. However, whether we are aware of it or not, theoretical assumptions about how the world works, and how health care, illness behaviour or doctor–patient interaction are organized, do frame the kinds of questions that are considered important, or legitimate, to ask and how we choose to answer them. There are several ways in which theory does this. First, there are what could be called large-scale, or macro, theories about the social world and how it works.

Macro theory

'Macro' theoretical perspectives frame particular issues as 'puzzles' or questions requiring research because they entail particular assumptions about the way the world is, and how people behave within it. These might include questions such as: 'Is it inevitable that wealth is unequally distributed?' 'Is there a real world of physical objects that exist separate from and independent of our perceptions of them?' One well-known example of macro-theory is the *materialist approach*, which is built on an assumption that the material sphere of life (such as economic relations) determines other aspects, such as culture. In this tradition, Karl Marx developed his theory of class relations to explain both the contemporary situation and to predict future social patterns. The basis of his theory was the inevitable conflict produced between those who *own* the means of generating wealth (the means of production) – that is, the ruling class – and those who have to sell their labour – that is, the working class. This is an economic theory of production using generalizable concepts.

It is, nevertheless, not the only way of explaining that particular set of social relations, and other economists, Adam Smith for example, observed the same phenomena (the effects of industrialization) and theorized that the division was not only inevitable, but also that it was uncontentious. Other social theorists (rather than economists) working at a similar period to Marx also produced explanations of these conditions but proposed that the social processes to which they gave rise were a matter of consensus between the different interest groups. Thus one of the major divisions in social theory has been between those who take a 'conflict' and those who take a 'consensus' perspective. Clearly this initial position about the way in which the social world works will lead to very different ideas about how to make sense of other social phenomena, and indeed whether they are even framed as puzzles or problems at all. Thus, if you take a Marxist view of industrial relations, conflict between workers and bosses, for example in the form of strikes, would seem entirely expected – and harmonious periods of production would be puzzling and might suggest a modification of the theory was needed. In contrast, a consensus theorist would feel that a period of dispute was an anomaly. Large-scale, or macro, theory allows questions to be asked at the higher level of social organization. Examples would include questions about the relationship between social class and ill health, or indeed poverty and ill health, or about the effects of globalization, or if 'globalization' is a phenomenon that exists.

A larger set of presumptions or particular world-view will, then, frame any social inquiry. For the most part, however, these remain implicit. Few researchers state the assumptions they have about the social order, and why these have shaped their particular research question as a legitimate one, or as a puzzle that needs explaining. Nevertheless, we believe it is important to bear in mind that all researchers will have a particular world-view, or theoretical perspective, which both underpins and shapes their project and its findings.

Middle-range theory

As well as shaping inquiry at the most abstract level, macro-theory also generates what we could call 'middle-range theories' that link concepts together, and sometimes generate hypotheses to be tested, or interesting questions to address. Middle-range theories are the link between the general, abstract concepts of macro-theory (social class, gender, globalization and so on) and the grounded, observable behaviour of people in everyday settings. Thus, in understanding specific social issues, such as ill health, the concepts of 'health' or 'illness' that are employed will generally be derived from a larger scale – if taken for granted – theory about the way the world works. These might lead to questions such as: What is the relationship between employment and health? Or, are women's experiences of health care different from those of men? In Box 1.1, for instance, the aims of Hardey's (1999) study of how people use the internet to access health information explicitly cite debates about 'deprofessionalization and consumerism'. These are middle-range theoretical concepts that he has drawn on to generate research questions. How users of the internet use the information they find becomes an interesting question in the light of theories about deprofessionalization (that, for instance, the power of medicine is in decline because of the public's greater access to health knowledge) and consumerism (that treating health as any other commodity may change the ways in which we access health care). As another example, the study by Geneau el al. (2008) in Box 1.1 aimed to understand how decisions were taken in Tanzania about patients' willingness to pay for surgery for cataracts. The authors begin their paper with a discussion about economic theory related to the concept of 'willingness to pay', much of which arises from utility theory, which assumes that people act to maximize the most 'rational' outcomes. Such a theory would predict that for sight-saving surgery with minimal risk, patients would have a high willingness to pay, in order to maximize a valued state (good eyesight). The qualitative research conducted for this study questions these theoretical assumptions, as the researchers found that in practice decisions about paying for health care in Tanzania were household, not individual decisions, and willingness to pay was related more to the resources a patient might reasonably expect to muster across the extended family than it was to their own individual assessments of utility.

So middle-range theory generates the particular questions we ask, and the findings of qualitative studies may add to the body of theory at this level, as in the case of Geneau et al. (2008), who suggest a significant limitation in the ability of utility theory to explain health care decisions in settings such as Tanzania. Middle-range theories are often rooted in particular disciplines, and we acquire our knowledge of them through training as nurses, doctors, sociologists, psychologists, economists and so on. For example, if we take the study listed in Box 1.1 by Maggie Evans and colleagues on how parents make a decision to have their children immunized, there are a number of theoretical approaches that might have had relevance within different disciplines. Each would imply a rather different research question, with preferred ways of finding out the answer. Box 1.2 suggests, in summary form, some 'middle-range theories' associated with particular disciplines or professional knowledge that might influence other studies on this topic.

The suggested questions in Box 1.2 are all potentially interesting and legitimate, but our professional and academic training means that we are more familiar with some of these bodies of theory than others. When we are considering a particular topic, we draw upon these explanations (of how professionals and clients relate, or how individuals make decisions) to shape specific questions that are interesting because they relate to a broader body of theory. Social science disciplines such as sociology and psychology tend to be more explicit about these kinds of theory than biomedical sciences, but health professionals also have a set of more or less formal explanatory models they can draw on to make sense of topics as research questions. The advantages and challenges of working across disciplines, when we are often combining not just methods of data collection, but also these kinds of theoretical approaches, are discussed in Chapter 9.

As an example of how middle-range theory informs both the framing of particular issues as research problems, and the ways in which we can understand them, consider the example of Rachel Jewkes and colleagues' (1998) work on nurse–patient interactions in South Africa's obstetric public health services. Jewkes et al. found evidence of widespread abuse of patients by nurses, including clinical neglect, scolding, humiliating, and even slapping women in labour. Although widely recognized as a 'problem' in South Africa, and commonly talked about by both patients and nurses they interviewed, it had not been recognized as a policy problem by professional organizations, nor had it been the object of research aimed at finding solutions. That the researchers could frame what is presumably an everyday feature of normal life as a research question ('Why do nurses abuse patients?') relies first of all on a body of nursing theory that constructs the nurse's role as one of caring, nurturing and compassion. Without a normative theory of how things 'should' be (that is, nurses should be caring, not abusive), the behaviour they documented could not be constructed as a problem to be understood. Second, although participants' accounts focused on the personal characteristics of individual nurses as the cause of the problem, the researchers could draw on a number of theoretical perspectives to make sense of the problem in a way that suggested particular solutions. These included accounts of the ethnic and class basis of the South African social structure, which makes the nurses' social position precarious; in this kind of social context, abusing patients may be one route for symbolically stressing the social distance between themselves and their patients.

Box 1.2	Researching parents' decisions about childhood immunizations: possible theoretical starting points for research	
Middle-range theory	**Possible research questions**	**Main discipline**
The *health belief model* (Becker 1974) suggests that the likelihood of an individual engaging in a particular behaviour results from their assessment of the costs and benefits of that action, and their perceived vulnerability to illness	What risks and benefits do parents associate with the immunization? How susceptible do they think children are to measles, mumps and rubella?	Psychology

Lack of 'compliance' with health advice reflects, in part, failures of health professional-client communication	Are parents more likely to 'comply' with immunizations if they have an opportunity to discuss their worries with a health professional?	General practice
There is 'lay epidemiology' (Rogers and Pilgrim 1995) of risks associated with immunizations that may be different from that of experts	What sources of knowledge do parents draw on to assess the risks of immunization? How do experts and non-professionals explain these risks?	Sociology

Theories of knowledge

A third level of theory that researchers have to consider relates to theories of knowledge, or ideas about how we come to *know* the world, and have faith in the truth, or **validity,** of that knowledge. The theory of knowledge belongs to a branch of philosophy called **epistemology.** As research is essentially about producing knowledge about the world that we can claim as valid, some attention to epistemology is vital. Different epistemological traditions imply different ways of 'knowing' the world, and rather different accounts of the status of that knowledge. Most societies, for instance, include healers from a number of traditions who base their work on very different epistemologies; that is, different understandings of what leads to health or illness, different understandings of how the body works, and different understandings of how the healer can diagnose a problem. An illustration comes from a series called 'Second Opinion', that ran in the *Observer* newspaper, which used this contrast in a weekly article from two practitioners, one a general practitioner with a biomedical training, the other an Ayurvedic practitioner. Box 1.3 illustrates how the different epistemological assumptions of the two approaches lead to very different advice for potential clients.

There are clear implications for health research in these contrasting understandings of 'health' and what it is. If, for example, these two practitioners wanted to research the efficacy of their remedies, they would be asking slightly different questions. The biomedically trained general practitioner may be more interested in how the drugs reduce symptoms framed by a biomedical understanding of the 'disease' of arthritis, whereas the Ayurvedic practitioner might be interested in how well remedies detoxify the body. Understanding how different disciplinary traditions generate different legitimate research questions and different ways of convincingly answering them is key to working in multi-disciplinary settings. However, it is not always as easy to identify the different frameworks used by researchers as it is to identify the kinds of differences outlined in the box between different healing traditions, because they are rarely explicitly discussed, or set out as an obvious contrast. *Many debates about the value of research findings are rooted in epistemological differences between researchers in terms of what kind of knowledge they believe research should produce, or what counts as adequate evidence for conclusions to be drawn.* For this reason, it is worth outlining some of the main epistemological starting points of research, to help unpack the assumptions on which research knowledge is built. These will help you understand the kinds of knowledge produced by qualitative research, and the particular contribution they make. Many of the epistemological assumptions of qualitative research arise from a critique of **positivism**; that is, an approach to knowledge rooted in what early social scientists saw as the methods of the natural sciences.

Positivism

Over the last few hundred years the natural sciences, and many of the more quantitative social sciences, have developed a broad view of science and knowledge

Box 1.3	**How to deal with rheumatoid arthritis: different epistemological approaches**	
	Biomedically trained general practitioner	**Ayurvedic practitioner**
Cause	'the body produces antibodies to its own immunoglobulins'	'aggravated vata [air element] combined with an increase in ama or toxins in the body'
Advice	'rehabilitation programme of exercise, physiotherapy and patient education designed to improve muscle strength, encourage mobility and prevent depression'	'Panchakarma, a detoxification and rejuvenation treatment ... oil massage with mahanaraya oil ... a vata balancing diet with rice, vegetables and lentils'
Prognosis	'... there is no cure ... and a high incidence of serious side effects from drugs'	'good results ... [from] an anti-arthritic formula [of] anti-inflammatory herbs'
Source: *Observer Magazine, 30 June 2002*		

that has been described as 'positivism'. A positivist philosophy is one that assumes that there is a stable reality 'out there' – that phenomena (such as diseases, bacteria, villages, health) exist whether we are looking at them or not, and that they exist in exactly the same way whether we understand them or not. Thus, human understanding may be flawed (in, for instance, believing malaria to be caused by 'bad air'), but there is a potential 'right' explanation. There is also an implicit notion of progress in positivist accounts, that suggests that as knowledge gradually increases, we progress towards a better understanding of health and disease. The implications of this starting point for research methods are threefold. First, there is a stress on *empiricism*, or studying only observable phenomena. At the beginning of the 'scientific revolution', this was an innovation, in terms of replacing the philosophical speculations of pre-Enlightenment scientists with a science grounded in the experimental method and on observations of the natural world. The second implication is known as the *unity of method*, the idea that eventually, when mature, all sciences will share the same methods of inquiry. At this point of maturity, the proper object of scientific inquiry is the establishment of relationships of cause and effect and the generation of laws about the natural world. That many of the social sciences focus on other questions is, in this view, evidence of their immaturity. Because we understand, as yet, little about human behaviour, we have not got to the point where we can look for relationships between cause and effect. A third element of a positivist approach is the emphasis on *value-free inquiry*. Science is held to be separate from society, and as objective, rational and neutral. In this view, knowledge derived from proper scientific inquiry is not bound up with emotional, subjective or political viewpoints, and is 'true' for all times and places.

This model of scientific inquiry has come under considerable criticism, from both those who see it as an idealized model of how scientific progress happens and those who see it as an inappropriate model for research, particularly social research. In the qualitative social sciences, research is often rooted in rather different epistemological traditions, which depart from one or more tenets of positivism.

Interpretative approaches

Some have seen a positivist view as an unachievable and inappropriate goal for research into human behaviour. Human beings differ in some essential respects from the objects of natural science inquiry. Unlike atoms (or plants or planets), human beings make sense of their place in the world, have views about researchers who are studying them, and behave in ways that are not determined in law-like ways. They are complex, unpredictable, and reflect on their behaviour. Therefore, the methods and aims of the natural sciences are unlikely to be useful for studying people and social behaviour: instead of explaining people and society, research should aim to understand human behaviour. This is the starting point of the *interpretative approach*. In this view, the most interesting questions are not about the 'reality' of the world, but about people's interpretations of it. Thus, if we were interested in how people took medication for their asthma, we might be more interested not in any objective reality of the severity of symptoms, but rather in patients' interpretations of their symptoms, since these may tell us more about how they use medication. This interpretative tradition characterizes much qualitative work in health research, which focuses on the meaning of phenomena (such as symptoms, health behaviours) for people. Case Study 1.1 illustrates an example of research in this tradition, and many other case studies throughout this book draw on interpretative approaches. Case Study 5.2, for instance, summarizes a study of how people interpret media messages about HIV and AIDS and Case Study 8.1 describes research on the meaning of glaucoma diagnoses and symptoms for patients. The aim of interpretative research is an understanding of the world from the point of view of participants in it, rather than deriving an explanation of the world.

Phenomenology

Many interpretative traditions are rooted in the philosophical approaches of **phenomenology,** and the writings of the philosopher Edmund Husserl (1970) and sociologist Alfred Schutz (1964, 1970) (see also Holstein and Gubrium 1998). Husserl, writing in the first decade of the twentieth century, posited that the distinction made by natural science between subject and object was false as everything was subject to the act of perception. He argued that objects in the world were not passively understood, but were actively constituted through consciousness and subjective experience. To understand the 'essence' of phenomena, one had to understand how the 'life-world' was directly experienced. The **methodology** he described for doing this was called 'reduction', by which he meant a process of attempting to 'bracket off' the conceptualizations, prejudices and theories by which we come to understand phenomena and attempt to get to their universal and essential nature, which is experienced directly. Schutz is associated with bringing these philosophical ideas into sociology, and his approach focused on the ways in which the 'life-world' (the everyday world which we experience and take for granted) was actively constituted by 'members' (social actors within that world). In terms of epistemological position, this is clearly a departure from positivist social science, as the 'life-world' is not merely there, passively experienced, but is created through talk, interaction and behaviour. Following Husserl, Schutz's methodological stance is also one of 'bracketing' (or setting aside) taken-for-granted assumptions about the world (whether they are from 'common sense' or grand theory) and attending closely to how members themselves orientate to phenomena. This is not the same as attempting to be 'objective', in the positivist sense, but rather an attempt to open up to how the life-world is experienced. In this approach, then, phenomena are real because they are treated as real; whether they 'really' exist, objectively speaking, is irrelevant, as the 'essence' of objects can only be understood through studying subjective perceptions of those objects.

Therefore, a phenomenological researcher interested in studying medical dominance on a hospital ward might be interested in questions such as 'What is the lived experience of medical dominance?' and might focus on how dominance is created, at an everyday level, through the talk and inter-action of members such as doctors and nurses, with the focus of enquiry being how 'dominance' as a phenomenon is actually constituted through what people say and do, through the stock of common-sense understandings that members draw upon in their day to day lives. Social life on the ward would be seen as a 'taken-for-granted' accomplishment, one that happens because in general we all assume that others routinely share our under-standings and perceptions of phenomena. Unless there is some obvious breach in this sense of shared understanding, we are often oblivious to the 'taken-for-granted' nature of the life-world.

Phenomenological approaches have been particularly popular in qualita-tive research in nursing. The appeal lies in part in the focus on subjectivity, and perhaps also on the possibilities of identifying the 'essences' of what can be diffuse concepts used in nursing practice, such as 'caring' or 'comfort'. As illustrations, these aims are taken from three published qualitative nursing studies that overtly situate themselves as phenomenological research to:

- 'describe the lived experiences of men and women who suffer from psori-asis' (Watson and Bruin 2007)
- 'explore the meaning of comfort care for hospice nurses' (Evans and Hallett 2007)
- 'investigate the meaning of living with cancer in old age' (Thomé et al. 2004).

The focus of each of these studies was on experiences and meanings, and attempting to identify what was unique about those meanings. Thomé et al. (2004) suggest that in investigating the experience of living with cancer in old age, their aim was to identify: 'What is it that makes this lived experience what it is?' and 'What is unique about this?'

Social constructionism

The interpretive and phenomenological approaches overlap considerably, in that they focus explicitly on either interpretations or experiences of the world as it is subjectively understood, rather than attempting to explain the objective reality of the world. A second criticism of positivist assumptions that has informed much qualitative work is a more extreme questioning of the view that there is one stable, pre-existing reality 'out there' waiting to be discov-ered. The *social constructionist* (sometimes called 'constructivist') approach instead assumes that reality is socially constructed. How we divide up the world in order to comprehend it (for instance, how we see the systems of the body, or how we classify diseases) is the result of historical, social and politi-cal processes, rather than an inevitable result of our greater understanding of the 'reality' of the body, or disease. The proper object of research from this perspective is thus how phenomena are constructed: what are the processes by which diseases become classified in particular ways, who has the power to produce legitimate classifications, and what are the implications of such classifications? There is a strong tradition of constructionism in the qualitative social sciences in health, which has had a vital role in questioning common-sense assumptions about the categories we use routinely, as if they were 'natural' categories, rather than social ones. One example is described in Case Study 7.1, which shows how Sudden Infant Death Syndrome can be analysed as a socially constructed category.

The **constructionist approach,** although an influential one in qualitative research, has not been without its critics. Mike Bury (1986), for instance, takes issue with the **relativism** implied by an extreme constructionist position, claiming it poses a logical difficulty. If phenomena such as disease categories are merely 'social constructions', he argues, rather than categories of the natural world, how are we to derive knowledge of them, other than through similarly constituted social categories? There is no rational basis to make a claim for producing valid knowledge of socially constructed phenomena, as there is no sense in which the researcher can 'stand outside' the constructions that he or she is analysing. Bury warns that an extreme agnosticism about the natural world can mean that 'reality is portrayed as a contingent and haphazard affair' (Bury 1986:155). In the arena of health and illness, where research deals with phenomena such as distress, pain and death, such an extreme view, he suggests, is untenable and unhelpful.

Case Study 1.1   Using qualitative research to explore patient understandings of asthma

(Source: Adams, S., Pill, R. and Jones, A. (1997) 'Medication, chronic illness and identity: the perspectives of people with asthma', *Social Science and Medicine*, 45: 189–201)

Asthma is a common condition, and from the perspective of health professionals, there is a problem in that many patients don't take medication as prescribed: the medication intended to prevent symptoms (the 'preventor') may not be taken at all, and the medication intended to relieve symptoms (the 'reliever') is often over-used. Adams and colleagues note that such apparently irrational behaviour is understandable if we look at the patients' perspective – how they understand symptoms and medications, and how these are managed within everyday lives. The study used in-depth interviews with a sample of patients on preventative asthma medication. After analysing patients' accounts, the researchers identified three broad groups in their sample.

First were the 'deniers'. These patients, about half of the sample, denied that they had asthma, although they had been identified from general practice records as people diagnosed with asthma and prescribed preventative medication. However, these patients did not see themselves as asthmatic, but saw their problems as 'chest trouble' or bronchitis. They also claimed that symptoms did not interfere with everyday life, despite at times using quite complex or drastic strategies to manage symptoms, such as complete avoidance of going outdoors. This group also hid their medication use to a large extent, reporting only using inhalers out of sight of others, and had negative views of asthmatics – an identity they did not accept for themselves. Most did not use preventative medications at all – partly because of worry that they would become dependent on drugs that have to be taken daily, but also because taking medication regularly, whether there are symptoms or not, relies on accepting an asthmatic identity, which these 'deniers' did not. Given that they didn't see themselves as having asthma, they did not attend special clinics for asthma patients.

A smaller group within the sample accepted both the diagnosis and their doctors' advice completely, using medications as prescribed and taking pride in doing so. For this group, the route to 'normal life' was gaining adequate control over symptoms through medication. Their definitions of asthma coincided with those of medical professionals. For them, 'asthmatic' was not a stigmatized identity, and they used inhalers in public.

The final group was identified as the 'pragmatists'. This group did use preventative medication, usually not as prescribed, however, but only when their asthma was particularly bad. They also had a pragmatic approach to disclosing asthma diagnosis; for instance, in telling family but not employers in case it prejudiced their employment prospects. This group accepted they had asthma, but usually perceived it as mild, or as an acute rather than chronic illness.

Looking at medication use from the point of view of patients enabled the researchers to see how health behaviour was tied tightly to people's beliefs about asthma and what kind of chest problems they had, as well as social circumstances and the threat of an asthmatic identity to other social identities. For service providers and health promoters, this kind of information is very useful. First it suggests that providing designated asthma clinics may not appeal to the majority of sufferers, since they don't identify themselves as having asthma. Second, professionals can see that what appears to be irrational use of medication, and the result of ignorance, is actually deeply embedded in complex social identities that have to be managed. For patients, health, defined in medical terms, may not be the top priority all the time, and the meaning of symptoms for professionals may be rather different from the meaning of symptoms for patients.

The 'constructionist' approach could, then, be seen as the opposite end of a continuum to the positivist one in terms of assumptions about the nature of reality, with positivism assuming that reality is entirely separate from human perception, and stable, and constructionists assuming that reality is an outcome of human processes, and impossible to separate from the processes from which it is constituted. Where an individual researcher stands on this continuum is largely a matter of their *a priori* assumptions about the nature of reality. It is impossible to 'test' the extent to which phenomena exist independent of our attempts to study them. There is no right approach to research, but these perspectives do generate rather different possible questions about a research topic. To follow on from the example of asthma in Case Study 1.1, for instance, rather than asking 'How do people cope with asthma?' or 'How do patients interpret symptoms?', a social constructionist research study might start with questions such as 'How and why did "asthma" emerge as a category of disease?' (see Gabbay 1982 for one perspective on this) or 'How do some people come to be defined as "asthma patients"?' Even if questions like these are not core to the research, they can be very useful for sensitizing researchers to be critical of the categories they do use. They would suggest, for instance, that we treat statistics about asthma rates with a critical eye. If rates of asthma diagnosis are rising, this might represent a growing number of cases of asthma, but it also might represent the different ways in which the category 'asthma' is being constructed by the patients, health professionals, researchers and record keepers who create those statistics through social processes.

Interpretative and phenomenological approaches, then, start with a different aim from positivist ones – that of understanding, rather than explaining, reality. Constructionist approaches go further, in taking issue with the very concept of a pre-existing reality.

Critical approaches

A third set of criticisms of positivism has questioned the third tenet of positivism: that scientific enquiry should properly be 'value-free'. These criticisms are of two sorts:

1 First, is the criticism that the notion of science being 'value-free' is an *idealistic* view: 'scientific research' is in itself a social process, carried out by humans within specific social contexts, so it cannot be separate from or outside our social world (that is, research *can't* be value-free).
2 Second, there is a criticism that 'value-free' enquiry is a morally indefensible position. There are some perspectives, for example some feminist and participatory approaches, that explicitly assume research should have a political goal as well as a purely knowledge-generating one. In these models, science should not stand outside society, but should acknowledge that it is inextricably bound up with the social order, and be striving to improve that social order (that is, research *shouldn't* be value-free).

A rejection of the 'value-free' aims of research is central to the *critical tradition* in social research, which Lee Harvey described as having the following elements:

> [The critical tradition] regards the positivistic scientific method as unsatisfactory because it deals only with surface appearances. Instead, critical social research methodology cuts through surface appearance. It does so by locating social phenomena in their specific historical context ... within a prevailing social structure. Critical social research analyses this structure ... and its ideological manifestations and processes. ... Critical social research includes an overt political struggle against oppressive social structures. (Harvey 1990: 19–20)

For Harvey, the distinguishing element of critical methodology is that epistemology and critique are intertwined: there can be no pure knowledge, and the task of methodology is to unpack the status of knowledge, and the processes by which it comes to be accepted. This perspective covers a number of traditions in the social sciences. One is the feminist approach, which has had a significant impact on the development of qualitative methodology in terms of positing rather different goals from the traditional ones of value-free inquiry.

Feminist approaches

The advent of 'second wave' feminist activism in the late 1960s has been mirrored by the development of feminist theory and research both within and outside the academy. This was notable in that it highlighted the relationship between knowledge and power, not just that knowledge enables empowerment but that the legitimation of knowledge claims is tied to social structures of domination. To this end, feminist theorists demonstrated that what counted as 'knowledge' reflected a masculine world-view – for example, reflecting only male experiences or concerns. Underlying this perspective is a notion of *difference*, whether it was to claim that men and women are *essentially* different (i.e., that, to some extent, biology is destiny) or that men and women occupy different *social* positions and therefore have very different world-views and experiences. This caused the claims of natural science to objectivity to be called into question. If knowledge supposedly mirrors an independently existing world, how do we account for the different subjectivities of women and men? This led to the development of the feminist 'standpoint theorists'. These included Sandra Harding (1986), who argued that all knowledge is produced by social subjects, and knowledge that is being produced predominantly by men about a world that is predicated on male experiences and views cannot be held to be objective. What this therefore implies is the need for an explicitly feminist science.

However, one of the earliest tensions within feminist theorizing arose from this. Feminism as a social movement is (in common with other social movements such as the black, gay, peace or ecological movements) an emancipatory project. It has its roots in Enlightenment ideals of justice and freedom; that is, a commitment to social change. Nonetheless, it also shares with the theories that underpin these other social movements a critique of these ideals. Notions of 'justice' and 'freedom' imply an absolute, objective existence independent of any power relations, but this becomes untenable in the face of the critique of 'objectivity' and the commitment to making the subjectivity of knowledge claims explicit. A further debate in feminist theorizing was over the principle of essentialism or relativism. This called into question the very existence of the categories 'male' and 'female'. Feminist theorists such as those of the French psychoanalytical school (see, for example, Irigaray 1985; Wittig 1992) attempted to examine the processes by which subjects came to have a gendered consciousness. Others, from more sociological traditions, such as Judith Butler (1990) and Donna Haraway (1991), have addressed the concept of gender as a social construction as part of the 'postmodern' turn in social theory.

In research terms it is clear that the particular feminist epistemological framework adopted, whether standpoint or constructionist, will determine both the research question and the subsequent research design.

Participatory research

This brief review of positivism and the alternatives that have informed qualitative methodologies illustrates the range of epistemological starting points of qualitative enquiry. These different perspectives shape the kinds of questions the researcher is likely to ask about their topic of interest, as well as the methods they will employ. They also, as we have seen, imply some rather different approaches to the overall aims of research, with the critical traditions in particular often having an explicit political aim as well as one of generating knowledge. This section takes this final critique of positivism as noted – that research *shouldn't* be value-free – in outlining some of the participatory approaches that are used in health research. Participatory approaches are often rooted not just in an epistemological critique of positivism, but also in an ethical critique of the relationships generated by traditional scientific practice. From this perspective, one consequence of striving for an objective and neutral scientific method, as positivist researchers do, is a consolidation of knowledge within a small elite, and an unhealthy separation of scientists from the wider society. Following on from this, researchers from participatory traditions see research as ideally a cooperative enterprise, involving working with communities as co-investigators. For some, this has liberationist aims, and the purpose of research should be to engage in dialogue with oppressed people in order to further emancipation or critical awareness.

This liberationist philosophy often cites the work of Paolo Freire, the radical Brazilian educator who believed that education should be empowering and liberating, rather than a process of teaching passive subjects to accept their place in the world. These ideas have been taken up by health workers and researchers in a number of settings (see for example Wallerstein and

Bernstein 1988), with the starting point being a dialogue with the community, such that knowledge (whether the product of education or research) is the outcome of a process of sharing, reflection, and experience, rather than a process of experts either inserting or extracting information. Wallerstein and Bernstein describe how this approach informed an alcohol and substance abuse prevention programme in New Mexico, and discuss the implications of a participatory approach for their evaluation of the programme. This worked with school students, involving them in visits to an emergency room and in interviewing people in jail about the role of substance abuse in their lives. The young people were included as co-learners, rather than passive subjects of health education, and were encouraged to develop solutions to community problems through peer support and a three stage process of listening, dialogue and action. In terms of evaluation, the researchers used an experimental design (with the random allocation of students to the programme) to measure changes in such outcomes as students' risk perceptions and reported behaviour. The researchers note that this rather positivist research design (with its assumptions that an intervention will have a measurable, objective effect on an outcome) sits uneasily with the participatory need to be responsive to the needs of communities engaged in the project, as some were unwilling to participate in an experimental evaluation. These tensions between the different aims of large programmes are discussed further in Chapter 9.

Peter Reason (1998) has identified three strands in participatory inquiry, which he labels cooperative inquiry, participatory **action research** and action inquiry. Cooperative inquiry assumes first that all actors are self-determining – in any research project, all involved are both researchers and subjects, cooperating by reflexively drawing upon their own experiences. Participatory action research is explicit about the relationship between knowledge and power, seeing the role of the researcher as liberating communities through research activities that shift the balance of knowledge. The aims are thus to produce understanding that is useful for the group that is being worked with, and to empower those people, rather than to do research 'on' them. Action inquiry is primarily orientated towards change, but involves a conscious approach to action, in which an organization or community develops a collaborative and reflexive awareness. The three approaches, he argues, share an epistemological focus on experiential knowledge, and an orientation towards change (in both understanding and social reality). They differ in the relative emphasis they place on psychological or small group processes relative to macro-structural factors.

Although the emancipatory aims of participatory approaches are perhaps more associated with research in developing country settings (see, for instance, Case Study 2.2, which used participatory methods as part of an evaluation of a sexual health programme in The Gambia), the collaborative and action-orientated elements of these approaches have influenced health care researchers in developed country settings as well. Julienne Meyer, for instance, has written widely on the challenges of using action research methods in nursing research in the UK (Meyer 1993, 1997) and argues that, despite challenges (such as the difficulty in integrating these methods with current frameworks of research funding), the role of action research is likely to be greater in the future, with a growing focus on interdisciplinary knowledge production and an emphasis on more 'porous' research structures that are less constrained by elitist university research and more open to partnerships with practitioners. In the UK, with an increasing focus on patient and public involvement in research, there have been initiatives to include representatives of the public on funding committees and project steering groups, and many funders of health research now expect some level of involvement from the 'users' of research. However, to date, these initiatives have been largely consultative rather than truly collaborative. Action research is discussed further as a type of research design in Chapter 2.

The orientations of qualitative research

There are, then, some very different theoretical, epistemological and political starting points in qualitative research, although many of them share a rejection of one or more of the elements of a positivist tradition in social science. These starting points will influence the kinds of research question that researchers address, and how they go about generating knowledge. Clearly, what counts as a 'proper' research question, and what counts as valid knowledge, will depend on macro-theoretical assumptions about the world, middle-range theories that are often rooted in specific disciplines, and epistemological assumptions. This might suggest that to talk of 'qualitative research' in general is impossible, given the plurality of perspectives researchers bring to bear on health. However, there are some broad orientations to methodology that are shared by many researchers, although not of course by all, or at all times. They are: a commitment to naturalism, **reflexivity,** a focus on understanding, and a flexible approach to research strategy.

Naturalism

'Naturalism' refers to a preference for studying phenomena in their 'natural' environment. We know that behaviour, including health behaviour, is contextual. It is, for instance, a common experience that we take more 'risks' with our health when on holiday than at home. Similarly, we are likely to behave differently while being studied than when not. This was a key finding of the famous Hawthorne studies, in which researchers found that human behaviour (in this case productivity in a factory) altered as a result of taking part in the study, rather than because of any of the specific interventions being tested. Rather than continuing with experimental methods, the Hawthorne researchers turned to ethnographic methods such as interviewing and observation to understand worker behaviour (see Schwartzman 1993 for a discussion). Studying health behaviour in a 'natural' environment allows us to study how, for instance, people manage medication regimes in the busy context of their everyday lives, rather than as part of a drug trial. Talking to people in depth, allowing them to tell their own story, provides us with access to their world-view rather than that of the researcher. Ethnographic methods (see Chapter 6) are perhaps the most 'naturalistic' in that they attempt to generate in-depth knowledge about a setting (whether it is a small village, or a hospital ward) over time, in order to understand how and why people believe and behave as they do. The aim is for the researcher to become part of the setting for long enough to minimize their impact.

For some social scientists, it is this 'naturalism' that defines a distinct qualitative methodological approach, and separates it from the methods of inquiry used in the natural sciences. Norman Denzin (1971), for instance, uses the term 'naturalistic behaviourism' to describe an empirical approach to studying the social world, with its own logic. For Denzin, social research should be closely tied to the everyday, routine lives of the people researched, aiming to understand their perspective and then 'reproduce in a rich and detailed fashion the experiences, thoughts and languages' of those studied. What distinguishes this enterprise from common-sense accounts of the same world is that the researcher 'attempts to impose order on the social world'. Naturalistic research is not merely the production of detailed, empathetic accounts of social worlds such as those of a hospital clinic or small village, but the theoretical analysis of them.

An orientation towards naturalism means that the qualitative researcher is more likely to be interested in everyday, or 'real life', contexts than in ideal situations (such as the laboratory setting of a drug trial), and is also more likely to explicitly reflect on how the research setting has in itself had an impact on behaviour. However, 'naturalism' is of course an idealistic notion, as there is in practice no 'untainted' research field observable by the researcher. Any act of observation will impact on the field, however 'invisible' the researcher becomes, and the researcher needs a reflexive approach that takes into account their interrelationship with the field studied. The second orientation of qualitative research, that of reflexivity, is an essential adjunct to a focus on naturalism.

Reflexivity

In essence, the principle of reflexivity is that researchers should subject their own research practice to the same critical analysis that they deploy when studying their topic. This extends to all aspects of the research process, and it is essential in qualitative research. In many quantitative traditions, the assumptions of positivism imply a striving for 'objectivity', in which the researcher attempts to minimize the kinds of political values, subjective impressions and partial accounts that might 'bias' their findings. In qualitative traditions, as we have seen, it is accepted that these values are inevitably part of the research process. It is impossible to have a field for study that is untainted by values, and impossible for the researcher to stand outside those values and subjectivities. Both research and researchers are part of the world, and there is no privileged place we can occupy from which to study that world objectively. However, this does not imply an extreme relativism, which would hold that any account is as good as any other and that research studies are merely another subjective story about a topic with no greater claim to legitimacy than any other. Reflexivity is one of the ways qualitative researchers have of taking subjectivity seriously, without abandoning all claims to producing useful accounts of the world.

First, reflexivity involves reflecting critically on the research itself. Why is it possible to ask this research question, now? Reflecting on why particular questions are legitimate, and why they can attract funding, or interest in the findings, enables the research to be situated within a social and political field. The reflexive researcher considers the broader political and social context of their research, in order to help to unpack any assumptions they have brought to the research, and to identify the ways in which this context might shape what they find. To illustrate, one of the studies listed in Box 1.1 was Leydon et al's (2000) study of the information needs of cancer patients. This study was reported in the *British Medical Journal*, which publishes short articles of interest to medical professionals, and does not generally give much space to theoretical concerns. However, Leydon et al. suggest in their introduction to this paper some of the reasons why they are able to ask 'why cancer patients do not want information' as a research question. They review the growing literature and health policy that addresses communication and information needs, and note the growing focus on ensuring that patients are as well informed as possible about their illness. That the researchers could ask this research question derives in part from this current assumption in Western health care that patients want, and ought, to know as much as they can about their own illnesses. There is a body of middle-range theory that addresses communication in health care settings and the needs of patients for information, and this generates a set of possible research questions around patients' needs for information and how these needs are met. This illustrates the kind of reflexivity that accounts for the research itself, in this case in terms of current health policy concerns, and ensures that the researchers do not uncritically work with taken-for-granted assumptions (such as greater information being universally a 'good thing').

The second level of reflexivity needed in qualitative research is more personal, and involves a consideration of the role of the researcher him or herself in generating and analysing their data. Who you are and where you are as a researcher (your gender, your social status relative to those interviewed, your institutional base) will inevitably shape the kind of data generated. Again, this is not to assume that those data are merely subjective impressions that would have been different if generated by a different researcher, but to attempt to account explicitly for the fact that data are 'produced' rather than merely 'collected'. The example in Case Study 4.1, on the differences between the data generated in studies with male and female interviewers, is an example of this in that the researchers used the differences actively in their analysis to identify something about the presentation of gender in interviews. This is not the same as addressing 'bias', which would assume that there was one account that could be 'true' if only we could collect it untainted by gender, but rather of assuming that all accounts are inevitably shaped by gender, and that reflexive practice attempts to account for this explicitly. In Chapter 4 we discuss further the implications of the ways in which social and cultural factors shape the kinds of data produced in a study.

A focus on meaning and understanding

Following on from the interpretative tradition in the social sciences, much qualitative research focuses on understanding the world from the point of view of the participants in the study. The starting assumption is often perhaps a generous one: that most people, most of the time, are rational and sensible in their choices if we can understand the constraints they are under, what their priorities are, and what they are trying to achieve. As the American sociologist Erving Goffman (1961), who studied behaviour in psychiatric hospitals, put it:

> any group of persons ... develop a life of their own that becomes meaningful, reasonable and normal once you get close to it ... a good way to learn about any of these worlds is to submit oneself in the company of the members to the daily round of petty contingencies to which they are subject. (1961: ix–x)

Thus, the best qualitative research starts by asking not what people get wrong, or don't know, or why they behave irrationally, but instead seeks to identify what they *do* know, how they maintain their health, and what the underlying rationality of their behaviour is. In the example in Case Study 1.1, for instance, apparently irrational behaviour (not taking medication as prescribed for a potentially disabling disease) becomes understandable if we see it from the point of view of those diagnosed with asthma. This is equally true of research with health workers. Doctors who refuse to implement evidence-based guidelines or nurses who don't wash their hands between caring for different patients are unlikely to be acting merely ignorantly or 'irrationally', and the aim of a qualitative study on their behaviour should be to focus on what they are achieving, and how, rather than what they are not doing, and why. Qualitative research attempts to understand the world (or the part of it we are interested in) from the perspective of the participant, not the researcher. So the most productive question may not necessarily be 'Why don't doctors implement evidence-based guidelines?' but 'How do doctors use evidence? How do the assumptions of evidence-based guidelines resonate, or not, with their assumptions about evidence, practice and health care? What kind of evidence is used in their work? How are guidelines in general integrated into the day-to-day work doctors have to accomplish?'

The benefits of this orientation towards understanding for health research are clear. Public health and health promotion, for instance, are often concerned with changing behaviour. Without an empathetic understanding of why people behave as they do, we are unlikely to identify the possibilities for change.

Flexible research strategies

In carrying out a large-scale survey or an epidemiological study, it is usual to plan most of the research in detail before beginning, including the sample size, the precise data to be collected, and the statistical tests likely to be used in analysis. Although qualitative studies also need careful planning, it is more common to have a flexible research strategy, which can be adapted as early data are produced and analysed. As a model it may be helpful to divide up the research process into stages such as literature review, research design, data collection, analysis and writing up, but in practice these stages are much more likely to overlap in qualitative work, and will inform each other. Early data analysis may suggest, for instance, a more refined (or even completely different) research question that will influence later sampling, and may send you back to look for more literature. As we shall see in Chapter 10, the process of writing up is an essential part of the analysis in most qualitative work.

The degree of flexibility required depends on the demands of the study and the perspective of the researcher. In some studies, flexibility may mean simply adding to the intended sample in order to add more depth to one finding. In others, the research design is developed as the study continues, utilizing a number of different methods and approaches as the researcher unearths new clues to the answers they are seeking. One metaphor that is sometimes used to describe the qualitative researcher in this approach is the French term 'bricoleur' (Lévi-Strauss 1966) or professional 'do-it-yourself' person. This is a kind of skilled Jack or Jill of all trades, who can utilize, adapt and devise methods of inquiry and bodies of literature as the need arises throughout a project (Denzin and Lincoln 1998). This approach has great appeal in health research, where so many aspects of everyday life impinge on the topic of interest, and we are often required to shift perspectives throughout a project, or utilize unexpected opportunities for data collection. It may, however, be difficult to pursue in funded research, with most sponsors wanting clear protocols at the outset of a study.

Added to naturalism, reflexivity, interpretation and flexibility, Bryman suggested two other characteristics of qualitative approaches: description and process (Bryman 1988: 63–6). By 'description' he meant a tendency towards detailed (or 'thick') description, rather than a focus on explanation. Detailed description allows the broader context of social behaviours to be delineated. Following from the emphasis on context in qualitative research, Bryman argued, is an emphasis on process. This, he believes, is both a consequence of an orientation towards wanting (historical) context and a reflection of an underlying belief that participants perceive the world as an unfolding sequence of changes, so research should capture this. Qualitative studies therefore emphasize the processes underpinning social activity through detailed descriptions of the participants' behaviours, beliefs, and the contexts within which they occur.

Together with the epistemological traditions outlined above, these orientations towards naturalism, reflexivity, understanding and flexibility imply some other common assumptions that qualitative researchers work with. The recognition of the contextual nature of knowledge and behaviour, and an emphasis on understanding, implies an acceptance of different world-views. In studying the organization of a rural clinic, we should not be surprised if the accounts given by patients and nurses are very different. It is not that one group is misinformed or mistaken, but that each provides an account that is rooted in different worlds. The task of the researcher is not to adjudicate between competing accounts, or to undermine the 'truth' of one, but to understand, from the perspective of those participants, how the world is the way they describe it. This is not an easy task, particularly when researching topics that are close to the researcher's own professional experience.

A second implication is that qualitative research is properly sceptical of received wisdom; that is, common-sense accounts and assumptions, whether these are from academics or participants in the field. Treating an account of clinic organization from a nurse as a valid account, given his or her perspective, is not the same as treating this as the 'truth' about clinic organization. The researcher is not merely a reporter, taking down stories from the field to report back. They must also analyse those accounts, and link the empirical findings with a theoretical understanding of health care organizations, of nursing work, or of professional–client encounters. Equally, the 'common sense' of health care knowledge must be questioned. Qualitative research properly questions the categories it is presented with, rejecting the normative assumptions built into many research studies. Thus, in studying the introduction of 'patient-centred care' to a ward, we should be careful not to assume that 'patient-centred care' is inevitably a good thing, or that it means the same thing to different actors. In studying the 'barriers to evidence-based practice', it is important to remember that these are only likely to be 'barriers' from the perspective of advocates of evidence-based practice.

Criticisms and limitations of qualitative research

We have suggested a range of approaches to qualitative work, and some orientations many traditions share. Despite a growing interest in multidisciplinary research in health care (see Chapter 9) and an acceptance of the value of qualitative methods for addressing questions of understanding and process, these orientations do not always sit easily with the more positivist assumptions of other health research disciplines, such as epidemiology. It is also not always clear to policy makers, managers or clinicians whether qualitative research can provide anything useful. We discuss further in Chapter 9 some of the opportunities and challenges of working across disciplines in health research, but by way of summarizing some of the discussion in this chapter, we review here some of the common criticisms users have of the limitations of qualitative methodologies, and point to where in this book these issues are covered in more depth.

Qualitative research is not 'scientific'

Murphy and Dingwall (2003) argue that a number of myths have grown up around qualitative research, arising in part from debates between sceptics, who reject qualitative methodologies for being unscientific and anecdotal, and romantics, who have rejected the entire attempt to be scientific. Setting out a realist programme for qualitative research, which they hold to be essential if health policy and practice is to gain from the outputs of qualitative research, they take issue with these myths, as well as what they call 'the romantic turn' in qualitative methodology. The first myth is that qualitative methods are more *inductive* than quantitative methods, meaning that they use a logic of 'theory generation' rather than 'theory testing'. Inductive approaches are those that start from the data, and from those data, search for regularities and patterns that suggest general laws. Deductive logic, on the other hand, starts with a theory, from which hypotheses are derived, and then tested against a body of data gathered to test that hypothesis. In practice, of course, all research uses elements of both logics, and it is perhaps impossible to be purely inductive or deductive. We cannot analyse our data with a completely blank slate, as there are always theories and assumptions made that shape the ways in which we read it. Similarly, theories and hypotheses do not come ready formed, and there are inductive processes at work which mean that researchers select particular theories to test, and have 'hunches' about how to test them. The potential polarization – which identifies quantitative methods as deductive and qualitative methods as inductive – is unhelpful, note Murphy and Dingwall, because it contributes to the separation of disciplines in health research, and the view that they are incompatible, whereas there is much potential for creative interplay between qualitative and quantitative methods. The essence of the realist programme they advocate is that qualitative methods can be 'scientific': that we can, and should, be disciplined and rigorous in the collection and analysis of data, and be thorough in subjecting our own assumptions to the same critical scrutiny as those of others. This echoes the positivist tradition of neutrality. The point is not so much to attempt to stand outside values (as we accept we cannot do that) but to approach research with a genuine striving for critical distance. This is not only an ethical stance, but also a pragmatic one. If researchers are overtly partisan, they have perhaps undermined the grounds from which they can claim to produce credible, rigorous accounts that have any status beyond merely 'one more account'.

Methodologically, though, this does create some tensions with the more critical approaches, such as action research. To be researching explicitly 'for' one group, or to decide, *a priori*, to privilege one set of accounts, is difficult to reconcile with an even-handed, reflexive critique of the researcher's own assumptions. This tension is discussed further in Chapter 3 as an issue of research ethics and values.

To engage in a debate about whether qualitative methodologies can be 'scientific' obviously relies on coming to a definition of science. If we take a narrow positivist view, then we have seen that most qualitative traditions do depart from this. However, if we take the logic of a scientific approach, as Murphy and Dingwall do, then we can argue that qualitative methods take subjectivity seriously, but do produce more than merely 'subjective' impressions. There are a number of strategies for maximizing the rigour and credibility of qualitative findings, which are discussed further in the chapters on analysis and writing, but reviewed briefly here.

Does qualitative research produce only subjective accounts?

Most qualitative traditions, as we have seen, take subjectivity seriously, given that it is subjective experiences which are seen as the important ones in thinking about health care (in interpretive approaches), or those that constitute the 'essence' of phenomena (in phenomenological approaches). However, qualitative research does not merely report these subjective experiences, but analyses them, and aims to produce accounts that have some value beyond reproducing anecdotes, or colourful examples. There are a number of strategies that perhaps differentiate research from other activities that seek to describe social life (such as novels or journalism). These include:

- *An attention to evidence*. Although any account of a social field (be it a hospital ward, or an asthma patient's experience) can never be complete, or the only one possible, qualitative research aims to provide evidence for descriptions and interpretation.
- *A critical approach to subjective accounts*. The subjective accounts generated through research are not simply taken as 'truth' about the world, but as situated, contextual accounts. The researcher's task is not to reproduce those accounts as if they offer a privileged representation of social reality, but to ask: why, and how, do people here come to think, behave and talk as they do? The aim is for an analysis that attempts to produce an understanding that may not be available to those we are researching, as we are often asking about taken-for-granted aspects of reality.
- *A critical approach to analytic accounts*. This principle of critically addressing the taken-for-granted and implicit rules of the social world applies to the research itself. Qualitative research should properly be conducted by constantly testing the assumptions built into the research question, and the emerging assumptions about interpretation. This involves a reflexive attitude, as suggested above, and also close attention to disconfirming evidence.
- *Careful and rigorous analysis*. The analysis of data should be done in a way that defends against cherry-picking evidence that confirms the researcher's assumptions, and ensures that the researcher does not see merely what they were hoping to see. Some methods for strengthening the reliability and validity of qualitative analysis are discussed in Chapter 8.

Although we have suggested, then, that qualitative methodologies often depart from positivist assumptions, it is clear that the *logic* of social enquiry is, in practice, very similar across different epistemological traditions, even if the style and assumptions about social reality are rather different. Specifically, doing good quality research involves both empiricism (even if the nature of that 'evidence' is rather different to that in the more quantitative sciences) and neutrality (we accept that research cannot escape values, but do subject those values to reflexive scrutiny so they do not determine research outcomes).

Does qualitative research contribute anything useful for understanding health and health services?

Finally, there is a question that, even if qualitative researchers do not ask it themselves, may be asked of them by others: what are the results of a qualitative study likely to contribute to policy or practice? The examples throughout this book illustrate some of the contributions that qualitative research findings have made to professional practices in areas such as public health, health promotion, health service planning and policy, and they suggest a number of pragmatic answers to this challenge.

Case Study 1.2 Evaluating an intervention to improve TB care in South Africa

(Source: Lewin, S., Daniels, K., Dick, J., Zwarenstein, M. and van der Walt, H. (2002) *A qualitative evaluation of the Kopana TB training intervention.* Internal Report, Health Systems Research Unit, Medical Research Council of South Africa)

Cape Town, South Africa, has high rates of tuberculosis (TB) and clinics face problems in persuading patients to complete the long course of therapy needed to cure it and bring the epidemic under control. Previous research suggested that one barrier to patient compliance could be poor support from staff, who have a 'task orientation', rather than patient orientation, focus to their work. The Kopana project aimed to deliver a participative, experiential training intervention to clinic staff that would lead to improved communication with patients through patient-centred care and an orientation towards quality improvement. An experimental design, in which clinics were randomly allocated to either receive or not receive the Kopana training package, was used to evaluate the intervention. This used quantitative measures, including TB treatment completion rates, to look at the effectiveness of the intervention, and a qualitative evaluation to look at the process. The aims of the qualitative evaluation were to explore how the intervention was developed and implemented, and what impacts it had on staff, clinic organization and patients.

   Simon Lewin and colleagues used ethnographic approaches to study the process of training and its impact on clinic organization.

This included observations of TB clinic routines and the Kopana training sessions, interviews with staff, and analysis of transcripts of the training sessions. The findings from this ethnographic study first helped identify why Kopana did not have the anticipated outcomes; that is, it did not reduce TB cure rates significantly in the intervention clinics. A key reason was that in many clinics what the researchers call the 'integrity of the intervention' was difficult to maintain. For various logistical and organizational reasons, it was impossible to deliver the training package (which involved six facilitated sessions with clinic staff leading up to them identifying changes in practice, plus a follow-up session) in line with intention. This is perhaps typical of training interventions: although they may work well with enthusiastic advocates in initial projects, when rolled out as realistic interventions in randomly chosen settings, they are resisted and adapted by recipients in unpredictable ways. Other findings from the qualitative evaluation were that 'task orientation' was deeply entrenched as a pattern of provision in this setting, and was hard to shift through the process of Kopana training; that a lack of middle management involvement may inhibit change; and that extensive health system restructuring at the same time as the intervention had created uncertainty among clinic staff and a high rate of turnover of experienced nurses. Qualitative interviews enabled the researchers to look in detail at staff concerns. In some clinics, staff fears about local gangsters causing trouble in the waiting rooms, or worries about catching TB themselves, meant that an intervention designed to increase patient-centred care raised concerns about reducing the amount of control they had over patients. In others, deep-seated interpersonal conflicts between staff members or inadequate management limited the impact of any intervention that relied on building on team-working. Nurses did not necessarily identify themselves as part of a clinic team, so an intervention addressing 'the team' did not resonate with their perspectives.

The qualitative study therefore helped unpack the results of the quantitative evaluation, in explaining why the intended outcomes had not occurred. It also suggested some issues to consider in future attempts to change the delivery of care for TB patients in primary level clinics. The ethnographic study also produced findings of wider significance, given the paucity of data on the organization of care in settings such as this one. Detailed accounts of how clinic organization is achieved from the perspective of staff involved, and why apparently irrational organization structures (such as 'task orientation') persist, are useful for building future interventions that take account of the motivations and behaviour of staff, rather than making assumptions about why nurses act in the way they do.

First, there is the argument that qualitative methods 'reach the parts other methods can't reach'. Thus, Green and Britten (1998) argue that qualitative research has a potential role in contributing to the 'evidence base' of medicine because it can answer questions that experimental methods cannot address, such as the meaning of medication for patients, the social processes by which 'evidence' is utilized, or the interactional processes at work in the health care consultation. Thus, the deficit model suggests that the specific contribution of qualitative methods to public health lies in their ability to answer important questions that cannot be answered from a quantitative perspective. Case Study 1.2, an example of how qualitative methods are used in an evaluation, illustrates this. Here, qualitative methods are needed to answer questions about process and the meaning of interventions for those providing and receiving them: they answer questions that cannot be addressed by the quantitative evaluation.

A second potential response is to appeal to the epistemological positions outlined above. Questions in qualitative work are largely about *understanding* different perspectives, or examining how reality is constructed, rather than explaining one 'reality'. Qualitative designs thus provide 'better' answers to questions located in less positivist epistemologies. Nick Black (1994), for instance, cites a study of doctors' views of audit. Although most surveys suggested that doctors were in favour of audit, observation showed that little was carried out. A qualitative study identified a raft of reasons why doctors were uncertain or even unsupportive of audit, few of which had been raised in surveys. Designs that maximize access to these different perspectives are more likely to generate useful information for policy making than those that merely ask for respondents' views in an unsophisticated way. Qualitative methodologies, then, can be presented as generating 'better' data on beliefs and behaviour.

Third, for individual professionals, qualitative findings are often useful for 'sensitizing' them to patients' views. In Case Study 1.1, for instance, several possible orientations towards asthma medication are described. It is less important to quantify what proportion of the population would share these views than to sensitize professionals to these as possible viewpoints. The 'usefulness' of this study lies in part in its potential to alert practitioners to possible patient perspectives, and how they affect health behaviour. At the policy level, qualitative studies have the potential to provide evidence for population needs, the development of appropriate policy, and evidence for how to implement policy with health care staff. To return to the examples of qualitative health research studies given in Box 1.1, looking at the conclusions of the studies listed illustrates what their contributions to policy or practice might be:

- The study of willingness to pay for cataract surgery identified a realistic amount that families could pay for surgery, and found that 'willingness to pay ... concerns not only the elderly patients but also their relatives', and important finding for those conducting surveys on similar topics in these settings (Geneau et al. 2008).
- Understanding why cancer patients may not want information at particular times helps inform a national cancer information strategy that is based

on understanding patients' needs, rather than common-sense assumptions about patients' needs (Leydon et al. 2000).
- Interviewing those seeking health information on the internet demonstrated some benefits for users: the ability to ask embarrassing questions, information about a wide range of health provisions, and access to information that could then be discussed with their doctor. Understanding how people use health information provides guidance for those interested in providing information for the public on the internet (Hardey 1999).
- An ethnographic study of Limba views about leprosy was used to evaluate the effectiveness of a leprosy control programme and to aid communication between health professionals and their patients, as both groups had misunderstandings about the beliefs of the other (Opala and Boillot 1996).
- The study of parents' views about the MMR vaccine found that parents felt more information from health professionals, shared in an open manner, would have helped their decisions and concluded 'only by fully appreciating the concerns of parents will health professionals be able to ... restore their confidence in the MMR' (Evans et al. 2001).

Conclusion

Qualitative health research in general, then, aims to answer 'what', 'how' or 'why' questions about social aspects of health, illness and health care. Although the contribution of qualitative research to our understanding of such activities as health behaviour and health provision is now broadly welcomed, qualitative researchers do still face some scepticism from those rooted in other research traditions. We have suggested this arises in part from differences in epistemological assumptions, with the preference for non-positivist approaches in qualitative methodology. We have also suggested the range of approaches covered by qualitative methodology, including interpretative, constructionist and critical traditions. While these approaches generate different research questions, there are perhaps some shared perspectives, including preferences for naturalistic studies, reflexivity, a focus on meaning, and flexible research strategies.

KEY POINTS

- Research questions arise from particular theoretical frameworks.
- Most qualitative research rejects a positivist epistemology, and instead adopts interpretative, constructionist or critical methodological approaches.
- Common orientations in qualitative methodology include: naturalism, reflexivity, a focus on meaning and understanding and flexible research strategies.

EXERCISE

Look at the abstracts of qualitative health research papers in a social science or biomedical journal. Identify any theoretical assumptions made by the authors, either explicitly or implicitly. What other theoretical frameworks could have been used to address the topic?

FURTHER READING

Murphy, E., Dingwall, R., Greatbatch, D., Parker, S. and Watson, P. (1998) Qualitative research methods in health technology assessment: a review of the literature', *Health Technology Assessment*, 2(16). For those interested in methodological theory, Chapter 1 of this review has a good discussion of the foundations of qualitative research perspectives, the philosophical underpinnings of the main traditions in qualitative research, and a brief history of two disciplines, medical sociology and social anthropology.

Pope, C. and Mays, N. (2006) *Qualitative research in health care* (3rd edn) Oxford: Blackwell Publishing. A very useful introductory reader, with chapters on the key methods of data collection and analysis. Many chapters are based on articles originally written for the *British Medical Journal*, and aimed at those with little familiarity with qualitative research.

2 Developing Qualitative Research Designs

CHAPTER SUMMARY

The 'logic' of developing research protocols suggests first identifying a specific research question and then developing an appropriate research design to generate data that will answer the question. Some guidelines for developing research designs in this way are suggested, and five general types of design (experimental, survey, observational, case study and action research) are described. In practice, qualitative research design is often an iterative process, with theoretical concerns shaping the kinds of questions in which a researcher is interested, and methodological preferences influencing the research design and type of data collection methods chosen. The term 'qualitative research' is also used to refer to those components of larger studies that use qualitative data collection methods, and this chapter concludes by identifying how qualitative methods are incorporated into broader programmes of health research.

Introduction

There are a number of tasks associated with research design, including refining the research question to be addressed, deciding what sort of study it will be, how the data will be identified, collected or generated, and how they will be analysed. There should be coherence between these elements such that the type of study and data collection methods chosen are capable of addressing the question. In qualitative work, research design has traditionally been very 'loose', in that the precise aims of the study may not be known at the outset, and decisions about how to collect data or what the data will be 'about' may emerge as the research progresses. Indeed, if the topic is one with little previous research, the aim may well be a purely exploratory one of identifying some interesting issues to follow up, or 'furthering our understanding' of a setting or a social group. Decisions such as what data collection methods to use, who will be included in the sample, or how long fieldwork will last may well change in the light of early fieldwork experience, and the relevant research question may only emerge in the later stages of data analysis. In Chapter 1, this kind of flexibility was identified as a characteristic of much qualitative research.

However, for most studies, whether small unfunded student projects or large programmes, you will need a research proposal or protocol early on which sets out the key elements of the study: what you want to know, how you will find out, and why. The protocol is a kind of map of the study, and will include practical considerations such as resources needed, ethical issues and time scale. This will need to be much 'tighter' than merely an outline of why a particular topic looks like an interesting one to explore. Most funders of health research, understandably, expect research protocols to demonstrate that the proposed study is both feasible and likely to produce findings that will be useful for public health. This chapter discusses the issues researchers need to consider when developing protocols for qualitative studies.

Research questions

The first element of research design is the 'what' – the question you want to answer. It is not common to have a formal hypothesis to test in qualitative work, but this does not mean that research questions should be vague or unrefined. A research question is more than the title of the study or description of the topic you are interested in. Ideally, it frames fairly precisely what question will be answered, and identifies clearly how it will be addressed. Good research questions are 'researchable' in that they are contained and specified enough for the proposed study to produce the data to answer them. They identify the key indicators that will be used to gather empirical evidence for the concepts of interest. Refining such questions from the 'problem' or vague topic of interest is a skill that takes time to develop. The first problem for many beginning researchers is to identify a broad topic, and there are a number of ways of generating ideas. Some productive sources of potential research questions include:

- Puzzles about the social world – everyday life generates a number of puzzles about health beliefs and behaviour that give rise to potential research questions: Why are suicide rates higher for men than for women? Why do many people consult with 'alternative' practitioners in countries where biomedical care is free? How is information technology such as the Internet being used by the public?
- Professional practice may also throw up puzzles – why does our unit have trouble recruiting enough nurses? Why don't patients take the medicines we prescribe? Why do some ward teams seem to function better than others?
- Reading the literature may reveal interesting 'gaps' in our knowledge of particular topics – we know a lot about how parents view adolescent mental health services, but how do adolescents themselves feel? Most of the research on hospital organization has been done in industrialized countries – how generalizable is it to other settings?
- Commissioned research – sponsors, such as government departments or health authorities, propose specific questions that they want answering to inform policy development or implementation or to evaluate service provision.

Ideally a researcher's curiosity and a sponsor's need will coincide and there will then be a sponsor willing to fund a study. Turning these initial areas of interest into researchable questions is the next stage. Even when the topic has been dictated by a funding agency, there a will be number of steps to take to develop a research question and identify whether that question requires a qualitative approach. One set of questions that should be considered at the beginning of the process might include the following.

Is this a problem that research can address?

Health care throws up daily problems for those delivering and managing it, but not all of those are research problems. If drugs are too expensive locally for most people to afford, you may not need to waste time and resources on researching the barriers to drug use, although such research is sometimes done for political gain, for instance to convince policy makers that a 'problem' does exist. If a hospital is understaffed, dirty and overcrowded, an ethnographic study is not needed to identify the major causes of patient dissatisfaction. However, beware of 'common-sense' answers to such problems. It may be, for example, that patients are *not* particularly dissatisfied as they realize staff are delivering the best care possible in circumstances beyond their control. It may be that 'patient dissatisfaction' is related more to the attitudes of staff towards patients, or certain groups of patients, than to the material circumstances. Indeed, some of the most interesting research can arise from the questioning of taken-for-granted 'common-sense' explanations. It is perhaps particularly important not to rely on common-sense answers to 'problems' when they rely on explanations of 'ignorance', given that most people, most of the time, behave in rational ways once their perspective is understood. Case Study 2.1, on women and smoking, illustrates this; although irrational from a health perspective, Hilary Graham's (1987) study shows how smoking could be a rational coping strategy for low-income women. However, in general, a question that research can address is one where there is some genuine uncertainty, and where research, properly done, could add to our knowledge or understanding.

Is a qualitative approach appropriate?

If you want to understand the perspectives of participants, explore the meanings they give to phenomena, or observe a process in depth, then a qualitative approach is probably appropriate. However, if you need answers to questions such as 'How many people are likely to use this service over the next year?' or 'What proportion of primary care physicians prescribe this medication?', a quantitative design, or at least a quantitative element in the study, will be required. As suggested by the discussion of theory and orientations in Chapter 1, qualitative approaches are ideal for questions that require an answer about understanding participants' views, or for questions that address the meaning given to phenomena.

What are the key concepts of interest?

'Concepts' are the building blocks of theory, the 'high-level' or abstract terms in which we frame our understanding of health. These refer to macro-theoretical constructs (see Chapter 1), such as 'inequality', 'globalization', and 'power', but also the middle-range theories in which our research questions are usually embedded. Here, concepts such as 'lifestyle', 'medical autonomy' or 'compliance' may be used as part of the common stock of knowledge within a particular discipline, but carry within them a set of (often implicit) assumptions.

It is worth thinking in some detail about the concepts referred to in your research study. This thinking should clarify two questions:

- First, what are the different *components* of these concepts? For something like patient 'compliance' with prescribed medication, these might include:

  ○ understanding the doctor's instructions
  ○ collecting the prescription
  ○ taking all the medicines at the time of day the doctor recommended
  ○ taking the medicines in such a way as to produce the desired effect.

- Second, what are the *assumptions* you are making in using them? As Chapter 1 discussed, theoretical assumptions are always made in research, whether explicit or not, and it is worth unpacking those that frame your particular question. The notion of 'compliance' implies a number of assumptions about patients and professionals: that, for instance, professionals are the 'experts' in the partnership; that not taking medications as prescribed is a 'problem'; that it is *non*-compliance that must be explained (rather than why patients *do* take medicines in line with professionals' advice).

Case Study 2.1   Using interviews and diaries to elaborate the meaning of statistical data on women and smoking

(Source: Graham, H. (1987) 'Women's smoking and family health', *Social Science and Medicine*, 25: 47–56)

Survey evidence suggests that those women in Britain most likely to smoke are on low incomes, with children but no work outside the home. At a superficial level, this is a surprising finding, as these are the women least able to afford cigarettes and most likely to want to make lifestyle changes to promote their own and their children's health. There is also good evidence that most of the population accepts the links between smoking and poor health: lack of knowledge is unlikely to explain the prevalence of smoking in this group.

Hilary Graham designed a study to explore these findings in the context of the 'everyday world of informal health behaviour'; that is, the day-to-day routines of housework and child care with which women were engaged. Her aim was a qualitative one, to explore these worlds 'through the eyes of the mothers', and she sampled a group of low-income and single parents. To collect data on daily experiences, she first conducted interviews, but found that these provided only a snapshot of women's lives. The focus on the women's own perspective also made it difficult to gather precise information on the details of everyday life, which Graham saw as essential for providing the context of health behaviour. To collect this fine-grained detail, she also asked participants to complete a 24-hour diary, with space to record their main and other activities over the day, and the presence of others.

There were important differences in the data from the interviews and the diaries. One was that smoking was significantly under-reported in the diaries, compared with interviews: in the diaries it was reported only if it was the 'main activity' at the time. Typically, only those cigarettes that marked significant breaks in the daily routines of housework and caring were reported. Graham suggests that cigarettes were the one luxury many low-income women could afford, and that they played an important role in reducing stress and structuring the daily round of caring and housework. Having a cigarette was one way to claim some 'adult time' in the

(Continued)

context of a busy life looking after young children, and could be a legitimate way of generating some physical space away for a short time. Thus, what appeared to be irrational behaviour (spending money on smoking when it potentially damages the health of yourself and children) was comprehensible when seen in the context of women's everyday lives.

Here, the study design is essentially a qualitative one (of exploring the meaning of health behaviour from the perspective of women themselves, in the context of their everyday lives), used to shed light on a relationship between two variables (poverty and smoking) found in the quantitative data. Within her study, Graham uses a mixed method approach to collect the data. This has the advantage of providing different perspectives on the topic of interest (smoking behaviour), and the different findings play an important role in the analysis in alerting her to the meaning of cigarettes in these women's lives.

Thinking about these assumptions can help clarify early on some of the potential limitations in your research design, particularly if the 'assumptions' of those you are researching are not the same as yours. Once you have identified the assumptions built into your research question, it can be a useful exercise to identify alternatives, and frame questions in terms of those. For instance, if we have identified an assumption that 'non-compliance' with medication is a problem in the question 'Why don't patients comply with medications?', we can turn the research question round as 'Why *do* some patients comply with medication?' Even if it is not a perspective you (as a practitioner or a researcher) share, it might turn out to be a more useful way of producing knowledge about patient behaviour than exploring non-compliance.

Refining indicators for these concepts

Abstract or theoretical concepts are good for thinking with, but need refining for use in empirical research (that is, research that relies on primary data being collected or generated). It is impossible to go into the field and 'see' or record compliance, or globalization, or medical autonomy. Once the components of each concept have been identified, *indicators* can be developed for those that are crucial to the research question. Indicators are events or phenomena that reflect (or provide evidence of) components of the underlying concept of interest. These indicators need to be empirical, in that we can generate data that capture them. In quantitative work, this process is perhaps more obvious than for qualitative. If, for instance, we are interested in measuring the health status of a given population, it is possible to specify some relevant components of health (perhaps including self-reported health status, or blood pressure) and then identify researchable indicators (questionnaire items asking for self-reports, sphygmomanometer readings) that can be used to 'measure' these in the field.

The concepts used in qualitative work are often less easily 'measurable', and indeed the aim of the research may well be to 'unpack' the concept, to further our understanding of it, rather than to pin down components for measurement. Suppose the researcher is addressing the topic of 'clinical autonomy in surgical wards'. Part of the research question might involve *identifying* the components of clinical autonomy, so it is difficult to define at the outset what the research will look for. However, the work of thinking through the assumptions embedded in the research is still vital. Here, we would be interested in identifying the components of the rather nebulous concept of 'autonomy'. Does it include control over treatment decisions? Control over the decision to admit patients? Responsibility for the work of other professionals? Once these components have been delineated, it is possible to think about how the research might generate empirical evidence for them, for instance by looking specifically at how clinical decisions are made on the ward.

Refining indicators helps specify what questions the research can and can't answer. Take the example of compliance again. If we have identified 'taking the medicines at the time of day recommended by the doctor' as one component, we can then think about what would constitute evidence for that. Observation of behaviour (watching patients to see when they took medicines) might provide good evidence, but of course is unlikely to be feasible, and anyway would only provide evidence of what happened when a researcher was watching. More feasible possibilities might include asking patients to complete a diary each day, noting when they took their medicines, or interviewing them, and asking for self-reports of when medicines were taken. Neither of these are particularly good indicators for the *behaviour* of taking medicine, as they are really evidence of patients' records of that behaviour, or patients' accounts of that behaviour. The research question would have to reflect this, perhaps asking 'How do patients report compliance?' A key element in refining indicators for qualitative studies is, then, to pay careful attention to the method of data collection and to make sure the data generated by the proposed study are capable of reflecting these indicators.

Defining a research question

The different theoretical starting points outlined in Chapter 1 clearly shape the way in which researchers frame research questions, and which kinds of questions they are drawn to in the first place (see Box 1.2 in Chapter 1). These are often implicit, in that the reports of the research may not refer to them, but they nonetheless influence the kinds of issues or problems in which researchers are interested and how they turn them into research questions. It is worth asking yourself right at the beginning of a project which theoretical frame is implicit in your research question and then deliberately considering how alternative perspectives might have generated different questions, different types of information (data) needed to answer the question, and different ways of acquiring that information (data collection methods).

As an example from Box 1.2 in Chapter 1, on different possible approaches to researching the topic of immunization, if we wanted to address the question 'What sources of knowledge do parents draw on to assess the risks of immunization?', we might want to refine that in the light of a discussion about the components of 'sources of knowledge' and 'risks', and how we might identify evidence of these (indicators). We would need, for instance, to consider what would be evidence of 'drawing on a source of knowledge'. Suppose one potential source of knowledge was a newspaper report. Potential kinds of evidence for different components of this might include: mentioning newspapers unprompted in an interview about immunizations; saying 'yes' to a direct question about whether this was a source of knowledge; and using citations of newspaper reports in everyday conversation with others as a way of legitimizing beliefs about immunization risks. These kinds of evidence will imply different data generation methods (**in-depth interviews,** survey interviews, and perhaps focus groups or observation, respectively). The next step is then a balancing act between what is needed to answer the original question and what is feasible. One outcome might be a study that used interviews with parents, asking them about their views of immunization risks and asking directly about how they have come to know about these risks. The research question might then be refined as: 'How do parents account for their knowledge of immunization risks in interviews?'

The aim of refining the research question is, then, to generate a feasible question that it is possible to answer with the methods proposed and within the resources available. Inevitably this involves a number of 'trade-offs'. There is no 'perfect' design, and in refining the research question, most researchers have to leave out some components of interest to ensure that the study is feasible, or accept that the data generated may not provide a complete answer.

Research designs: some examples

Research design refers to the logic of the study: the what, how and why of data production. It will include the type of study proposed (such as an experiment or a case study) and the intended methods of producing data (such as interviews or observation). Clearly, the design should be appropriate to the research question. This sounds obvious, but many (even published) studies progress with a design that cannot possibly answer the proposed question. This may be because of inadequate work at the design stage, or because resource restrictions limit the scope of the study. The research design, and therefore the question, may, then, have to be tailored to meet resources. There are many ways of classifying research designs. Some take the experiment as the ideal, or prototype, research design and describe others in terms of how they resemble an experiment. Most qualitative researchers take a rather different starting point

Measurements at time 1	Intervention?	Measurements at time 2
Experimental group	✓	Experimental group
Control group	✗	Control group

Figure 2.1   The logic of experimental research design

in selecting an appropriate design, and begin by considering the kind of data that will be generated. Those trained in ethnographic methods, for instance, may begin by thinking about what kinds of questions these methods might help them address in a given setting. The following list is, therefore, not a definitive typology of all research designs, but rather suggestive of the kinds of design you are likely to come across in health research.

Experiments

An experiment is perhaps the 'classic' design of the positivist tradition, as it sets up a study capable of answering a question about cause and effect. Essentially, an experiment involves an intervention, with comparisons of observations before and after to identify the effect of that intervention. Ideally, experiments should have a 'control' group, who do not receive the intervention, as well as an 'intervention' group who do, to allow the researcher to separate those changes that would have happened anyway from those resulting from the intervention. Figure 2.1 illustrates the logic of experimental research design. This is perhaps a design most familiar in the natural sciences, but qualitative methods are sometimes used within experimental designs. In medical sciences, the 'randomized controlled trial' (**RCT**) is considered the 'gold standard' design for testing interventions. This kind of experiment randomly allocates participants to the control and intervention group, to eliminate bias from differences between the two groups. RCTs are used extensively in trials of new medicines, where it is important to identify precisely what the effect of the intervention is. However, there has been recent interest in extending this kind of methodology to complex health service interventions, such as training schemes for staff, or new modes of treatment delivery. In these studies, sometimes called 'pragmatic trials' to suggest that they are testing 'real world' effects, qualitative methods may be used to generate data from 'before' and 'after' the intervention.

One example is Ann Oakley's (1990) evaluation of an intervention designed to increase support for new mothers. She used in-depth interviews in an experiment designed to evaluate whether social support in pregnancy (provided by research midwives) had an impact on outcomes such as mothers' satisfaction with care and infant birth weight. Oakley makes a strong argument for using experiments more widely in health research, given that they are the most appropriate design for evaluating interventions, and produce the strongest evidence for policy makers. She also notes many of the problems facing those trying to implement pragmatic trials in health service settings. First, frontline staff may be very resistant to the process of randomization. Professional ide-ologies stress the value of offering services based on need, and allocating ser-vices randomly may seem perverse to practitioners, especially if some clients are apparently in greater need, or the professionals have strong feelings about the worth of the intervention. Much work is needed to demonstrate that there is genuine uncertainty about whether clients would benefit from the inter-vention or not. Second, the process of gaining **informed consent** from par-ticipants needs considerable thought. If consent is to be truly 'informed', then the trial risks being 'contaminated' by those allocated to the control group attempting to gain support from outside the trial. Another example of the use of qualitative methods to evaluate an intervention with an experimental design was described in Case Study 1.2, and Case Study 9.1 describes a large qualitative study conducted alongside a trial.

In summary, experimental designs are the strongest ones for demonstrating cause and effect relationships, and thus for evaluating the effect of interven-tions. Qualitative methods can have a role in studying the process of trial implementation and in collecting the data needed. Increasingly, large trials are established with a qualitative component (see Case Study 9.1). However, few qualitative studies utilize an experimental design because the aims of qualitative methodology are usually around understanding or interpretation, rather than determining cause and effect relationships.

Surveys

Survey is the general term for a design that aims to collect the same set of data for every 'case' in the study. Classic surveys include censuses of the popula-tion, which collect a set of information about every person in the country. More usually, health researchers will use *sample surveys*, which collect a set of data from a sample of the whole population of interest. Surveys are the design of choice for descriptive quantitative research questions about preva-lence (how many people in the locality need this service, or have had this kind of experience?), or when we want to look for associations between two mea-surable variables, such as health care experiences and demographic charac-teristics. Although we usually think of quantitative data when we think of surveys, in which questionnaires or structured interviews are used to collect information, many interview studies utilize survey designs. The study in Case Study 1.1, in which the researchers interviewed people about their asthma, can be thought of as a survey design, in that a similar set of data (beliefs about asthma, use of medication, demographic details) has been collected for all of those interviewed. However, the aim of this study was not to examine the interviewees as a sample of the whole population of asthma patients, or to look for statistical associations between the variables, but a rather more qualitative one of looking at patient narratives.

To some extent, the logic of experimental and survey design is rooted in a positivist epistemology, in which the aim of research is explanation, and there is an assumption that, ideally, a stable 'truth' about the world (whether causal relationships or descriptions of population) can be discovered. Not all research questions are about cause and effect and, following from the orientations outlined above, many studies will begin with quite different aims – to understand the social world, rather than to explain it. The remaining designs are more rooted in a qualitative style of research, rather than those that just use qualitative methods within other designs.

Observational studies

If the aims of the research are describing and understanding what is going on in a particular social setting, then observational designs are called for, which allow the researcher to document social life in its 'natural' state. Many qualitative studies utilize the logic of observational design, in that they aim to document everyday life, or explore some aspect of life in its 'natural' context. Observational designs include ethnographic studies that aim to provide a rich, 'thick' description of a particular setting, and studies of naturally occurring data such as videos of health service consultations. These are described in Chapter 6. The key characteristic of an observational design is that the researcher does not intervene (or at least not deliberately) and seeks instead to document what happens in everyday contexts, rather than research ones. The 'data' are thus the naturally occurring talk and behaviour of those being studied. Examples of observational studies include Rosenhan's study of psychiatric hospitals described in Case Study 3.2, in which researchers became patients to observe hospital admission procedures and routines, and the study summarized in Case Study 6.2, which utilized tape recordings of consultations between doctors and their patients.

Case studies

For some writers on methods, describing a study as a 'case study' merely identifies the way in which the sample for the study is selected (Hammersley 1992a) or the data reported (Wolcott 2002). Martyn Hammersley (1992a: 184), for example, defines a case study as research investigating a small number of naturally occurring cases, as opposed to an experiment (in which the cases are created by the researcher) or a survey (in which a large number of cases are investigated). For Hammersley, there is no specific logic implied by a 'case study', nor do they have any specific theoretical or methodological characteristics, so we should not define it as a type of design. In this view, selecting a case study design rather than a survey or experiment involves decisions about what the aims of the sample are. If the need is for empirical generalizability, then a survey will be appropriate; if depth and accuracy are needed, a case study will be. If the need is for evidence of causal relationships, an experiment will be preferable; if we want to examine naturally occurring rather than artificial phenomena, then a case study will have advantages.

However, others have argued that case studies represent a distinctive research design and methodological approach, with implications beyond those of sample selection. Robert Yin (1994) argues that a case study is the research design of choice when 'a "how" or "why" question is being asked about a contemporary set of events over which the investigator has little control' (Yin 1994: 9). A case study involves studying a phenomenon (such as a change in health service management structures, or the health practices of rural villagers) within its context (the hospital, the village). Yin distinguishes case studies from other designs by noting that they explicitly include context, unlike experiments (which attempt to 'control out' context) and surveys (which can only include the context considered at the outset, when designing the questionnaire). Classic case studies include traditional ethnographies, in which the researcher spends many months, or years, in one 'field' and aims to write an in-depth account of the community (see Chapter 6). They typically involve a combination of data collection methods, such as observation, documentary analysis and interviews.

One particular type of case study is the *life history*, based on the story of one individual. Ken Plummer (1983) sees the life history as acting as a 'humanist' corrective to the more positivist and generalizing traditions in the social sciences, through its focus on individuality, subjectivity and the particular. Although perhaps not widely used in health research, there are some interesting examples from the literature that illustrate the potential of this approach. Plummer cites life stories collected from heroin addicts, a woman dying of terminal cancer, and prostitutes, which could all be used to provide an individual perspective on policy issues, some insight into change over time and, in many cases, invaluable information about the impact of social structures on individuals that could not be accessed in any other way. One illustration from the health field is Pauline Prior's (1995) case study of a man, 'Samuel', who spent 40 years as a resident of a large mental hospital in Northern Ireland. Using an analysis of case notes and interviews with professionals, Prior used Samuel's life history to illuminate changes in mental health policy and the impact of institutionalization on individuals. Despite his residence in a long-term institution, Samuel maintained a strong self-identity, and resisted a stigmatized identity as 'mentally ill' and isolated, partly, Prior argues, through his involvement in the local church and as a reliable manual worker. Drawing on theoretical perspectives on the impact of institutions on self-identity, stigmatization and deviance, Prior shows how this life history is an 'atypical' case, which can develop our understanding of institutions through exploring how some individuals resist the effects of institutionalization.

Action research

Action research, a term that is increasingly used in health research, has different meanings among its many exponents but is often rooted in a participatory approach (see Chapter 1). The distinctive element of action research design is that the research aims to *change* practice as well as studying it. The aims may not be as explicit as 'emancipation', but rather a more open and equal relationship with research participants, who have a role in setting the research agenda and contributing to design. Action research has a number of historical roots, including community development projects, where research questions arise clearly from social problems, such as poverty, drug use or social exclusion, as well as early twentieth century industrial sociology and psychology, where research was orientated towards methods to improve working relations. The first use of the term 'action research' is often attributed to Kurt Lewin (1946), a psychologist who attempted to join up a scientific approach to studying social groups with a method for addressing social problems (see Hart and Bond 1995, for a discussion of the history of action research).

In developed countries in recent years, nursing professionals in particular have seen action research as a particularly appropriate type of design for allowing researchers to address the power relationships inherent in other research designs (Meyer 1997), and as a method for addressing problems that arise from professional practice, rather than those imposed from outside. Julienne Meyer suggests that action research designs may become increasingly utilized in health care settings with the greater emphasis in many health care systems on getting all practitioners involved with research as part of their professional development, and as a way of improving health services (Meyer 2000). Hart and Bond (1995) discuss the potential of these strategies for frontline health professionals interested in improving practice or changing organizations. Rather than engaging in research with the aim of changing practice in the future (through, for instance, influence on policy, or incremental shifts in cultural understanding that might result from 'pure' research), action research combines the production of knowledge with the process of changing practice in the short term. It is essentially problem-orientated and research, action and evaluation are linked within one process. Findings are shared with participants throughout the process of the study, so that discussion can inform the subsequent stages. This leads to a cyclical research design (which Lewin called a 'spiral of steps') in which planning, observing, acting and reflecting feed back into the next planning cycle. Thus, the core research topic may throw up many other issues for participants, as reflection on findings generates new questions. Case Study 2.2 (Paine et al. 2002) uses an 'action research' design in developing a sexual health programme in The Gambia.

One criticism of action research has been the difficulty of balancing the two aims of 'action' and 'research'. A clear focus on changing practice in one setting, and adopting the priorities of those in the field, means it can be difficult to make a contribution to knowledge beyond the local site of the project. Many reports of action research studies are perhaps weak on how their findings have contributed to theoretical knowledge in the area. Tina Koch and Debbie Kralik (2006), in their book on participatory action research, are clear about their priorities: 'Whilst our participatory action research approach is primarily concerned with practical outcomes or change, theory is a bonus ...' (2006: 4). Clearly, there are difficulties in generalizing from one setting in which the 'problem' for research has been defined essentially as a local issue, although as Koch and Kralik show, in their development of a theory of transitions in chronic illness, it can be possible to build up theory from an engagement in a range of projects. However, whether or not 'action research' should be considered as a 'research' design, rather than a model for development or reflective improvement, it is an approach that increasing numbers of practitioners are utilizing, and for which they draw on qualitative methods to aid in the steps of identifying problems, finding solutions and evaluating action.

Problems with design typologies

The typology of research designs outlined above suggests the difficulties faced in attempting to classify designs. First, the divisions between different designs are not clear-cut. An 'ethnography', for instance, could be described as being an observational design or a case study. Second, it is impossible to develop an exhaustive typology – there are some studies that do not quite 'fit' any of the descriptions of the designs above. Indeed, the typical qualitative health research study is often an in-depth interview study based on a small sample. Many of the case studies in this book draw on this kind of data (see, for instance, Case Studies 1.1, 2.1, 4.1, 4.2, 5.1, 5.2, 8.1 and 8.2). The 'design' of a small-scale interview study is perhaps midway between an observational study and a survey. The small-scale interview study does depend to some extent on the logic of observational work, in that the aims are often to access the 'everyday' knowledge or talk of interviewees, although of course there are limits to how far a research interview can capture naturalistic talk, as is discussed in Chapter 4. Although qualitative interviews do not aim to collect exactly the same set of data from each respondent, there are also elements of survey logic, in that the analysis might look for regularities and typologies within the interview accounts (see Chapter 8). It would be difficult to argue, though, that the interview study constitutes a separate design: there is nothing specific about the logic by which it addresses a research question, as this borrows from both the naturalism of observational designs and the format of the survey.

Most importantly, this discussion of research design in terms of logic and aim demonstrates that there is *no necessary relationship between the design of the study and the methods of data collection.* Although quantitative methods may be more associated with surveys and experiments, and qualitative with observational and case study research, this is not always the case. Oakley's experimental study of the impact of social support on pregnancy outcomes used interviews to collect some data on outcome measures, and a case study might use a mix of qualitative and quantitative methods of data collection. The *methods* of data collection used in a study should not be confused with the *design* of the study. Following from this, it is clear that the term 'qualitative research' is used in practice in two rather distinct ways:

- to describe the orientation and design of a study (qualitative methodology); and
- to describe the data collection methods used (qualitative methods).

Case Study 2.2   A participatory evaluation of the 'Stepping Stones' sexual health programme in The Gambia

(Source: Paine, K., Hart, G., Jawo, M., Ceesay, S., Jallow, M., Morison, L., Walraven, G., McAdam, K. and Shaw, M. (2002) '"Before we were sleeping, now we are awake": preliminary evaluation of the Stepping Stones sexual health programme in The Gambia', *African Journal of AIDS Research*, 1: 41–52)

Stepping Stones is a programme that aims to 'enable participants to increase control of their sexual and emotional relationships' through a project involving community-level workshops that cover relationship skills as well as information on sexually transmitted diseases and condom use. It works with both men and women, and addresses their concerns as well as those of the research team. The research team aimed to evaluate the impact of Stepping Stones in two villages in The Gambia. Although HIV infection was relatively low in The Gambia, it was slightly higher in the intervention site and there were reported to be other negative consequences of sexual behaviour, such as subfertility and unwanted pregnancy. Intervention villages were chosen randomly from a list matched on the basis of key geographic and socio-demographic variables. The overall design of the study was, then, an experimental one.

The evaluation used a multi-method approach, including a participatory evaluation by the study villagers, in-depth interviews, focus group interviews, surveys of knowledge, attitudes and practices, and a monitoring of condom supplies. The participatory evaluation was based on a series of workshops (with separate groups of old and young men and women) carried out over ten weeks, which invited participants to consider broad topics (such as 'relationships') but in ways that facilitated them, rather than the research team, to set the priorities and to decide on action. An early way in which participants set the priorities was in shifting the focus away from 'family planning' to 'infertility prevention', which was in line with the community's own values.

The first workshop was used to prioritize health problems, and to decide which were the most urgent. Some of the sexual and reproductive health problems identified included: sex when the woman was unwilling, jealousy over co-wives, domestic violence and lack of financial support from husbands. The themes from the four groups (old and young men and women) were presented to the whole village. At the one-year follow-up, the groups were asked what had

(Continued)

changed as a result of the programme. In both intervention villages, participants listed better communication between wives and husbands, less domestic violence and safer sex outside marriage. The villagers reported enjoying the programme techniques, such as role plays.

The results of the interviews and surveys suggested that there were some important increases in the intervention villages in knowledge about sexually transmitted diseases, especially HIV, and how to prevent them. Collecting valid data from surveys on sexual knowledge and behaviour is a challenge, and the researchers drew extensively on interview data to determine the impact of Stepping Stones on issues such as condom use and knowledge about transmission of infection. Interviews suggested women had been empowered by the project to be more able to insist on condom use. However, one of the most significant findings for the project team was the broader change to relationships between men and women that emerged from the programme. Almost all interviewees reported a reduction in dissent between men and women, and the development of more effective strategies for discussing difficult issues without arguments.

This case study demonstrates how, in practice, research designs are often mixed: an experimental intervention is evaluated with a multi-method approach, utilizing a range of tools to access attitude and behaviour change. The underlying approach of the intervention and evaluation was that of 'participatory research', with the research team aiming to include participants in the programme, rather than researching 'on' them. The aims, then, are rather broader than disease reduction, and reflect a more holistic view of health including empowerment and the capacity for community development.

Although this book is primarily concerned with qualitative studies in the first sense, the principles of 'good practice' of course apply equally well to qualitative components of other studies, or to the use of qualitative data collection techniques in other kinds of study. However, in practice there is often some tension between the epistemological traditions when qualitative methods are used in multidisciplinary studies. Chapter 9 discusses some of the problems as well as the possibilities of mixing methods and disciplinary approaches.

Influences on research design

In principle, then, the main influences on research design are the research question, adequately refined as a researchable question, and the aims of the study, such as assessing an intervention, exploring a process, or involving users in the research and changing practice. Theoretical perspectives, as introduced in Chapter 1, will also frame both the kinds of questions a researcher will ask and what legitimate kinds of answers can be generated. It would, however, be idealistic to assume that only these methodological concerns will influence research design. Political factors impact on what is likely to be funded, but also on what kinds of research are currently seen as worthy of public funds, how easy it will be to get findings published, and how influential the findings are going to be. There are also 'fashions' in particular methodologies, which make some kinds of study easier to fund at times than others.

Feasibility is also a constraint on designing the 'ideal' study. It is not always possible, ethically or practically, to do observational work. If we are interested in 'private' behaviour, such as sexual behaviour, we may be restricted to interview methods to collect accounts, rather than methods that would generate direct empirical evidence. Time may restrict a study to looking at documents when we would ideally like to interview people as well. Feasibility is also a function of who the researcher is, and what institutional affiliations and networks they can draw upon. These are to some extent opportunistic – a specific professional network and access to particular settings are likely to generate particular research questions, and also provide the resources to answer them. In some cases this relies on personal characteristics. Here, for example, is Lee Monaghan's description of why it was feasible for him to undertake an ethnographic study (see Chapter 6) of the risks faced by 'bouncers' (door staff in night clubs):

> As a reflexive ethnographer I know my male gender, relative youth (under 30 during the main study period) and bodily capital (muscular, weighing approximately 16½ stone at six-foot), represented resources for getting in and getting on with this study ... my embodied social history consisting of lifting weights and boxing ... rendered me willing and able to assume an active membership role [as a doorman]. (Monaghan 2003: 21)

Monaghan presumably developed an interest in the health risks faced by these workers in part because of his personal network of contacts, which in turn facilitated an entry to the field that would have been extremely difficult for anyone without his physical attributes or life experiences. Although this is an extreme example, practical issues of feasibility are likely to impact on most study designs, and any protocol should demonstrate that a study is practically doable with the resources (both material and personal) available.

An idealized logic?

So far, we have described the process of framing a research question and developing an appropriate research design as if it were both rational and time-ordered, constrained only by external factors such as available funding and feasibility. Although this is the way in which research studies are

often written up (the author formulated a question and then decided how
to collect data in the light of this), it represents an idealized and often post-
hoc logic. Given the flexible and evolving nature of qualitative research
design, it is possible that the precise research question will not emerge until
quite late in the study. It may be that the researcher has a 'hunch' that a
particular field is interesting, and that initial exploratory data analysis will
generate a fruitful line of more detailed inquiry.

Jennifer Mason (1996) suggests a rather different logical order in research
design, which perhaps better reflects the 'real' evolution of many qualitative
study designs. She poses five questions that researchers should address in
moving from a broad area of interest to a workable proposal for research. In
summary they are:

- What is the nature of the phenomena that I want to investigate?
- What might represent knowledge or evidence of those phenomena?
- What broad topic is the research concerned with?
- What is the intellectual 'puzzle'?
- What is the purpose of my research? (Mason 1996)

This is an interesting approach to research design, as it highlights ontological
and epistemological concerns at the outset, rather than assuming that they follow on from the research question. The 'nature of the phenomena' refers to the
essence of the researcher's interests – whether it be individuals, perspectives,
narratives, collectivities, cultures, order, disorder, or some other phenomenon.
These, notes Mason, are located in very different social places, and presume
very different assumptions about the nature of the world. Only through clarifying their own perspectives (from the range of alternatives that are available)
can researchers identify what their research is really *about*. To take an example,
suppose we were interested in the development of the nursing profession in one
country. Identifying the precise phenomenon for the research would involve
thinking about whether that meant we were interested in nurses' own views of
the profession; the relative status of the profession in the health policy arena or
how well nursing in that country measured up to some set of international criteria on issues such as educational levels, influence, registration and so on.
Although these topics are clearly related, each implies a very different phenomenon of interests: perhaps nurses' perceptions, influences on health policy
and the 'reality' of nursing development respectively.

The second of Mason's questions relates to epistemological concerns.
Once the phenomena of interest have been clarified, the researcher can identify what would represent evidence of them. If our interest in the nursing profession is around its status in the health policy arena (whether nursing leaders
are involved in the Ministry of Health, for example, or whether they are consulted routinely by policy makers), then we would probably not use an interview study with junior nurses to generate data. Although that might provide
data on their perceptions of nursing leaders, it would not furnish good data
on what actually happens in the health policy arena. We might instead look
at documented meetings and conferences, or interview policy leaders.

The aims of the study come much later in the process for Mason, and can be addressed only in the light of answers to the first two questions. If we identify that the phenomenon that really interests us is not nursing leaders' influence, but the perceptions of those on the ground, then we could frame our research question more carefully now – perhaps as 'How do junior nurses in this country perceive the status of the nursing profession?' Mason's final question, on the purpose of the research, relates to both the immediate aims (such as contributing to knowledge, completing a PhD thesis, or developing a health promotion intervention) and the 'purpose' in terms of the precise research question that is to be answered. This is worth thinking through at the outset, in terms of who the research is 'for' in the most general sense. If you are interviewing nurses, is this a project that is ultimately for them, in terms of representing their voices, and trying to understand their worldviews? Or is it a project that is speaking to 'the profession' of nursing more broadly, which seeks to inform nursing educators or policy makers about what would improve the status of nursing? These are of course not incompatible, but clarity about the overall purpose of the research can help ensure there is a clear line through the design, methods, and through to writing up at the end.

In practice, much health research design is a circular and iterative process, involving a mix of the idealized logic of formal research design, the more qualitative approach of Jennifer Mason, and the many incremental and opportunistic decisions we make on the way. Some researchers are more comfortable with thinking through from the general (what is the big theoretical problem this research addresses?) to the specific (what research question will shed light on this theoretical problem?), whereas others are more comfortable thinking the other way round, and starting with the specific question and then thinking through the theoretical framework that may be most appropriate for making sense of the question. To some extent this is also constrained by the context of the research. For student projects, the researcher may have more leeway to think abstractly about the kinds of theoretical problems in which they are interested, and can then move down to a feasible question that will contribute to our understanding of these problems. Professional researchers employed in applied settings may have to work with questions defined by other people, and work 'backwards' from these, although of course much qualitative work will end up reframing these initial questions.

For instance, in a study commissioned by a UK health authority to identify the 'problems' general practitioners in single handed practice faced in providing good-quality care, Green (1993a, 1993b) found that in practice the general practitioners interviewed did not see themselves as facing 'problems'. From the perspective of the health authority, the working conditions of these doctors clearly presented them with 'problems', such as having to provide 24-hour-a-day care to their patients without colleagues with whom to share the burden, or being unable to take holidays. However, from the perspective of the doctors, these were not 'problems' but rather sources of pride in their ability to cope, and the 'problems' for them were located in what they perceived as their marginalization by the health authority. Their perceptions of 'good-quality care' were also rather different from those of both the health authority and their colleagues in larger practices, as they were more likely to stress the quality of the doctor–patient relationship than technical aspects of care such as the range of services provided. The research question thus changed from 'What problems do single handed GPs face in providing good-quality care?' to 'What is "good-quality care" from the perspective of single handed GPs, and how do they provide it?'

Qualitative research design is by necessity flexible, in that the research question may well shift throughout the process of doing the research, and the 'stages' of planning, fieldwork, analysis and writing up are rarely sequential. Each feeds into the others, as the concepts identified at the beginning are refined through analysing the data, and further through writing up the analysis. Designs in qualitative research are inevitably provisional to a large extent. However, this does not mean that the work involved in designing a project is redundant: developments in conceptual thinking do not happen in a vacuum, but in the context of particular questions, framed by a theoretical understanding of the problem. These need to be carefully considered at the outset.

Data collection/generation and analysis methods

The decision about which data generation and analysis methods to use can also be described as a logical one deriving from the needs of the study, but in practice the majority of researchers are most 'comfortable' with or skilled in particular styles of data collection, whether ethnographic observation, in-depth interviewing, or less intrusive measures such as analysing documents. These preferences are likely to lead to particular kinds of research topics and questions being selected. The chapters in Part 2 of this book describe some of the possibilities and limitations of four ways of generating qualitative data (interviewing, group interviewing, observation and documentary analysis). These cover the major methods, but of course there are many variations on these and some we don't address. Particularly hard to reach groups or sensitive topic areas might require imaginative methods of collecting data. Rachel Baker and Rachel Hinton (1999), for instance, describe the use of video in a study of street children in Nepal, in which they chose activities to film and enacted sketches showing events in their everyday lives, such as rag picking and sleeping on the streets. The development of novel data collection methods may in itself be an aim of a study, in which case the researcher may not know at the planning stage how well they will work.

However, at the planning stage, it is essential to think through in general how the data you are likely to generate will answer your research question. This goes back to Mason's question about specifying carefully the phenomenon of interest, and ensuring that the data generation method you propose really will furnish the kind of data that could shed light on these. What will interview transcripts, or the documents you will collate, tell you, and will this address your question? Although it may be inappropriate to detail precisely how you aim to analyse the data, it is also worth thinking through, at a theoretical as well as a practical level, what the analysis will entail in general. If the aim is to interview 80 individuals, will all of these be transcribed? What kind of analysis will you undertake? Some types of qualitative analysis are time consuming (see Chapter 8) and you may need to undertake a small pilot to estimate the time needed. This is the point at which you should consider carefully the likely number of cases you will include, and should check that this is both feasible within the resources available, and sufficient to address the question as you have framed it. If not, you may have to return to the research question and either narrow it down or reframe it such that your proposed methods can address it.

Practical issues

Once the fundamental questions about what the research is aiming to do, and how, have been addressed, planning can move on to the more practical questions and a protocol, or plan, for the research can be drafted. The main headings used in most research protocols are summarized in Box 2.1. Different organizations and funders have different formats for writing protocols, but most will require descriptions in varying detail of *what* you will do, *why* and *how*.

The 'methods' and more practical issues should follow on logically from the work described in the first part of this chapter. The data collection methods should be capable of producing the kind of information that will answer the research question, and the protocol should deal with issues of feasibility. This might include references to pilot work or discussions with collaborators to show that you can gain access to the fieldwork site, or anticipate being able to recruit the required number of interviewees. Even if the final sample size will be theoretically determined (see Chapter 4), the protocol should give some indication of the likely scope, in order to cost the study. For case studies, such as ethnographies, the choice of site needs to be justified in terms of its usefulness for answering the research question.

Multi-method designs: the place of qualitative work in larger health research studies

Qualitative social science studies of health topics typically use one research strategy, and address a single qualitative question. However, in health research, the use of multiple methods of inquiry is becoming more common, and is encouraged by many funding bodies. This means that qualitative methods of data collection are not only used in qualitative studies. In much health research qualitative approaches are used in combination with others, or as part of a larger programme of study. For instance, the study described in Case

Box 2.1 Main headings for research protocols	
Aims and objectives	The 'what' of the study, including the broad aim (what you are going to do) broken down into measurable objectives
Background	The 'why': why this is an interesting question, an important question or a policy-relevant question
Methods	The 'how': a detailed description of the data you will collect and how, including sample sizes, if appropriate, and issues of access
Ethical issues	Particular ethical issues raised by your study, including whether you need and have ethical approval, and how you will address them
Resources	Costings for staff, travel and materials
Time scale	This should include important milestones, such as commencement and completion of fieldwork, draft report completion
Dissemination and outputs	How will you inform others, including participants, of the findings? What outputs are you expecting?

Study 5.1 (on Bedouin views of maternal and child health) is from a larger, five-year programme of work on interventions to improve child health in the area. Case Study 1.2 is an example of qualitative research done in the context of a larger evaluation of an intervention, which included clinical outcomes as well as organizational ones. Chapter 9 discusses the issues raised by collaborative working on these kinds of multidisciplinary programmes, but here we outline three ways in which qualitative methods might combine with other research strategies in terms of research design, either within one programme of work or as a series of studies. First, qualitative studies can be used in exploratory (or pilot) work. Here, qualitative work is logically the precursor for other designs. Second, qualitative work can follow other research, with the aim of adding 'depth' to findings from quantitative studies, or exploring the meaning of quantitative findings. Third, some projects use qualitative and other approaches in tandem, with the aim of addressing different aspects of the same research question.

Exploratory or pilot work

Qualitative work can precede quantitative work in multi-design projects for two reasons: as preparatory, or pilot, work when the aims of the proposed quantitative study are already known, or as 'hypothesis-generating' studies, in which the aims of the quantitative work will be refined when the qualitative data have been analysed.

Most projects involve some initial pilot work to look at feasibility and predict problems with implementation, and qualitative methods are often used at this point. For instance, if a large-scale trial of different treatment options was being considered, some ethnographic study of the clinical sites at which decisions were made would be sensible, to outline the possible barriers to random allocation, and the views of the staff involved. In developing a questionnaire for a survey, qualitative interviews would be used in the initial stages to identify salient issues for respondents and to develop questions that used the vocabulary of intended respondents.

One example is a large national survey of sexual behaviour in the UK conducted by Kaye Wellings and colleagues, in part to provide essential information for planning health promotion activities and health services to reduce HIV infection (Wellings et al. 1994). The aims of the survey included quantifying aspects of individuals' sexual histories, measuring the prevalence and distribution of different patterns of sexual orientation, and measuring attitudes towards sexual behaviour. As a large amount of personal information was needed from respondents, a face-to-face interview survey was planned. The first phase was a qualitative one, including 40 in-depth interviews. These interviews were used to explore how much sexual information people were willing to disclose, what vocabulary people commonly used to discuss sexual behaviour, and how various terms were understood. The research team found a wide diversity of terms used to describe sexual experiences, and wide variations in how particular expressions (such as 'having sex') were understood. They also found that interviewees were uncomfortable with the use of vernacular terms in a research context, although these terms were used in private conversation. This is all essential information for designing a survey interview that is acceptable to respondents, and capable of generating reliable and valid data across the population.

Adapting existing survey instruments for new populations also requires qualitative research to improve the validity, **reliability** and sensitivity of the instrument. Annabel Bowden and colleagues (Bowden et al. 2002) discussed the challenges of developing a culturally sensitive measure of 'health' for use in studies evaluating the impact of interventions, in their case in Kenya. This kind of instrument would be largely used in quantitative studies, in order to measure the self-perceived health status of the target population following an intervention. However, as the authors argued, considerable qualitative research is needed to facilitate this. Many individual components of their study used qualitative methods to improve the survey instrument design. First, they drew on extensive anthropological **participant observation** studies to conceptualize 'health' from the perspective of the Kamba community in eastern Kenya.

Second, they used interviews to assist in pre-testing potential questionnaire questions. In these, respondents were asked the survey question, and were then prompted for their comprehension of key phrases and for their views on how appropriate the question was for respondents of different age and gender. Third, group interviews were used to generate discussion around some key issues in the survey. These allowed the researchers to access not just individual interpretations of questions, but also how opposing suggestions were debated. One such issue was what a 'family' comprised of. The researchers used the local word for 'homestead', but found that even this had different meanings for different members, or even across different survey questions.

One contribution of qualitative methods to research programmes is, then, in the development phases, to provide data on feasibility, to generate hypotheses, or to do the developmental groundwork for new, or adapted, survey questionnaires.

Adding 'depth' or understanding findings from quantitative data

The second logical position a qualitative study can have within a broader programme is as a successor to quantitative work. Survey data might identify a relationship between variables, for instance, but may not be able to uncover the mechanisms – that is, *why* they are linked. Case Study 2.1 is an example of qualitative research contributing in this way, to explore the reasons why women living on low incomes in the UK might smoke. Case Study 1.2, on the use of ethnography within a process evaluation, also used qualitative data to explore the meaning of quantitative data on outcomes. Similarly, qualitative research has had a vital role in understanding the 'meaning' of quantitative records, in terms of uncovering the processes by which the statistics that are used routinely in public health are produced. Data such as mortality rates, birth weight, population data and health service utilization statistics are often used routinely in health service planning, with only a superficial consideration of the problems with reliability and validity. Qualitative work can identify the social factors that shape how these are both produced and used, providing some understanding of how valid they are.

Gillian Lewando-Hundt and colleagues (Lewando-Hundt et al. 1999; Lewando-Hundt 2001), for instance, used observational methods to examine the social context of birth registration in Gaza. Having intended to use information recorded on birth certificates for identifying a sample of mothers to interview, they found that the address listed on the certificate was always either incomplete or inaccurate, although the date and place of birth of babies were recorded correctly. Following the pathways information took to get recorded officially on a birth certificate, the researchers found that clerks actually used the father's registered address for the birth certificate, even if this was different from the baby's, as the birth certificate would be rejected by the Ministry of the Interior if the two addresses were different.

Other social and political incentives for not recording addresses accurately also suggested that interventions to improve registration would be unlikely to work. There were, for instance, few street names or house numbers at that time in the Gaza Strip, as most had been removed during the *intifada* and the Palestinian population might be cautious about any records that made them easier to locate. A second problem was recorded birth weights. These were often missing from hospital discharge sheets, as doctors reported being too busy to complete them, so some clerks would leave a blank on the form. Another, though, said he would fill in a nominal weight of 3kg. Accurate birth weights are essential information for epidemiological research, yet this study suggests likely systematic biases in its collection mean that the low birth weight in Gaza is underestimated. This example demonstrates the value of qualitative methods as a way of unpacking the meaning of statistical records.

Parallel studies

Finally, qualitative and quantitative research questions on the same topic may be undertaken simultaneously, with the aim of extending our understanding of a phenomenon. Brent Wolff and colleagues (1993) argue that even though surveys and focus groups (see Chapter 5) are rooted in different theoretical approaches, they can be used as complementary methods within a single research study. They illustrate the benefits from their own study of the consequences of fertility in the decline of families in Thailand. This study aimed to explore the relationship between family size and three outcomes: educational attainment of children, wealth accumulation, and the economic role of women. Wolff and colleagues discuss three ways in which the two elements added to the study. First, data from the focus groups illustrated survey findings, providing 'colour' to the statistical associations found in the quantitative data. Second, focus group findings helped clarify the survey results. For example, one apparently contradictory finding from their survey was that although the majority of respondents felt that smaller families enjoy a relative economic advantage, a significant number also felt that if their family was larger, they would own more consumer goods. Focus groups enabled the researchers to see that one's position in the life course was critical to understanding the role of the number of children in wealth accumulation (whether they lived at home or were married and had left) and the role of children in persuading families to buy consumer goods. Third, focus groups raised new explanations that would not have arisen from the survey data. One example was the impact of child care on women's productivity in agricultural work. Even though variables such as number of children and length of time away from agricultural work for each could be quantified, the impact of child care on productivity could not, so the qualitative study provided this kind of detail. Here, qualitative and quantitative designs are used simultaneously to contribute different perspectives on the same problem.

Conclusion

Designing feasible, interesting and useful qualitative health research projects is probably the most difficult part of the whole research process, and one that is often inadequately done. In part, this is because it is difficult to develop clear guidelines for many of the important steps, such as refining the research question. Martin Bulmer, for instance, discusses the problem of describing how concepts in research questions are formed and refined. Noting that many of the concepts that social scientists use are complex and rich in meaning, he says:

> Concept-formation ... proceeds neither from observation to category, nor from category to observation, but in both directions at once and in interaction. The distinctive character of concepts in empirical social science derives from this dual theoretical and empirical character. (Bulmer 1984: 44)

The work that goes into thinking about the concepts of interest (such as health behaviours, beliefs, health service utilization or communication) involves both reflecting on theory and on empirical evidence. This chapter has outlined some starting points for this process, in suggesting some questions that researchers can ask themselves when starting out on designing qualitative studies. A final suggestion is that working with others can be a productive way of developing your own design. Colleagues can suggest other theoretical and epistemological starting points and, in doing so, may help to test your assumptions. Explaining the logic of your design to them will help you clarify exactly what it is you are hoping to do. Once the research design has been adequately developed, you should be able to explain to a non-specialist what you want to find out, how you will do this, and why.

KEY POINTS

- A good research design is a coherent argument for how the data generated will answer a research question.
- Although many qualitative studies use flexible and less formal designs, in health research relatively formal protocols are usually required.
- Refining your research question involves reflecting on the concepts of interest and how you will generate data that can reflect components of these (indicators).
- There are a number of dimensions along which research designs could be classified. We suggest a pragmatic typology based on the aims of the study: experiments, surveys, observational studies, case studies and action research.
- There is no necessary relationship between the design and methods of data collection.

EXERCISES

1 From your own experiences of health care, either as a patient or a provider, identify some potential research topics, based on any 'puzzles' you have about patient or provider behaviour.

2 Take one of these that relates to qualitative questions, and refine it as a research question. Consider the concepts of interest, what components of these concepts would be researchable, and how you would find evidence of them.

3 Design a small research project that would enable your research question to be answered. What factors do you need to take into account? What assumptions are underpinning your design? Which methods would be most suitable for generating the data you think necessary?

FURTHER READING

Patton, M.Q. (2002) *Qualitative research and evaluation methods*, (3rd edn). Thousands Oaks, CA: Sage. Originally written for qualitative research in evaluation, the third edition of this textbook expands to a full discussion of qualitative methods, with an emphasis on the practical decisions around everything from design and sampling to reporting qualitative studies. In a readable style that would appeal to many students, this includes many case study examples, and is a useful guide to all stages of the research process.

Silverman, D. (2004) *Doing qualitative research: a practical handbook*, (2nd edn). London: Sage. This draws on students' diaries of their research experiences to look in a grounded way at the decisions that have to be made about the design and choice of methods. Includes chapters on the research experience, selecting a topic and writing research proposals.

3 Responsibilities, Ethics and Values

CHAPTER SUMMARY

Ethical research practice requires a consideration of responsibilities to research participants, professional and academic colleagues, research sponsors and the wider public. Although ethical guidelines exist for most disciplines, qualitative health research often generates ethical dilemmas, which are not easily solved by reference to codes of practice. This chapter discusses the kinds of decisions qualitative health researchers have to make in designing studies that address their often conflicting responsibilities to different stakeholders.

Introduction

Any research study involves a number of different stakeholders, potentially including the research team and the institution for which they work, the professional organizations they may represent, the participants, the sponsor, policy makers who may use the results, various groups affected by those results, and the wider public, who pay for much health research. Meeting the diverse needs of these stakeholders generates a number of questions and (sometimes) conflicts about responsibilities and values. Who is the research ultimately for: the participants who helped generate the data, the wider community, knowledge for its own sake, or the research funder? How should it be conducted: is the researcher the expert, who should decide all aspects of methodology, or should participants have a role in shaping the research questions and data collection methods? How should findings be disseminated, and whose interests must be protected while doing this? What happens when our contractual obligations to sponsors (for instance not to publish until they have approved a report) conflict with our professional obligations to disseminate widely? What happens if we come across cases of poor clinical practice while doing fieldwork – do our professional obligations to protect patients override our responsibilities as researchers to protect the confidentiality of our informants? There are no clear 'rules' for deciding how to deal with these kinds of ethical dilemmas. However, researchers do have a duty to be informed about areas of ethical conflict, so that they can engage in open debate about the issues their research is likely to generate at the outset of the study. This chapter discusses the key issues of values, responsibilities and ethics raised by conducting qualitative research on health.

A first source of potential tension arises from different models of what research is *for* at a general level, which each imply some rather different ideas about the proper responsibilities of researchers.

Values in research

A positivist view of science is of investigative endeavour that somehow lies outside human values, and searches for an untainted 'truth' without reference to political or social influences. This is of course an ideal, as all science is rooted in social values. The topics that are held to be worthy of research, the kinds of questions that emerge as 'problems' to be addressed, the ways in which they can be legitimately researched, and the likelihood of publication of the findings are functions of the current social, political and cultural interests. However, the notion of the 'ivory tower' researcher who can pursue research questions to produce knowledge for its own sake, without the constraints of policy and politics, persists as one ideal to strive for, and as a pervasive influence on some approaches to research ethics. In this view, the responsibilities of the researcher are to conduct research in a scientifically sound way, and questions about what happens to the results are less important: the policy implications of findings are not the task of researchers, but of other social actors. To some extent, many disciplinary codes of ethics lean towards this model, and often focus on ensuring the scientific soundness of research, rather than considering its social implications. The statement of ethical practice of the British Sociological Association, for instance, although mostly dealing with responsibilities to participants, also contains several exhortations to members on professional integrity. Members, it says, should

> strive to maintain the integrity of sociological enquiry ... and to publish and promote the results of sociological research ... they should not accept work of a kind they are not qualified to carry out ... they should satisfy themselves that the research they undertake is worthwhile ... [they] should be careful not to claim an expertise in areas outside those that would be recognised academically as their true fields of expertise ... members should have regard for the reputation of their discipline. (BSA 1992)

As a 'scientist', then, of whatever discipline, the researcher has an obligation to 'do good science' and the primary responsibility is to 'knowledge' in an abstract sense, and perhaps to future generations of researchers. The implications this has for research practice are secondary. For instance, it would be important to carry out research in a way that is sensitive to the needs of participants in the field – but primarily so as not to 'spoil the pitch' for future researchers.

A weaker liberal approach holds that ethical values cannot be absolute, and that therefore ethical practice is relative and dependent on the moral professionalism of the researcher. Just as 'science' is not the value-free, objective system it is often claimed to be, so 'ethical principles' are not universals. In clinical medicine and public health, for example, ethical debate often takes the 'four principles' of Tom Beauchamp and Jim Childress (1983) as a starting point, which are rooted in health care ethics:

- autonomy – respecting the rights of the individual;
- beneficence – doing good;
- non-maleficence – not doing harm;
- justice – particularly distributive justice or equity.

These are, for most of us, laudable aims, but the language used to formulate them suggests they are somehow ancient and natural laws, rather than the constructions of a particular historical and cultural setting, such as Western liberal democracy (see, for instance, Gillon 1994 for some perspectives that differ from these as foundational principles). These principles arise from a consideration of medical practice and the individual patient, where it is perhaps relatively straightforward to balance potential good against potential harm, or to respect autonomy. They may be less useful as guides to decision making in complex health research settings, when the 'good' for future patients may have to be measured against the autonomy of current participants, for instance. In the liberal view, decisions about what to research, how to do it and how to publish must be made at the discretion of the researcher, whose conscience should be the primary guide. Roger Homan, in his (1991) book on social research ethics advocates one version of this position: that social research needs to develop what he calls a 'professional morality' around 'quality control ... and a commitment to truth and knowledge' (1991: 183). For Homan, there will always be conflicts between the individual scruples of researchers (over, for instance, from whom they will accept funding, or what methods they think are justified) and the public need to know. It would be impossible for ethical codes to legislate effectively for all eventualities and potential conflicts of interest, and in any case professional codes are likely to be in the interests of the profession, rather than the public. It would, then, be difficult to determine any normative ethical principles for social research, and we need instead, argues Homan, to develop a professional commitment to ethical practice built on an understanding of the dilemmas involved.

A third position is an overtly partisan one, believing that research should be carried out with the explicit aim of contributing to social justice, or emancipation. As Howard Becker put it, in a classic statement of the partisan position, 'The question is not whether we should take sides, since we inevitably will, but rather whose side are we on?' (Becker 1967: 239). His answer was that we should take the side of 'the underdog'. He argued that society is marked by what he called a 'hierarchy of credibility', which makes the views of those of higher status more 'credible' than those further down the social scale. The assumptions of a common-sense view of the world are that those at the top of any established order have a less biased view than those at the bottom. Thus the views of adults are believed over those of children, those of chief executives over the shop-floor workers, and those of medical professionals over patients. Therefore, argues Becker, the job of the social scientist is to query the established order, reveal the hierarchy of credibility for what it is and, in our research, give more credence to the views of the 'underdogs' to redress the bias that goes unremarked in most accounts of the social world.

Although perhaps attractive to some for its overtly political stance, there are considerable problems with Becker's position. First, there are of course multiple and complex hierarchies in most social settings. If we are to take the side of patients rather than their doctors, we must ask 'which patients?' Annette Lawson (1991), for instance, in taking issue with Becker's account, discusses her experience of doing research for a voluntary organization representing those with multiple sclerosis. Although as patients these participants would be the 'underdogs' of Becker's hierarchy, the voluntary organization was in fact a well-funded and relatively powerful one, which meant they had considerable power over the research agenda. In addition, different patient groups had very different views on the research aims, so it was not possible to identify one homogeneous 'underdog' perspective. Lawson also notes the institutional changes that have happened over the decades since Becker's account was published, which have shifted the focus of research towards a more obviously policy-relevant agenda. Continued funding, and thus employment for researchers, relies on being seen as producing 'useful' and credible findings that are not obviously tied to the interests of one group or another.

In short, the debates around the proper responsibilities of researchers could be summarized as three broad positions that can be adopted as starting points for ethical decisions. These positions contain rather different assumptions about the relationship between research and society that is either possible or desirable. They are:

1   *The 'neutral outsider'*. Researchers should strive to be disinterested in political and social values, given that their role is to produce knowledge for its own sake. The implications of that knowledge, and the impacts it has on society, are not the proper concern of the researcher.
2   *The 'liberal relativist'*. As ethical standards are differently constructed across different settings, researchers should follow their own (professional) conscience in deciding what to research and how to do it.
3   *The 'radical'*. The proper role of research is to improve society, and the researcher should be explicitly partisan about their practice, striving to redress inequalities and increase social justice through their research practice. Of course, researchers can be partisan from conservative political positions as well, although more generally research from the position of the status quo is able to position itself as 'neutral'.

In practice, few researchers would locate themselves exclusively within one of these positions, and the approach taken may well shift between different projects. In reviewing these various positions on the proper role of researchers in relation to social and political values, David Silverman (1985) criticizes all of them for what he calls a 'self-righteousness' about the role of social research. Instead, he suggests a more modest question around values that should be the starting point. Rather than asking whether or not we should take sides, we should, he suggests, ask what we can contribute. This is in many ways a neat side-stepping of the issue, and certainly a more answerable question. As the previous two chapters have suggested, the potential contributions of qualitative research to our understanding of health and health care are diverse, and at a number of different levels: the key issue about values becomes one of identifying the potential contribution, rather than positioning the research in terms of political standpoints. However, the question of identifying potential contributions does not absolve the researcher from considering often difficult issues around the ethics and responsibilities that are raised by all research. The particular 'contribution' is of course usually tied to specific political or policy positions. We still have to consider various sets of responsibilities, and are sometimes faced with difficult decisions about the 'right thing to do'.

Deciding on the 'right thing to do' in research practice involves a consideration of the immediate impact on research participants and colleagues, longer-term potential impacts on communities that could be affected, and responsibilities to both research sponsors and to professional and academic colleagues. These various stakeholders in the research process might have rather different interests, and the various models of ethical practice outlined above imply that those of different stakeholders would be stressed. The 'neutral outsider' would see the primary stakeholder as the discipline, and the primary responsibility of the researcher is to contribute knowledge to that discipline. The 'liberal relativist's' primary responsibility is to their own conscience. That of the 'radical' is to the participants and society more widely.

If we follow Silverman, and instead ask where our contribution lies, then we will see our primary responsibility is to the users and funders of research. The various stakeholders have different, sometimes conflicting, interests in the research process, and one task of ethical reviews is to adjudicate between them: to balance society's need for knowledge against the rights of individuals involved in the research, or obligations to professional colleagues against the needs of sponsors.

Ethical review and codes of practice

What constitutes 'ethical practice' is different in different places and times, and across different disciplines. It is, then, impossible and perhaps even undesirable to develop a set of criteria that will ensure that a study is 'ethical' if they are met. Instead, there are a number of issues raised by doing qualitative work that must be considered in the context of each particular study. First, this context will include a number of more or less formal frameworks that determine what kinds of research activity can and can't be done:

- *Legal frameworks*. National law may have an impact on issues such as confidentiality of data, and responsibilities to particular groups of participants, such as children.
- *Disciplinary codes of practice* governing research activity. The research activity of those in professions such as nursing and medicine is usually governed by professional codes of ethics. The professional associations of social scientists in many countries also issue ethical guidelines, which are usually advisory rather than mandatory.
- Local *cultural norms of ethical conduct* in both the fieldwork setting and the researcher's institution.
- Formal *ethical review*, through ethics committees.

In many institutional settings, ethical review is a formal process, requiring approval from an ethics committee before any study can start. This is part of research governance, in which institutions monitor standards of good practice and ensure that the relevant codes of practice are upheld. In the UK, for instance, the Department of Health issues guidance for local Research Ethics Committees, which are responsible for approving any study that involves users or staff of the National Health Service. Their role is primarily to consider the interests of research participants, but also to ensure that any proposed studies use appropriate designs for reaching sound conclusions (DOH 2001). Difficulties arise when there are conflicts between these various frameworks. Within the NHS, for instance, local Research Ethics Committees are primarily concerned with clinical research, and may have little experience in judging the appropriateness of qualitative designs. The local norms of the fieldwork setting may be very different from those of the institution, and the ethical guidelines of professional associations may not be in line with those of the institution's ethics committee.

In health research, many researchers are working within health care institutions or medical schools that are concerned primarily with the implications of medical research. Medical research is in general more tightly governed than other kinds of research, and guidelines developed for the conduct of research on medical subjects have a long history, starting from the Nuremberg Trials of 1947. This trial of the 23 doctors accused of atrocities committed during the Second World War resulted in the Nuremberg Code, which established principles of medical research including voluntary participation, informed consent and the justification of any risks expected (Homan 1991). Since then, issues of confidentiality and privacy have been added to most ethical codes. Internationally, for instance, the Declaration of Helsinki (WMA 2000) sets out ethical principles for medical research for the World Medical Association. This begins by placing the well-being of the 'human subject' above the interests of science and society. Researchers have a duty to protect the life, health, privacy and dignity of the human subject and to seek ethical review for all research protocols.

To carry out any work within health care settings may require the approval of an ethics committee, which will usually use criteria based on these principles taken from medical research guidelines. Social research in many countries has been less regulated, with fewer formal mechanisms to vet the ethics of proposed studies. As ethics committees are more familiar with medical research such as drug trials, the criteria they apply may work less well for qualitative social research on health. Even the language used may be rather inappropriate. Medical ethics committees, for instance, tend to refer to research 'subjects' rather than participants. The criteria may be very detailed on issues around potential biomedical risks, but less useful on the sorts of issues that are faced by ethnographers, or those using flexible research designs. Within the United Kingdom, as in many other developed countries, health research is (at the time of writing) heavily regulated, and all research involving patients or health professionals within the National Health Service must be approved by a Research Ethics Committee.

For social research, professional bodies such as the British Sociological Association (BSA 1992) and the Association of Social Anthropologists (ASA 1987) also have ethical guidelines, although in most countries these are more likely to be advisory and informative than mandatory. The ethical approval of social research is generally left to individual institutions rather than professional bodies.

Although medical and social research ethical guidelines have differing emphases, two key principles common to both, and included in most codes of ethics, are *informed consent* and *confidentiality*. Although both are perhaps uncontroversial as principles, they do generate some difficult decisions in practice with many qualitative designs.

Informed consent

Informed consent is the principle that individuals should not be coerced, or persuaded, or induced, into research 'against their will', but that their participation should be based on voluntarism, and on a full understanding of the implications of participation. Homan (1991: 71) suggests that there are four components to the concept of 'informed consent'. 'Informed' implies both that all pertinent aspects of what will happen are disclosed to the participant, and that they are able to comprehend the information. 'Consent' implies that the participant is capable of making a rational judgement about whether to participate, and that their agreement should be voluntary rather than the result of coercion or undue influence.

Informed consent has been a cornerstone of most sets of ethical guidelines since the Nuremberg Code. The first of ten rules for the ethical conduct of medical experiments sets out the principle of voluntary and informed participation (Homan 1991), and these have been endorsed by medical professionals through the various revisions of the Declaration of Helsinki (WMA 2000), which states that 'subjects *must* be volunteers and informed participants' (point 20, emphasis added). Similar criteria are a basic principle of all professional guidelines for conducting research, such as the British Sociological Association (BSA 1992), which states: '*as far as possible*, sociological research should be based on freely given informed consent' (BSA 1992, emphasis added).

The 'as far as possible' reflects the broad range of research designs in social research, whereas the stricter criteria of Helsinki and other medical codes assume perhaps an intervention design, in which the 'research' activity is easily separated from other areas of social life. In a traditional experiment, such as a drug trial, it is relatively easy to inform participants of the aims of a study, which are fixed at the outset, and for the participants to know when they are being experimented on. In many qualitative designs, data will come from a range of informants, and it may be difficult to know at the time whether an opportunistic interview in the field will be 'data' in a formal sense. Further, some observational designs are based on observing people in public settings, where it would be very difficult to secure consent at the outset. Local sets of guidelines (such as those of institutional ethics committees) often attempt to operationalize what 'informed' should mean. This might include guidelines that list the kind of information that should generally be given to participants, including the objective of the study, who is funding and conducting it, the risks involved, how the data will be handled, and who can be contacted for further information.

Despite a high degree of consensus that informed consent is a worthwhile principle, there is considerable debate over what this means in practice. Given the complexity of research designs often used in health care research, how far do we go in informing research participants about the study aims? Research on how participants understand terms such as 'randomization' and 'trial' has suggested that these can be understood very differently from how the research team might use them (Snowdon et al., 1997). In ethnographic studies, where the aims may shift during the process of data collection and analysis, how far should researchers go in keeping their participants informed about changing emphases? Increasingly, ethics committees require researchers to provide written evidence of informed consent unless there are good reasons not to (such as a non-literate population). However, the very act of asking someone to sign a form can, in many cultures, undermine the research relationship, as illustrated in Case Study 3.1.

A further problem for many ethnographic or participatory designs is that participants may not be recruited to a study as individuals, but as collectivities, such as staff on a hospital ward, or members of a patients' organization. Here, gaining informed consent can pose practical difficulties, in that the participants may change over the period of fieldwork, and new people can enter the field at various points. Carrying out participant observation on a ward, for example, may involve not only informing nursing, medical, clerical and cleaning staff but also those who may come onto the ward occasionally, such as physiotherapists or porters, and locum or agency staff, as well as patients and their visitors. Although regular meetings at shift hand-overs can be a useful way to renegotiate consent throughout the fieldwork period, it can be very difficult to make sure everyone contributing to the emerging data set is truly informed about the study.

Multiple **gatekeepers** present similar problems in situations where direct access to study participants is not possible. Gatekeepers are those who control the researcher's access to the fieldwork site or to other participants, either formally, in cases such as managers whose support will be needed to gain access to a hospital, or informally, to aid the recruitment of hard to reach groups or to legitimize the study. Examples might include community leaders who can help inform their communities about your study, or employers who can help recruit their employees. Although such gatekeepers are an essential route for gaining entry to many settings, they are, of course, also influential on the final participants, and indeed are often chosen for their persuasiveness or support for the research. Individual participants may find it difficult to refuse to take part if an influential community leader or their employer has encouraged participation. Research with young people in schools is a good example. Here, permission might be needed from a hierarchy of gatekeepers, such as the local authority responsible for schools in the area, head teachers, class teachers, parents, and only finally the children. Although consent from the participating individual should be secured, it may be very difficult for young people to refuse to participate if their teachers and parents have given their permission. If one potential danger of the use of gatekeepers is that of undue pressure to participate, the other (less commonly considered) is the opposite: that the use of gatekeepers can restrict who is invited to take part. In the school setting, for instance, there may be a requirement to have parental consent before children are approached, meaning some young people who may want to participate may not even be given the opportunity to consider it.

The use of gatekeepers to aid and legitimate access is a necessity in many studies, but the researchers should strive both to ensure that participants are truly voluntary, and that the voices of particular individuals or groups are not being silenced by a dependence on gatekeepers for contacts.

Confidentiality

The Helsinki Declaration notes that 'Every precaution should be taken to respect the privacy of the subject [and] the confidentiality of the patient's information' (WMA 2000). Social research ethics also stress confidentiality as a key criterion for ethical practice.

This first means not disclosing information gained from research in other settings, such as through informal conversation. Some research designs make this more difficult than others. In participatory designs, for instance, it may be difficult to separate out information provided by participants as 'confidential' research information from routine information that is to be shared. Doing research close to home also makes confidentiality a difficult issue. Many researchers will choose research questions arising from their personal or professional lives, and initial ideas for a project can come from everyday conversations with colleagues or friends. Clearly the ordinary social rules of confidentiality will apply to information given in this way, but once an area of interest has become a 'research study', there are perhaps additional obligations. If pilot interviews are carried out with colleagues or acquaintances, it is particularly important not to let information given here slip into everyday gossip.

Second, confidentiality relates to published accounts of the research, in which the identity of the sites and individuals should be protected where possible. Names and other identifiers can be changed to protect the privacy of participants. Case studies and evaluations of innovative service provisions present particular challenges in terms of anonymity. In straightforward evaluative studies, the site may well be named and consent will have been secured on the understanding that the final report will be of that site. In many settings, this means that individuals may be identifiable as well – there may only be one manager, or one health visitor, so qualitative accounts using quotes must be done very carefully, with the consent of those quoted. Research based on a single case, especially if this is an atypical one, is more problematic. To preserve enough detail to give the reader sufficient context to understand the findings may mean that anonymity, and therefore confidentiality, are difficult to maintain. Ideally, such issues need to be discussed fully with participants at the outset, so that any assurances of anonymity and confidentiality are realistic, or the researcher may find publication impossible. Some participants may not want confidentiality. Anne Grinyer (2002), for instance, reports how in her research with parents of young people with cancer many participants actively requested the use of their own and their children's real names. Otherwise, they felt, they lost ownership of a deeply personal story.

Another constraint on confidentiality comes from legal frameworks. It is difficult to give absolute guarantees of confidentiality, as there are situations in which there may be an obligation (moral if not legal) to break this. One example might be research with children, to whom the researcher has a responsibility as an adult, as well as a researcher. If a child being interviewed were to indicate that they were at risk in some way (for instance from parental abuse), many ethicists would see the primary duty of the researcher as one of safeguarding the child's safety, rather than their privacy. In some countries this would be a legal responsibility. If this is the case, researchers cannot offer complete confidentiality to young people in research settings. In settings where the researcher has no legal obligation to breach confidentiality, there is a difficult judgement call involving the degree of likely risk. For research with vulnerable groups such as children, it is good practice to establish protocols for these events at the beginning of a study, with a nominated person for the interviewers or research staff to contact in the first instance with concerns.

For many health care professionals engaged in research, there can be real difficulties in aligning the roles of dispassionate researcher and concerned professional. The discovery of very poor practice while doing fieldwork, for instance, can generate dilemmas in terms of whether to breach confidentiality. If patients are being abused, or professionals are incompetent, should the researcher disclose this information? The answer to this may depend on a fine judgement of the likely risks to individuals in the research setting and the likely benefits arising from the research findings. Confidentiality should not be breached lightly: future participation relies on a climate of trust, and the researcher is not an auditor of good practice (unless this is the aim of the study). In settings where, as a professional, a researcher may face these kinds of dilemma, there are a number of strategies to adopt. One is to provide participants will an information and consent sheet that makes clear what the limits of confidentiality will be at the outset, although of course this does potentially limit the validity of data likely to be generated. A second option is to consider action research designs, which would enable a more open relationship between the professional as researcher and those in the field.

Responsibilities to research participants

Consent and confidentiality are core principles that inform the responsibilities of researchers to the participants in research, but they are not the only issues to consider. Although social research is unlikely to generate risks to physical health, there are other, less obvious, impacts that need to be thought through, especially if the research is on a sensitive topic. This section considers the particular responsibilities to research participants raised in interview and ethnographic studies.

Ethics in interviews

The primary responsibility enshrined in most codes of ethics is to participants in the research: those who are interviewed, observed or who have contributed time and effort to the study. Although most qualitative research does not involve interventions that appear to impact directly on the lives of participants, we should not forget that involvement in research can have emotional consequences, particularly if the research concerns experiences of ill health, traumatic incidents, or issues normally considered 'private', such as sexual behaviour.

If qualitative research is built on respect for participants' world-views, data collection methods do have to convey this respect. This might involve, for instance, making sure interview questions reflect the concerns of interviewees, rather than merely pursuing the researcher's perspective. Kathryn Ehrich, a sociologist who reports on her experience of being on the receiving end of being interviewed, notes the discomfort she and her partner experienced as interviewees when an interviewer pursued a research agenda on the impact of chronic illness on families, without acknowledging the experiences that were most salient to them as 'respondents':

> ... we found that the research agenda was fully theirs, with no space for asserting our own experience of living with chronic illness. There was no dialogue, only the opportunity to answer questions co-operatively or not. My response was increasingly the latter, and I felt misunderstood, as though they thought I was presenting 'resistance'.... Our focus was simply not of particular interest. (Ehrich 2001: 23)

When interviewing is done with regard to the interviewees' agenda, with empathy and understanding, it can be a very positive experience for participants, with many people pleased that someone is taking an interest in their lives and concerns. In her study of the transition to motherhood, for instance, Ann Oakley (1981) reported that the majority of her interviewees felt that the interviews had been a good experience, giving them an opportunity to talk about concerns and to reflect on their experiences. One exception may be members of particular groups who may become 'over-researched', and asked to take part in multiple studies. This can be particularly distressing if researchers raise expectations of, say, service improvements that are never realized.

One ethical problem in interview studies is that the tenets of 'good' interviewing practice (see Chapter 4) are those of encouraging trust and disclosure, the very skills that may make it most difficult for respondents to refuse, or to withdraw, once the interview has started. Good interviewers build a sense of rapport, and encourage interviewees to tell personal and detailed stories about themselves. They are, in short, experts at exploiting and mining individuals for data. For this to be done ethically, it has to be done with respect for the interviewee as an individual, rather than merely as a carrier of 'good data'. The expert interviewer also has to remember to provide real opportunities to refuse, at any point. High response rates are often seen as an indicator of good-quality research, yet could just as easily be seen as evidence of the inadequate possibilities for refusal or withdrawal. The researcher may have to balance the 'scientific' needs of a representative sample with ethical needs to ensure proper consent is given, on an ongoing basis, to participation. They may also have to balance the scientific need for 'good data' against the possible risks to the participants of disclosure. Case Study 3.1, from rural India, is an example of a setting in which the research team had to be particularly careful of 'over-disclosure' on the part of their interviewees, in this case in focus group interviews.

Particular care should be taken when interviewing participants who are in a relatively powerless position compared with the researcher or those whose cognitive abilities are impaired. The latter may be less able to be 'informed' while the former may be less able to positively 'consent' to participation. Both situations may require imaginative steps to maximize true voluntary consent, but they do not preclude research with groups such as those with mental disabilities, limited language skills, or powerless social positions. Indeed, one might argue that researchers have a duty to reflect the voices of those who are least likely to have any other access to the public arena. Information about the project needs to be provided in ways that will be appropriate for the participants, and this may mean using video or photographs rather than written forms.

Case Study 3.1   Cultural sensitivity and ethical practice: an example from rural India

(Source: Vissandjée, B., Abdool, S. and Dupéré, S. (2002) 'Focus groups in rural Gujarat, India: a modified approach', *Qualitative Health Research*, 12: 826–43)

Bilkis Vissandjée, Shelley Abdool and Sophie Dupéré discussed the appropriateness of focus groups (see Chapter 5) for their research on women's autonomy and health behaviour in rural India, in part because of strong local oral traditions. However, they also noted that the method must be adapted for local conditions, taking into account the research topic, the participants, and the social, political and cultural context of the study area. This raises a number of ethical considerations for researchers, who must think through how to adapt research designs in order to facilitate relatively disempowered participants in expressing their views, and ensure that the research is conducted in an appropriate ethical manner – namely, that it is 'culturally competent'.

   The project setting for their study was a rural area of Gujarat, with 25 relatively small villages that had little contact with outsiders. The research team were aware that this posed potential problems in establishing good relationships. First, the villagers might be distrustful of outsiders, especially those from outside the country (there were Canadian researchers on the team) who might hold negative views of Indian society. Second, the topics they were asking women to discuss were not traditionally those on which women were encouraged to hold views, and some local men were concerned that the researchers were intending to 'change' the women. Finally, the presence of an overseas research team may raise (false) expectations of aid or policy action. To address these concerns, the researchers embarked on a period of field preparation, in which they built relationships with community leaders and members. They did this in partnership with a local Community Health Volunteer (CHV), who knew the local villagers well. The team were careful to match genders at this point, as it would not have been appropriate to have women walking unaccompanied through the villages, or for a male researcher to talk to the local women. The CHV also helped with focus group recruitment, assisting in door-to-door recruitment of potential participants. Recruiting door to door was essential in rural areas; not only did it facilitate communication in an area with no telephones and limited literacy, but it also enabled the researchers to ask women to participate in the presence of the men in the household, who might otherwise feel hostile about the groups.

The researchers had to take into account local power relationships, including those of caste and any family relationship. It was not culturally possible to hold separate group discussions for the different castes in the village, but in the groups higher-caste women inhibited lower-caste women from speaking. Similarly, mothers-in-law had more authority than daughters-in-law in discussions. Here, the composition of groups entailed ethical decisions that offset the need for cultural appropriateness (including everyone) with the need for hearing disempowered voices. Vissandjée and colleagues note that even if they had run more homogeneous groups that included only low-status women, in an area where 'everybody knows everybody' women may feel that anything they say will be reported back, and would therefore still be constrained in discussing their views.

Written consent to participation was inappropriate, so the research team gave only verbal assurances of confidentiality. Written papers, in this context, would be negatively associated with government documents.

The closeness of rural communities also has an impact on the researchers' ability to ensure confidentiality. The team had to consider how far they were responsible for any of the consequences of women's behaviour in the focus group, given that they would be seen as representatives of their families, and whether any disapproved behaviour or talk would probably be communicated back to the family. In these circumstances, the focus group moderator had to stress that the research team would treat the data generated with confidence, but also had to guard against 'over-disclosure' (participants feeling so comfortable that they revealed more than they had intended) in the group, given the possible future consequences for participating women. Given also that the researchers were asking women to reflect on their own lives in ways that were potentially very destabilizing, it was also useful to provide follow-up opportunities for private discussion and reflection on participation in the group discussion.

The authors were working within a participatory approach, where the key ethical dilemmas faced were the need to balance 'empowerment' for women in the community with the potential risks to individual women as a result of their involvement in the project. One ethical risk of this kind of project, they noted, is that once the researchers disappear, individual women may be left with a sense of developing awareness but with a dissatisfaction that there is nothing they can do, as they are too busy or isolated to discuss the issues raised with other women. An essential step to minimize the risk of this happening is to disseminate any findings from the study at a village level, and to work with local health care providers to develop follow-up local activities.

To offset the power imbalance between researcher and interviewee, the interview format may need to be thought about carefully. First, the location is important. Given that most interviewees will feel relatively more empowered in their own environment than yours (Green and Hart 1999), the interviewee's home or another familiar place may be more suitable than a university office or clinic room. This is, of course, context specific: in some settings the home enviroment may be too crowded or lacking in privacy for one-to-one interviews. Case Study 5.1, which describes a study of Bedouin views of maternal health services, is a good example here, as Susan Beckerleg and her colleagues describe the inappropriateness of trying to do a 'private' interview in the home setting. Here, an institutional setting might be preferable if the topic were one that required privacy.

A second consideration in thinking about power in the research process is the interview format. A one-to-one interview can be intimidating, and interviewing people in pairs or small groups may redress the power imbalance. This is particularly useful when working with young people, who can be asked if they would like to do the interview with a friend or sibling. However, it is worth remembering that few interviewees are entirely powerless. In practice, most participants will have a number of strategies at their disposal for declining to participate without actually having to refuse. Adolescents, for instance, may be monosyllabic in answering questions, or rural villagers may deliberately divulge only misleading stories. Baker and Hinton quote one of the participants in their research, who was resentful of the many interviews she had previously been asked to take part in. Rather than refusing, she said her approach was to 'give a quick answer to let them go away' (Baker and Hinton 1999: 88).

Ethics in observational studies

Participant observation (see Chapter 6) involves the researcher participating to some extent in a social field (a village community, a hospital ward) in order to research it. The first ethical issue raised by using these methods in health care projects governed by medical ethics is that informed consent is often problematic. In a bounded field (such as one small clinic) it may be possible to secure consent from all parties. Most health care settings, however, will involve changing shifts of staff and a rapid turnover of patients, and it is very difficult to ensure that all parties present at every point in the fieldwork are fully informed about the study and have actively consented to being research participants. Julienne Meyer (1993) discusses the limitations of informed consent in her action research study of lay participation in care in a London hospital ward. Finding a ward that would be willing to work with her for a year of fieldwork was a long task, but even with this careful preparation, Meyer had some reservations about consent. Once the project was underway, she noted, it would have been very difficult for an individual to withdraw as they were part of a group that had made a commitment to work together. If a few individuals were to become uncomfortable with a project, would it be ethical to call a halt, given the input and commitment of the rest of the team?

Joan Cassell (1980) discusses the wide range of models adopted by anthropologists doing fieldwork, and suggests that the key principle for informing ethical practice should be a respect for human autonomy. Medical research ethics primarily entail assessing the risks for harm to 'subjects', but this, she argues, is an inappropriate rubric for anthropologists. First, assessing the likely 'harm' is very difficult, and second, the kind of 'harm' caused by social research usually relates to hurt feelings, or invasions of privacy, rather than the kinds of injury or physical harm resulting from medical interventions. Although anthropologists should of course take all steps possible to remove the risk of harm, the more important principle should be the attempt to treat people as autonomous agents, rather than means to ends. Thus, research practice that involves coercing people to participate in an interview, or deceiving them, would be difficult to justify ethically even if confidentiality was respected and there was no harm to the participant. A focus on respecting autonomy would make most covert studies questionable.

Covert methods

Covert methods, in which the researcher does not disclose their role to those in the field, clearly raises a number of particular ethical dilemmas. Not only is the autonomy of the participants not respected, but informed consent is impossible to secure, at least before the fieldwork. The use of covert methods is discussed in Chapter 6. One classic example is Rosenhan's (1973) study of psychiatric hospitals in the USA, which relied on research assistants gaining admission as patients by pretending to have the symptoms of mental illness, described in Case Study 3.2.

Rosenhan's study of psychiatric hospitals raises some interesting ethical issues. It clearly violates the principle of informed consent, and it is unlikely that many ethics committees today would approve such a study. However, the findings from his study could probably not have been gained in any other way. Although it could be argued that there are many detailed 'insider' accounts from 'real' hospital patients, both autobiographical and literary, these have come from people stigmatized by the diagnosis of 'mental illness' and thus have less legitimacy than accounts from an academic team of researchers. Does this justify the deceit involved? One justification is the 'public interest' argument. Rosenhan's study may have had little immediate policy impact, but was part of the backdrop of cultural knowledge that influenced policies in many countries away from long-term hospitalization as a way of managing mental illness and towards community care. However, a real cost is the loss of trust between professionals and researchers.

Another argument that has been made in defence of these covert methods is that of cultural relativity: that ideas such as autonomy and privacy are tied to Western notions of individuality, and may be inappropriate in different settings. Justifying their covert study of a hospital ward in Ghana, van der Geest and Sarkodie (1998) argue that the very notion of 'informed consent' is a culture-bound one, and that in the Ghanaian context, especially in a rural environment, there is less concern with the notion of privacy. Although we would agree that notions of 'privacy' are of course culturally specific, and good research practice should involve identifying how they are locally constructed (as in Case Study 3.1), there are real ethical problems with the applying different *standards* in different settings. In their paper, van der Geest and Sarkodie suggest that their practice (although not in line with the anthropological codes of ethical conduct) is justifiable because the research may lead to better hospital conditions for patients in Ghana. In other words, the ends justify the means. In terms of Cassell's focus on respect and autonomy discussed above, this would not of course be justifiable.

Case Study 3.2   Covert observation of psychiatric hospitals

(Source: Rosenhan, D. L. (1973) 'On being sane in insane places', *Science*, 179: 250–8)

Rosenhan was interested in how reliable and valid diagnostic measures of 'sanity' were, and whether psychiatric staff were able to distinguish the sane from the insane. He devised an experiment in which eight 'normal' people got themselves admitted to US psychiatric hospitals by claiming to hear voices that said 'hollow', 'empty' or 'thud', but by otherwise presenting their 'real' medical and social histories to admission clinic staff. All were admitted with a diagnosis of schizophrenia, except one with a diagnosis of manic depressive psychosis. On admission, the researchers behaved normally and cooperated with hospital routines. Given that they spent considerable time in the hospitals waiting to be discharged, their undercover status provided an opportunity for **covert observation.** Rosenhan's paper reports on their experiences of being hospitalized, and the ways in which the diagnostic label they had received at admission shaped the interpretation of their behaviour by staff. None of the researchers were identified as sane pseudo-patients by staff, although interestingly many other patients challenged them, assuming that they were undercover journalists or researchers. In general, they were discharged with diagnoses of 'schizophrenia in remission'.

Rosenhan's findings were important. Not only did he contribute to the debate around the social construction of labels such as schizophrenia, but the reports of his pseudo-patients were an important contribution to our understanding of the effects of both hospitalization and labelling. Labelling someone as mentally ill shapes the interpretation of all their behaviour. As patients with a diagnosis, the everyday behaviours of the researchers, such as writing notes or being anxious in the new hospital environment, were seen as symptoms of their disease. Rosenhan's descriptions of many aspects of hospitalization, such as the low level of interaction between staff and patients, the occasional abuse of patients and lack of privacy, were a significant development in our understanding of how institutions lead to depersonalization and may contribute to mental ill health, rather than cure it. With other studies of long-term institutions, this pseudo-patient study was an influence in the gradual policy shift in many countries away from asylums and towards other forms of care for those with mental health problems.

However, the design of the study raises a number of ethical questions. First, there are the problems of deceit. Except in one case, neither the hospital staff nor other patients knew that they were participants in the research (though some patients did guess), and had not consented to take part. Rosenhan defends the concealment (though he does admit it is 'distasteful') on the basis that it was necessary. It was the only way that these data could have been gathered. If hospitals were warned that researchers would try to get themselves admitted, there would be no way of knowing whether the process of admission and experiences on the wards were typical or not. The hospitals and staff are not named in the report: Rosenhan is not interested in exposing poor practice (as an undercover journalist might) but rather in generalizing from his data to say something about the ways in which mental illness is dealt with in the American health care system. The defence against breaching normal expectations of informed participation is thus a public interest one, based on utilitarian principles. In short, the ends (furthering public knowledge with the aim of improving services for some of the most marginalized people in society) could be said to justify the means. Arguably, though, Rosenhan's study 'spoils the pitch' for future researchers attempting to study psychiatric services in more open ways, making mental health professionals defensive and less willing to consider change. If these disadvantages are taken into account, the benefit in terms of service improvements may be less likely. A final ethical consideration is the safety of the research team. Once admitted to the hospitals, most of the researchers wanted to leave very quickly, as they were unpleasant places to be. It is, however, difficult to get discharged at short notice, and they spent between 7 and 52 days as patients. This experience may be distressing, and there was also the danger of having to take unnecessary medications.

In terms of fieldwork practice, one source of debate over ethical positions is, then, between those who view the *process* as the key issue, and develop methodological strategies that maximize respect for human autonomy, and those who consider the *ends* to be the deciding factor. For the latter, decisions about ethics are made in a more utilitarian way, in terms of assessing the likely benefit to the people involved (such as improved services) or the wider community against the risks.

Anthropological research and representing the 'other'

The ethical issues of participant observation studies do not end with field-work. Responsibilities to participants continue in the writing up and dissemination of accounts, and researchers should consider carefully the likely impact not only on individual participants, but the likely policy impact of the study more broadly. This includes obvious considerations of confidentiality and being careful to disguise distinguishing characteristics. Circulating a draft report to informants can help identify any areas they feel may leave them vulnerable if identified.

Beyond the immediate concerns of embarrassment for individuals who may be identified in research reports, there are broader issues around representing communities. Nancy Scheper-Hughes (2000) gives a moving account of her attempts to write 'honest ethnography' whilst maintaining a respect for those she lived with for nearly a year. Returning to the Irish village community she studied 25 years previously, she is struck by how betrayed villagers still feel by the book she wrote of her experiences. The book, *Saints, Scholars and Schizophrenics* (1979), was an exploration of how particular social structures and family patterns could be functional for society, but dysfunctional for individuals, making some vulnerable to mental ill health. Like any ethnography, it was, she notes, a partial view – as much reflecting her political and theoretical concerns as the views of the villagers. Reacting against a 'functionalist' tradition in anthropology, which stressed only the positive and functional aspects of culture, she brought a feminist and theoretically eclectic approach to exploring the dysfunctional aspects of rural community life against a historical backdrop of British colonialism, famine and the decline of agricultural economies. Despite attempts to disguise the identity of the community in her ethnography, it was identified by a journalist, and became visited by a number of other researchers in the intervening years. Reflecting on the controversy over the book, and the anger of villagers years later at what they saw as an overly negative portrayal that said nothing about the positive aspects of rural Irish culture, Scheper-Hughes suggests some of her ethical decisions would be different now. First, she would avoid pseudonyms and anonymity. These protect the anthropologist more than the participants, she argues, and perhaps mean we think less carefully about what we write. Second, there are the positive aspects of village life that could have been addressed as well – the absence of violence, close and enduring friendships, and social equality between men and women. Scheper-Hughes' experience illustrates the balancing act that many researchers face in meeting obligations to both communities (in representing them faithfully and not betraying close working relationships that have been built up over time) and the discipline (in analysing culture in ways that move forward our thinking about, say, the cultural roots of mental illness).

Different models of the research relationship

Participatory designs are built on the assumption that researching with, rather than on, people can change the power relationships inherent in the research enterprise, such that a more democratic relationship is established. Action research, as discussed in Chapter 2, is one potential participatory approach, given that the problem and solutions are identified not by an outside researcher, but by those in the field, with the researcher acting as facilitator rather than 'expert'. Julienne Meyer (1993) questions whether, in practice, this approach is in fact more democratic. In some ways it can lead to greater exploitation than traditional researcher–subject models, as the relationships between those in the field and the researcher are likely to be closer and more collaborative, therefore putting the participant in a potentially more vulnerable position. Further, the very experience of taking part in research, and having an outsider encourage questioning and reflection, might make for uncomfortable group dynamics as people reassess not only their own roles but those of others in the organization.

When a significant power imbalance between the researcher and the research participants generates ethical challenges for research, then participatory designs may be a useful way of finding a more responsible way of conducting the research. Virginia Morrow and Martin Richards (1996), for instance, suggest that participatory methods may be a good way of working with children. This might involve training young people themselves as interviewers so they can help shape the process of data collection with their peers and including young people's representatives on steering committees. Rachel Baker describes working with a 15-year-old former street child when researching the health and lives of street children in Nepal (Baker and Hinton 1999). This young man was in a position to talk with street children in a more equal way than the Western researchers, or workers from local agencies, although of course he was not an 'insider' in an unproblematic way. As the study described in Case Study 3.1 suggests, though, a participatory design does not solve the difficult issue of power imbalances within communities. In a rural Indian setting, Vissandjée and colleagues were interested in women's empowerment, and designed a participatory study to involve local villagers at all stages in the process. However, they had to work within both patriarchal and caste relationships in order to facilitate the research, and take account of power relationships within families. Further, they had no way of ensuring that by 'empowering' women in making them conscious of their own positions they were helping to dismantle any of those power dynamics. In short, participatory designs have to be thought through very carefully to ensure that researchers do not just compound social inequalities. Research is a very different enterprise from community development, and researchers should be wary of making extravagant claims about 'improving' communities unless they are really prepared to work long term in particular settings, rather than just carrying out one-off studies.

With rather less lofty aims, it is becoming more common to include the participants (or the wider community from whom they are selected) as recognized stakeholders in the research process, even if the design is not a participatory one. In the UK, researchers are often asked to include users or community representatives on steering groups for the project, or to build collaborative links with likely end users of the research, such as patient groups or local communities. The Association of Social Anthropologists (ASA 1987) has the involvement, as far as possible, of those being studied in both the design and conduct of the research as an ethical principle. There is, then, a principle of 'involving' users, as a 'good thing' in itself, even if not making claims about the virtue of this in terms of empowering research participants.

The association between participation with empowerment, or even a more equal partnership with researchers, is being increasingly questioned by those who have critiqued what Bill Cooke and Uma Kothari (2001), for instance, have called 'the tyranny of participation'. In their edited collection of debates around participatory development, they point to a number of ethical problems with assuming that participation is inevitably, or even possibly, an empowering experience. First, there is a real danger that participatory research designs can usurp legitimate decision-making processes. The experience of many of those involved in participatory projects is not that local people shape the development agenda, but rather that they merely learn what agencies can and are able to deliver. 'Local knowledges' are simply a product of particular kinds of research contexts, just as any other research data are, and there is nothing particularly 'pure' or empowering about those generated through participatory methods. Second is the ethical problem of assuming that outsiders coming in to 'empower' people can do anything more than reinforce existing social divisions. Communities are rarely homogeneous groups with similar needs and interests, but are typically structured by gender, social status or other power imbalances, and it is unlikely that the needs of all can be included in 'the community view'. In terms of a debate about research methods, there are also real challenges in maximizing the most appropriate methods for the research question when there is a primary focus on communities collaborating in the research endeavour. Research is a specialised and professionalised activity (like most other occupations in modern societies), and there is a real danger that methodological quality suffers if the emphasis is on including participants in the design, conduct and interpretation of findings. We return to the methodological implications of combining development and research goals in Chapter 9.

Responsibilities to yourself and co-workers

We have considered how responsibilities to participants have to be balanced against those of the public's 'right to know' and the potential future benefits to others. One set of responsibilities that is less often considered are those researchers have to themselves and co-workers at a personal as well as a professional level. At its most basic, there is a responsibility of personal safety. Traditionally, social researchers have often been rather cavalier about risks, and many of those working in the health field are working with agencies that operate in what could be seen as inherently risky environments, such as post-conflict settings or areas with epidemic disease. A review of risks to the well-being of qualitative researchers carried out by Mick Bloor and colleagues (Bloor et al. 2007) concluded that, although physical harm to researchers was rare, emotional risks were more widespread and there was (in the UK, at least) poor support from most researchers' institutions for preparing and supporting research staff and students. Increasingly, though, the health and safety of researchers as employees or students is being taken seriously by institutions, many of which will require a risk assessment to be carried out prior to fieldwork. If the sponsor or employing institution does not require risk assessment as a formal process, it is worth working through some of the potential risks faced with other members of the team and supervisors, particularly if you are planning on conducting fieldwork in an unfamiliar setting. In a review of safety in research, Gary Craig, Anne Corden and Patricia Thornton (2000) suggest that researchers and those responsible for them think about the following sets of potential risks:

- physical threats or abuse
- psychological trauma, including that arising from real or threatened violence or from what is disclosed during fieldwork
- the potential for compromising situations, in which accusations of improper behaviour might be made
- increased exposure to risks such as infectious disease or accidental injury.

The aim of carrying out a risk assessment exercise is to identify and minimize the risks potentially faced by the research team, and to develop procedures for dealing with emergencies. The details will of course depend on the specific study: on the fieldwork environment, the data collection strategy and the support available in the study site. The risks faced by an ethnographer in a remote area of an unfamiliar country are rather different from those faced by an interviewer conducting research with managers in their own institution. Those planning projects in unfamiliar environments should consult widely with others who do know the setting. However, familiarity should not lead to complacency, as we are often less aware of risks on our home territory than we are in less familiar settings. Some common ways of minimizing the risks listed above might include:

- *Training.* Do fieldworkers need training in those interpersonal skills that are vital to avoid conflict, understand the cultural norms of the fieldwork site, or be aware of any particular areas of risk assessment to do their job safely?
- *Maintaining good contact with field staff.* Interviewers can leave itineraries with office staff or nominated individuals, and ensure that visits to interview sites are notified. The provision of mobile phones or phone cards to use to confirm arrival and departure from interview sites may be worth considering, although these need careful management to ensure fieldworkers do phone every time, and a consideration of appropriate protocols if they fail to do so. Regular email contact with those based away from the

host institution is advisable, both to update managers with itineraries and to ensure distance staff and students minimize their potential isolation.

- *Debriefing.* Returning from a period of fieldwork can be emotionally difficult, and some form of debriefing should be organized. Equally, interviewing on sensitive or emotional topics can be traumatic, and some kind of support is needed, whether from colleagues or the supervisor.
- *Travel advice.* Adequate advice on travel health for those doing fieldwork away from home includes the provision of appropriate health insurance, advice on immunizations and other health needs, and local transport risks.

Some of these considerations of personal safety have resource implications, and should therefore be costed in at the outset of a study.

Ethical dilemmas and conflicts

So far, we have outlined various sets of responsibilities that researchers have, and a number of principles on which ethical decisions can be taken. We have suggested that ethical principles are not absolute, but are shaped by wider cultural values such that they vary across time and place. Privacy, for instance, was not addressed by early codes of ethical practice in medical research, but is now a core component in many professional codes, reflecting general social concern about data on individuals and how these are managed. Further, the practicalities of putting even widely agreed principles (such as consent) into practice have to be adapted to local norms, as shown in Case Study 3.1. The socially determined nature of ethical values means that it is not unusual for conflicts to arise over the proper way to manage a project, or to disseminate findings, with different stakeholders stressing different principles or disagreeing about how they should be enacted. In qualitative research on health, the first source of tension can be the different cultures of social and health research.

Social research and biomedical ethical practice

Much qualitative health research is done in multidisciplinary teams, or across a number of institutions or countries, and these situations increase the chance that ethical dilemmas will arise about the 'right' thing to do. This chapter began with a reference to codes of practice for medical and social research. Although these codes of practice address the same issues, there may be differences across professions and research communities in what counts as ethical practice. One example is that of informed consent for young people. In medical research in the UK for people under 16 the consent of parents is required, but many community organizations working with young people would see this as undermining young people's autonomy to make their own decisions. Qualitative research designs themselves often generate difficulties for ethics committees that have been set up to review bio-medical research, in part because their flexibility and open-endedness can appear to be poor design, which would be difficult to justify in terms of the likely benefits to the participants. Biomedical ethics committees will often consider research in terms of risks and benefits, rather than respect for the participants' autonomy. Even though the risks of social research may be low, the benefits can be hard to judge in instrumental ways.

The differences between the expectations of medical research and social science research communities also present potential dilemmas around data archiving. In many senses, archiving data for future researchers to use is good ethical practice: it is an efficient use of resources, avoids duplication of the research effort, and leaves the study data potentially available for other analysts to look at, so increasing the **generalizability** of findings. In the UK, the Economic and Social Research Council (the main funders of social science research) encourages all researchers to retain/deposit in a national archive any qualitative data arising from their studies. However, many medical ethics committees will expect data to be destroyed at the end of a project to ensure confidentiality. Gill Backhouse (2002) advises researchers to deal with this dilemma by making sure data (such as transcripts) are anonymized, with all identifying material removed, before they are prepared for archiving. She also encourages researchers to secure written consent from participants for archiving, and for participants to see transcripts for approval. Of course, in many research settings this will be difficult or inappropriate.

Whose risks?

Risk assessments are another potential source of ethical debate. Precautions that minimize risk for the researcher may in themselves recreate social prejudices about 'risky environments' – environments that are the homes and communities of those we are studying. What may seem like sensible precautions for the researcher when interviewing in, say, a deprived inner-city estate (such as making contact with someone outside by mobile phone when entering or leaving, only interviewing during the daytime, or interviewing in pairs) could well feel like disrespect and suspicion to the resident of that estate. In addition, there is often a trade-off between 'safer' and 'more productive' data collection strategies. In participant observation studies in particular, the informal and opportunistic interviews and observations are often most useful, but of course these are the ones that might be avoided to maximize personal safety. Interviewing people in their own homes may be less safe than inviting them into the university, but may also mean there is more chance of developing a trusting relationship.

Whose truth?

Marina Barnard (2005) discusses the ethical dilemmas generated when researching sensitive areas when the accounts of different sets of interviewees might construct rather different 'truths' about the social world. Her example is perhaps a particularly ethically challenging one, but it does illustrate a general problem with naive attempts to solve ethical challenges in research. Interviewing parents who were drug users about the impact of drug use on child care, as well as on their children, Barnard found, unsurprisingly, different accounts of the effects of drug use. Parents were likely to present themselves as having managed to provide reasonable levels of child care, despite their problematic drug use, whereas children were more likely to report memories of having had to go without food, or experiencing a chaotic upbringing. Interviews, of course, have to be treated as situated accounts, rather than any simple representation of a reality (in this case, that of 'what life was like when the children were young'). However, Barnard notes that we do need to make some claims about the relative validity of the data as indicating something about an external reality (such as drug-using parents' ability to look after children). The ethical dilemmas come first from obeying the dictum of non-maleficence, as not doing harm to one set of respondents (in terms of how accounts are reported) may harm another set. Reporting the damaging effects of drug use on child care, although potentially contributing to a better provision of services or support for children, is also likely to add to the stigma of this group. This is an area where research reports may well be disseminated widely through mass media as well as academic publications, and the researcher may be responsible for further negative coverage of an already marginalized group. As Barnard concludes:

> A world that is neatly divided into goodies and baddies would present few problems for clear-cut recommendations. However, the problem as ever lies in the grey areas, those ambiguous spaces where people are neither so good nor so victimised as their representation; and furthermore where the representation of their interests is axiomatic with the downplaying of others. (Barnard 2005: 15)

Research in low-income settings

We have already touched on the problem of dealing with local cultural norms when researching across different countries, and suggested that a distinction must be made between exploiting such differences (in, say, carrying out studies that would not be approved in the researcher's own country) and respecting differences (in designing culturally appropriate protocols). The Nuffield Council on Bioethics (NCB) (2003) looked at the issue of health care research in developing countries, and highlighted a number of potential risks of being 'sensitive to the local social and cultural context, while [needing] to ensure that their clinical methods reflect the obligations imposed by relevant national and international guidance' (NCB 2003: 134). The key issue, they suggested, is a respect for difference, rather than necessarily adopting local practices if these would be considered unethical in most settings. One example might be that of senior members of a household consenting for, say, adult women. Sensitivity to local practice might suggest that heads of households are approached first, but ethical practice would require each individual's informed consent in addition. Although their report focused on the issues raised in clinical research, the general conclusions reached are perhaps also applicable to qualitative designs. They suggest four principles that should inform ethical practice: the duty to alleviate suffering, the duty to show respect for persons, the duty to be sensitive to cultural difference, and the duty not to exploit the vulnerable. Externally funded research in developing countries should, concludes the report, be ethically reviewed by a committee within the developing country which can ensure that the proposal fits with the health care priorities for that country, is scientifically valid and is ethically acceptable.

In practice, the requirement to be sensitive to local norms whilst not exploiting them can be more difficult than the guidelines imply. Catherine Riessman (2005) for instance, discusses the dilemmas she faced, as a researcher from the USA, in researching clinics in India where women were treated with no privacy. First, she felt complicit in researching in this setting, which felt disrespectful to the women. More acutely, though, she was aware that her own access to both the clinics and women to interview was facilitated by the relative lack of governance in hospitals settings, compared with the USA. This is a common experience for researchers from high income settings.

More practical problems will often arise from the competing demands of ethical review bodies and local cultural norms. The insistence on signed consent sheets by many review committees is a good example. Although these may be seen by some in high income countries as 'protecting' the interviewee, official forms are, in many parts of the world, intimidating and will signify coercion rather than protection.

Commissioners and researchers

The different stakeholders in the research process may well have very different agendas, which may generate tensions for the researcher. Those who carry out and those who fund and commission research may be working with rather different models of what the research is for. Research for health is often commissioned by organizations that need timely findings disseminated as quickly as possible to address policy-relevant problems. However, researchers in academic settings may gain more credibility from generalizable, theoretically driven work that takes considerable time to write up and publish (Wenger 1987). There may, then, be conflicts between obligations to commissioners, in terms of either quick publication, or sometimes (if the findings are politically sensitive) not publishing at all, and the demands of academic research. For Stephen Gorard (2002), 'quality' is the arbiter of these dilemmas: ethical research, he argues, is research that does not squander public money, and researchers have a responsibility to the general public (not just the participants), who may stand to benefit from any findings, to produce high-quality research with valid and reliable findings. In practice, however, the dilemma of responsibilities to a commissioner who wants the report withheld or delayed and the obligation to publish may be more difficult to manage than an appeal to quality might suggest. Publishing against the wishes of a commissioner is unlikely to encourage them to fund your work again, or to fund other work in your institution. In many fields with few sources of funding, that could be severely damaging to your chances of doing further research, and that of your colleagues, and any decision to publish 'in the public interest' would have to be taken carefully.

Participants and research users

We have noted the increasing encouragement to involve research participants and users in research. In the UK, an organization called INVOLVE (www.involve.org,uk) promotes public involvement in research at all stages, including commissioning, advising and designing research, with the aim of developing active partnerships rather than a relationship with the public as simply the 'subjects' of research. According to INVOLVE's website, the rationale for involving the public as partners is that of ensuring that the research priorities identified are those which are important to patients; that resources are not wasted on topics which are irrelevant to the public and that different perspectives are included in the research. Much of the literature on public, or patient, involvement is ideological, assuming that such involvement is a good thing, even if difficult to achieve in ways which are not merely tokenistic. It is rather difficult to take issue with the aim of involving user stakeholders without appearing elitist or protectionist about research activity, but research *is* a professionalized activity, involving a number of technical and craft skills. It takes considerable time to develop these skills in the various stages of research, and clearly the amount of support needed to involve non-expert users involves a trade-off in terms of resources. Are the gains, in terms of either research output, dissemination opportunities, or (if this is an important goal) social involvement and empowerment of users, worth this investment? Qualitative methodologies are often explicitly orientated towards gaining multiple perspectives and reflecting user views, and it can appear that these could be used by anyone, with little training.

Although it is obviously essential to include potential participants on project teams if the team needs a particular perspective, it can sometimes be difficult to see what would be added by involving a small number of users in steering committees or projects if they are recruited simply on the basis of being representative of 'the public'. George Martin (2008) points to some of the tensions inherent in having to 'represent the public' in his analysis of different rationales for participation in health care policy, arising from both democratic imperatives (that is, involvement should represent the public in the sense of reflecting the range and differences between the public) and technocratic ones (the public are involved because they have specific sorts of expertise to contribute, for instance as a diabetic patient, or mental health service user). He concludes that those involved have to become 'experts in laity': their 'non-expertness' is what is prized, but being a 'non-expert' turns out to be a rather burdensome and responsible task of mediating between the community and the health care system (or research system).

As well as generating practical dilemmas for researchers, taking seriously the involvement of public and user stakeholders also generates some rather more philosophical dilemmas that return us to the debate we started with about the 'proper' role of the researcher in society. If researchers see themselves essentially as 'neutral outsiders', producing knowledge for its own sake, the obligation to take user and public perspectives seriously and attend to them in framing research proposals and disseminating findings can be rather burdensome, as public views will be shaped by political needs and social values. The radical may feel more comfortable working towards an active partnership with users, but will also face dilemmas in terms of the inevitable conflicts between different users of the research. In practice, the research questions we ask, the findings of our studies, and their implications for policy and practice are rarely straightforward, and stakeholders – such as participants in the study and the various groups of users and potential users – are unlikely to have identical interests.

Conclusion

We have discussed ethical research practice as involving a balance between a number of responsibilities to different stakeholders. Doing qualitative health research may generate particular ethical dilemmas, because in addition to these (sometimes conflicting) responsibilities there may be divergent expectations from health research and social research communities. Some of these conflicts have their roots in the different models of ethical principles being utilized, whether that of respect for participants as the core principle, or whether it is a more instrumental one of balancing the risks and benefits of the study for participants. This means that checklists of 'good practice' are unlikely to be a sufficient guide to many of the decisions that have to be made in designing a study: they are more useful as guides to the kinds of issues that need to be considered. However, qualitative health researchers cannot take the stance that 'anything goes'. Apart from the moral responsibilities to the various stakeholders in the research process (participants, sponsors, their professional colleagues and the wider community), there are some practical reasons why any deviations from the 'good practice' checklists need very careful justification. One rather instrumental reason is that publication of findings may be very difficult if your study is not seen as ethical, and some journals will require evidence of ethical committee approval. A more public-spirited incentive is to maintain the good faith of all stakeholders in the research process, whose trust is risked by apparent breaches in good ethical practice.

KEY POINTS

- Research involves sets of (sometimes competing) responsibilities to participants, sponsors, colleagues and the wider public.
- There are different models of the proper role of research, which stress different stakeholders in the process.

- One division is between ethical models that focus on the ends (and whether these are justified by the means) and those that focus on the process (and how it can maximize the autonomy of participants).
- Ethical guidelines are a starting point for considering the ethical implications of a study. Given the diverse designs and approaches used in qualitative research, they are rarely a sufficient guide to ethical practice.
- Some key issues qualitative researchers should consider at the outset include informed consent, protecting privacy and the representation of research participants.

EXERCISES

1   For the project you designed for Exercise 3 at the end of Chapter 2, consider all of the potential stakeholders. What particular ethical responsibilities would you have to each of them in carrying out the study and disseminating the results? Do any of them conflict, and if so, how would you balance your responsibilities?

2   Imagine an ethnographer wants to come and live in your neighbourhood or work in your workplace to carry out a long-term study of health behaviours. What concerns would you have as a potential participant in this research? Outline the responsibilities you think the ethnographer has to you and your neighbours or colleagues in terms of:

(a) confidentiality;
(b) representing your views and behaviours;
(c) publishing results that might be critical of your behaviours.

FURTHER READING

Alderson, P. (1995) *Listening to children: children, ethics and social research*. Ilford: Barnardo's. Thought-provoking discussion of the particular issues raised by social research with young people, but many of Alderson's points are generalizable to other relatively powerless groups in the population.

Homan, R. (1991) *The ethics of social research*. London: Longman. A detailed and thoughtful discussion of the issues raised by social research, rather than health research. Homan's concern is with the tendency for guidelines to restrict debate, reducing ethical decisions to a checklist, rather than encouraging debate about moral decisions.

Part 2

Generating and Analysing Data

4 In-depth Interviews

CHAPTER SUMMARY

Interviews are a particular kind of conversation, and are probably the most common source of qualitative data for health researchers. Selecting interviews as the method of choice involves considering both the nature of data produced in interviews in general and reflexively accounting for the specific context of the study in terms of how this shapes the data generated. The issue of language is central in all qualitative work, and is particularly explicit in cross-cultural settings. The chapter concludes with suggestions for dealing with the practical issues interviewers need to consider, including sampling decisions.

Introduction

The interview is the most widely used method of producing data in qualitative health research. In essence, an interview is a conversation that is directed, more or less, towards the researcher's particular needs for data. How far the researcher directs the interview, in determining the topics covered and how they are discussed, is one dimension by which research interviews could be classified. At one end of such a scale is the *structured* interview, which schedules the kind of data produced quite tightly. In this type of interview, the interviewer must follow a specified set of questions, in a specified order, for each interview to generate comparable answers from each respondent. They are typically used in survey designs. At the other end of this scale, *informal* interviews are more like natural conversations that happen fortuitously in the field, in which data are gathered opportunistically. Perhaps the most commonly used interview types in qualitative health research are between these extremes, in the form of what are variously called *semi-structured, in-depth* or *narrative* interviews.

* In a *semi-structured* interview, the researcher sets the agenda in terms of the topics covered, but the interviewee's responses determine the kinds of information produced about those topics, and the relative importance of each of them.
* An *in-depth* interview is one that allows the interviewee enough time to develop their own accounts of the issues important to them. As an example, look at Case Study 8.2, which uses in-depth interviews to explore how women discussed their pregnancies.
* In a *narrative* interview, the researcher's aim is to facilitate the interviewee in telling their story. There has been an increasing interest in narrative in health research, both in terms of the stories people tell about their health and illness, and as an analytic device to make sense of data as narrative. The study described in Case Study 8.1 uses narrative interviews, as a way of encouraging participants to relate the 'story' of how they came to be diagnosed with glaucoma.

In practice these descriptions are used rather interchangeably, although they do suggest different emphases in terms of the amount of control the interviewer has over the encounter and what the aim of the interview is. This chapter is primarily concerned with these types of interviews, at the less structured end of the continuum, as these are properly qualitative interviews, aiming to produce rich, detailed accounts from the perspectives of the interviewees. However, many of the techniques discussed will be useful for more structured interview studies.

The research interview

In-depth interviewing is a distinctive, often frustrating craft. Unlike a pollster asking questions, the in-depth interviewer wants to probe the responses people give. To probe, the interviewer cannot be stonily impersonal: he or she has to give something of himself or herself in order to merit an open response. Yet the conversation lists in one direction; the point is not to talk the way friends do ... The craft consists in calibrating social distances without making the subject feel like an insect under the microscope. (Sennett 2003: 37–8)

In this passage, the sociologist Richard Sennett (2003) is reflecting on his early experiences as a field researcher, in which the 'craft' skills of establishing rapport are an essential element. To know when an interview is the appropriate method, to ask the right questions, and to listen carefully to answers, are skills that take time to develop, but are also skills which build on the everyday knowledge we have of social interaction.

The research interview, as a type of interaction, has some similarities to other interactions familiar in many cultures. The job interview, the clinical history-taking, the police interrogation and the celebrity interview on television are all ways in which one party (the interviewer) attempts to produce certain kinds of data from the verbal utterances of another (the interviewee). Like these general kinds of interview, the qualitative interviewer uses their skills in social interaction to get others to disclose particular kinds of information. Most of us have developed everyday skills in social interaction that are useful in research contexts, including skills in building a rapport, listening to the accounts of others, encouraging them to continue, and making people feel 'safe' to reveal their views and stories.

The qualitative research interview differs from these other kinds of interaction in that the kind of data generated are rather different. Unlike the job interview, the qualitative research interview is not 'testing' the account of the interviewee against those of others in the sample, but rather exploring their accounts, and comparing these with others to develop, say, a theoretical understanding of the underlying structures of beliefs. Unlike the clinical history-taking, where the health professional narrows down responses to obtain data useful for a diagnosis, the qualitative interview 'opens up' responses, and makes no *a priori* assumptions about the categories (such as symptoms or diagnoses) into which responses will fit. Unlike the police interrogator, the qualitative research interviewer does not assume that there is one version of the truth that can be uncovered, but that the interviewee's story will be valid as their *account* of events. By 'account' we mean the verbal report that an interviewee gives in an interview, which provides data not on their innermost feelings or beliefs (we have no access to these) but on what is said, and how it is said. In this chapter we shall develop this consideration of the aims of the qualitative research interview and the particular interactive skills needed to produce qualitative data from interviews. The first consideration is that of the nature of the data produced; that is, language data.

A word on language

In qualitative research, language is central. It is the most common form of *data* that researchers produce, first in oral form, then written as transcriptions or as excerpts in reports of qualitative work. At the same time, though, language is *method* – it is the strategy by which, through interviewing, data are produced. In qualitative work, then, language is central as both method and data, and a basic consideration is how we are to treat the language data that are produced. For language is fundamental to human understanding, to how we make sense of and shape the world around us; it is 'the most important sign system of human society' (Berger and Luckman 1967: 51). Unlike other sign systems, language is reciprocal, in that we think as we speak and think as we hear, such that in face-to-face conversations meanings are produced and reproduced in a continuous process. Through language we make sense of the world and ourselves, and then present these understandings to others. It is therefore vital that any qualitative researcher acknowledges both the theoretical and practical position accorded to 'language' in their work.

The ways in which we can think about language reflect the broad theoretical approaches to qualitative research outlined in Chapter 1. In positivist accounts, language is relatively unproblematic. It functions largely as the method of providing access to 'facts', as a window on the world, through which we can see the respondent's opinions, beliefs or behaviours. Thus, in a structured interview schedule, the question 'Do you always wash your hands before cooking food?' requires a simple, one-word answer, yes or no, which acts as an indicator of a behavioural variable. To say language is not problematic in these kinds of structured schedules is not to say that it is not an important issue. Rephrasing this question as 'In what circumstances don't you wash your hands before cooking?' would presumably generate very different answers, and elicit rather different accounts of hygiene behaviour. However, these considerations assume that an accurate picture of hand-washing is possible, though always potentially flawed by respondent failings. Such failings would include recall bias (problems of remembering accurately) and social desirability responses (the wish to appear as a morally worthy person to the interviewer). The interest in language in this kind of positivist approach lies in refining the language of questions to reduce such sources of bias, so that answers to questions act as the most 'accurate' indicators of behaviour possible. Sources of bias are seen as distortions to the potential of accurate representation, rather than of interest in themselves for what they tell us about the uses of language. If language is a window to the world, it is a potentially transparent one through which more or less accurate measures of human belief and behaviour can be taken, if we are careful with the linguistic prompts used.

In most qualitative work, language has a rather different role. As well as being the tool for generating data, language *is* the data. Language is the route to understanding how the respondent sees their world (in interpretative traditions) or as the route to understanding the categories that shape the world (in more constructionist traditions). Thus, in a qualitative interview, we might be less interested in responses to a closed question ('How many times do you wash your hands before cooking?') than in *how* people talk about their hygiene behaviour in the kitchen. We might, for example, be more interested in knowing: In what contexts do they stress their attendance to hygiene? How is hygiene prioritized against other outcomes (such as practicality, or speed)? How are cleanliness and dirtiness distinguished in the kitchen, and how are these categories constructed? Thus, the language used in this kind of interview tells us about the respondent, and how they interpret, classify and represent the world. Rather than using responses as a way of indicating behaviour around the pre-formed category of 'hand-washing', the data the interview produces are a method for building participants' own categories of hygiene behaviour. By comparing and contrasting the accounts of interview respondents, we hope to build up a picture of the underlying cultural categories that structure individual ways of interpreting and representing such concepts as dirt, cleanliness and hygiene behaviour.

Of course, there are many other ways in which language is analysed in interview data. One tradition in sociology derives from **ethnomethodology** – the study of how people make sense of what others say and do in everyday social interaction. Here, the focus is as much on the *form* as on the content of language, and attention is paid to the ways in which social actors make sense of the world. In health research, one method associated with this approach, **conversation analysis,** has proved valuable in analysing talk in encounters such as those between patients and doctors. Chapter 6 discusses this as an observational method, but of course it is also possible to see the research interview as an instance of 'real' social interaction, and to pay attention to how meaning is negotiated between interviewer and respondent, as well as to what content is produced (Rapley 2001).

All interviewers need to be at least aware of issues of how interaction itself produces meaning within an interview. This entails a sensitivity to the social context of the interview as experienced by both parties. It also assumes a cultural familiarity with the ways in which language is used in practice: how phrases, words and opinions are used in ways other than for their intrinsic content. As an example, consider this extract from an interview by Kathy Charmaz with a 61-year-old man who describes sharp chest pains he experienced on a walk with friends:

> [During the walk] I was white and sweating like crazy. I was in obvious pain. You didn't have to be a genius to figure out something was wrong. ... [Later] I lay on their couch for a couple of hours while they harassed me. ... They finally said, 'you're not going to die on my couch. Get out of here' [Laughing]. ... I was just so sick of listening to them. I was extremely uncomfortable, and they're just at me and at me and at me like pitbull terriers or something, so I thought, 'Okay, just to shut them up'. (Charmaz 1999: 371)

Charmaz is interested in the relationships between suffering and the self in her interviewees' stories of experiencing chronic illness. She argues that suffering is a profoundly moral status, and that the placement of the speaker in 'the moral hierarchy of suffering' affects whether and how an ill person's stories will be heard. In her analysis of interview data, Charmaz points to the strategies the speaker uses for preserving self-identity, and suggests that this has a gender dimension. In the men's stories in her sample, accounts are presented to demonstrate a certain degree of bravado and risk-taking, but she also suggests that they are told in a way that asserts their claims to moral rights: 'Their stories echo with their claims to moral rights and struggles to preserve their moral status' (Charmaz 1999: 371). Thus she is using the interview data as a topic – the language as data in their own right, looking at the phrasing, the nuances, the non-verbal communications. Note how in the extract above the pauses are represented and the addition of the descriptor 'laughing' in square brackets serves to illustrate the ironic tone implied by the words used. This then is more than using the language data as simple representation of behaviour (i.e., what this person did when he thought he might be having a heart attack, or how others treated him), but as a way of exploring the categories of risk, gender and moral status in the context of the experience of illness and suffering. This relies, though, on a sensitivity to the *ways* in which language is used, for instance in the rhetorical use of proverbial sayings, or as irony.

Language in cross-cultural settings

If language is problematic in general in qualitative research, it is of course particularly problematic where the researcher and interviewee do not share a common language. Qualitative work ideally requires fluency in the language and culture of the research setting. In anthropological fieldwork, the process of learning the language, and how different terms classify the world in the setting you are working in, is a key part of understanding the culture. Robert Pool (1994), working in Cameroon on a study originally designed to investigate reasons for the high rate of kwashiorkor (which in biomedicine is seen as resulting from protein-energy malnutrition) in one area of the country, discusses the role of interpreters. Reporting on one early discussion in the field, he notes that it was his assistant who actually conducted the 'interview', with Pool only contributing the occasional question. The discussion between him, his local assistant and the son of a local healer was carried out in English, almost as a performance for his benefit, with odd sentences in the local language, Limbum. Pool notes that in his reflections on the transcript of this discussion it became apparent how little fit there was between biomedical concepts of disease and its causes, and local accounts:

> ... the translation of illness terms seemed relatively straight-forward: kwashiorkor used to be called bfaa in Limbum, nowadays it was called ngang. ... Later, however, the meanings of the words 'bfaa' and 'ngang' were to become the central focus of my research, and I was to devote hours of discussion to trying to sort out their complex and inter-linked meanings. I was also to discover that the overlap between the meanings of these terms and that of kwashiorkor was only very partial. (Pool 1994: 18–19)

Pool notes that in traditional anthropological accounts, the role of interpreters is often not discussed in detail, even when the anthropologist must have been totally reliant on them, at least in the early stages of fieldwork. He argues that his local assistant was in fact a creative part of the ethnographic enterprise, not 'an unfortunate but necessary evil distorting reality and contaminating data' (Pool 1994: 21) as they are often seen. Their competence in the local language and culture needs to be made explicit, both as facilitator of the ethnographer's data-gathering and as sounding board for exploring understandings of the local culture.

In traditional ethnography, with an extended period of fieldwork, it is at least possible to learn local languages and recruit assistants. In shorter-term research, especially if it is being conducted in a number of different cultural settings, using interpreters and translators may be a necessity. A good interpreter should be able to translate not just the literal meaning of the words used by respondents, but the contextual information also carried, such as humorous use of words and phrases, sarcasm and metaphoric use. Ideally, of course, this relies on not just bilingualism on the part of the interpreter, but biculturalism, so that meanings, rather than just words, are being translated. The interpreter must be able to understand the emotional, cultural and lexical implications of each utterance and find an equivalent in the target language. This is not an easy process. Bogusia Temple (1997), reflecting on translation issues in her work with British-Polish families, points to the (often implicit) assumptions built into particular translations, and stresses the need for open and reflexive debate about how utterances are interpreted. One example illustrates how this process of debate is part of the data analysis itself:

My translator had written the following:

'Women can organise everything, but they cannot lead'

[G]oing back to the interview, I translated as:

'Women are allowed to organise everything but to take the lead on nothing'

Discussing the differences with my translator we agreed that from a word for word translation the statement could be translated either way. We discussed our views on women's position in society and discovered that they were very different [...] The interview meant different things to us. (Temple 1997: 616)

Through discussing with her translator the different emphasis they had put on the phrase, Temple was able to advance her own understanding of the role of Polish women in their community, and how this was seen by others (her translator) as well as herself. Thus, translation is not merely a technical service, but a vital part of the data analysis.

When translating written materials (such as survey questionnaires), best practice involves first translating into the target language, and checking this version with native speakers for comprehensibility. This version is then translated back into the source language to check that the writer's intended meaning has survived. In qualitative interview-based research this isn't possible, and there are two strategies for dealing with data collection. First, bilingual interviewers can be recruited and trained to carry out the interviews and the transcripts can be translated into the researcher's language. This of course reduces the researcher's flexibility in the data collection stage, and may mean a long delay between data collection and analysis. The alternative is simultaneous interpreting, with a bilingual interpreter used to translate each question for the interviewer, and then the respondent's answers. This requires a high degree of trust in the interpreter, who should ideally be fully involved in the study, rather than just hired for each interview. In many fieldwork settings, of course, ad hoc arrangements have to be made, and interviews may be carried out with the help of informal interpreters such as family members.

Noreen Esposito (2001) describes one strategy for managing the practicalities of translation in a study involving Spanish-speaking women in the United States. She conducted four focus groups (see Chapter 5) on women's beliefs about the menopause and their expectations of health care providers. Group interviews were facilitated by a Spanish-speaking graduate recruited from the local community who had some experience of running focus groups. She used a list of core questions developed by the research team. Esposito notes that, despite being bilingual, the facilitator was still not familiar with some of the colloquial Spanish used by participants, and that her 'communication style' was not that of the participants. In addition, the researchers recruited a trained professional translator for the group interviews, who sat in a sound-proof booth. She simultaneously verbally translated the ongoing discussion into a tape recorder into English. Once the (Spanish) tape of the research interview was also translated into English, the researchers thus had two translations available for analysis. These two tapes were, says Esposito, similar in content but had some interesting differences.

Esposito's example is of good practice when working with minority language communities in a developed country setting, with research resources including sound-proof rooms and the services of highly trained translators. She was able to use different translations to improve the validity of her data, but notes that this still restricted the kinds of qualitative analysis that could be done. Another example of using a multilingual research team to access views from minority language speakers is in Case Study 5.1 in the next chapter. In many settings, these kinds of resources will not be available, and it will be very difficult to find suitably skilled bilingual interpreters or researchers. Conducting an interview with an interpreter changes the social context of the interview, and the interpreter will have an influence on the data produced, just as the interviewer does. Whenever possible, interpreters (or translators of the transcript) should be fully involved in analysing the data to discuss how meanings should be analysed, and to debate the cultural implications of particular utterances. Ideally, they should not be just technical assistants, but a vital part of the research team.

Assumptions about our own language

Working with your own language does not eradicate problems of translation. To some extent all language use implies a translation, in which we assume shared meanings but cannot take them for granted. This is most explicit when interviewing those from other cultural groups, who may use particular terms in very different ways. Young people are an obvious example, as the meanings of vernacular words can change quite rapidly. The following extract, for instance, comes from a study of bilingual young people's experiences of translating for their parents in health care settings. The young people and the interviewer are fluent in English, but the interviewer (I) has to check on her understanding of an (English) term that the 16-year-old interviewees (R1 and R2) have used in relating the story of a health care encounter:

R1: I was translating for my mum, and he [the doctor] is like, screwing me as well

I: How did he do that?

R1: Just looks like [makes cross expression]

R2: A dirty look

R1: Yeah, dirty look. He most probably thought I was like cussing him because I started laughing when I was speaking to my Mum, translating, yeah, so that's probably why he started screwing me.

I: Screaming at you?

R1: Screwing me

I: Oh, screwing, is that what you said when he was staring at you, it's called screwing?

R1: Yeah

In this example, the context was enough to alert the interviewer that the young men to whom she is talking are not using the term 'screwing' in either its literal English meaning, or the slang meaning with which she was familiar (to have sex with), although she first mishears the term as 'screaming'. There are not always, though, enough clues to prompt the interviewer to check out their understanding of words and phrases in this way. Even when the use of language is apparently similar, we can't make any assumptions about shared meanings.

To some extent, the more social and cultural similarities there are between interviewer and interviewee, the more we are likely to assume shared meaning. It is much more difficult to prompt ('what do you mean by ...') in such situations, as this implies a breach of the communality which is often the basis of rapport and trust. To interrupt too often with requests for clarification risks disrupting the ordinary flow of a story. Thus, the existence, or otherwise, of shared language or culture can have advantages and disadvantages. On the one hand, shared meanings may mean taken-for-granted aspects of daily life are not problematized, thus missing out on analytical depth. But if the interviewer is a complete 'alien', and all aspects of the encounter are problematized, there is little opportunity to develop the trust and rapport needed for successful interviewing and for collaboratively generating meaning from the encounter. However, these unintentional misunderstandings also have the potential to enhance the data and their interpretation by providing the opportunity to pursue meaning (and consequently analysis) in more depth. Thorogood (1988), in a study in which she interviewed Afro-Caribbean women in innercity London, used a checklist at the end of her interview in which she asked the women to list some biographical details about their marital status, the number of children they had and so on. Even discussing these relatively straightforward seeming 'facts' generated obvious differences in how she and her interviewees classified families, with differences in who was included in a list of siblings (did this include those with whom you shared both parents, or either parent, or just the father? Did it include those who had died?). In realizing that the checklist answers were often different from those she had understood from the in-depth interview, Thorogood could problematize her taken for granted understandings of how people talked about their families.

In-depth interviews: what they can and can't do

The research interview can be seen, then, as a specific kind of interaction, in which the researcher and the interviewee produce language data about beliefs, behaviour, ways of classifying the world, or about how knowledge is categorized. These data consist of accounts of the world, not direct representations of that world. A commonly cited shortcoming of interviews is that they only provide access to what people *say*, not what they *do*. From a positivist perspective this is a problem, as interviews (people's accounts) are a poor substitute for empirical evidence. If, for instance, in a study of hygiene behaviour, we want to know about people's hand-washing behaviour, our information from an interview will be 'flawed' in that accounts of the frequency of hand-washing will not necessarily bear any direct relationship to how often people really wash their hands. In terms of research design, qualitative interviews would be a poor choice of method if our aim were to investigate the *rate* of hand-washing in a community. This does not mean that these qualitative accounts are not valid, or that interviewees are lying. Interview data are valid, so long as the interview is treated as a contextual account, not as a proxy representation of some other reality. Interviews in this study would be an excellent way of generating information on normative accounts, such as those relating to when people think they should wash their hands, or why they think they (or other people) sometimes don't. Sensitive interviews would be a good method for understanding how people talked about hand-washing, the cultural context of hand-washing, their beliefs about the relative importance of hygiene in different situations and the contexts in which their behaviour might differ from normative accounts.

Case Study 4.1   The gendered production of data: two studies of interviewing male nurses

(Source: Williams, C.L. and Heikes, E.J. (1993) 'The importance of researcher's gender in the in-depth interview: evidence from two case studies of male nurses', *Gender and Society*, 7(2): 280–91)

Christine Williams and E. Joel Heikes both carried out studies in which they interviewed male nurses working in the United States. They note that the impact of gender on the data generated is often commented on, but rarely explicitly explored in studies. When a study is carried out by one researcher, it is difficult to identify precisely how social factors such as the gender identities of interviewee and interviewer shape the data generated, but they were able to explore how gender made a difference by comparing transcripts and their analysis from the studies they undertook independently, but which addressed similar questions about their roles in what is a female dominated profession.

In terms of the content of the nurses' answers, there were many similarities between the responses the two researchers recorded. Male nurses in both studies talked about how they interacted differently with men and women, and about the types of speciality that were 'more appropriate' for female nurses, such as obstetric nursing. However, when they looked in more detail at what the men said in the two sets of interviews, there were differences in the style: the *ways* in which male nurses discussed gender with the male interviewer were different from how they constructed their arguments with the female interviewer. With the male interviewer, nurses were more likely to be direct and make claims to biological determinacy in accounts of why women were more suited to obstetrics (such as claiming 'there's just this mothering instinct'). This difference in how the male nurses expressed their views was evident in many of the topics related to gender. When they were asked about their views on the effect of the increasing numbers of men in nursing, they reported positive effects to both the male and female interviewer, but in much more direct ways to the male interviewer. Williams and Heikes suggest the more careful way this was expressed to the female interviewer reflects a social desirability bias, in that male nurses may well be reluctant to appear sexist to a woman, so are unlikely to make the very direct claims they did to the male interviewer, such as attributing current poor pay within the profession to the fact that it was dominated by 'divorced women or single women'. Similarly, in talking to a same gender interviewer, the men were less likely to report instances of being badly treated by male physicians. Such stories may lower their status in the eyes of another man, but are possible to discuss with a woman, who could be expected to be empathetic.

A superficial content analysis of the two sets of interviews would not have revealed the subtle differences not only in what was discussed, but in how these topics were discussed. These differences are an important contribution to the analysis, as they suggest some of the ways in which gender roles, as enacted in the interview, also influence gender roles as they relate to the topic of interest, that of the implications of being male in a female dominated profession.

(Continued)

These studies also illustrate some of the advantages of a qualitative approach to interviewing for relatively sensitive topics. The format of the in-depth interview allows the interviewee to frame their responses carefully, articulating their views in ways that maintain a valued identity in the eyes of the interviewer. In a more structured interview, with fewer opportunities for the interviewee to nuance their replies, they may only give the socially desirable responses, if there is no space to qualify their answer.

Interactions are inevitably gendered, although the precise ways in which gender operates to shape data depend on the cultural context of the study. In this example, the researchers had to reflect on their roles relative to that of the interviewee, as well as the status of their interviewees relative to others that they work with (female nurses, male physicians). This kind of reflexivity is part of the analysis of a qualitative study. This is not a matter of addressing 'bias' but of analysing how gender roles shape what can and can't be said, and what this tells us about the topic under investigation.

What interview data do less well is produce information about how people interact or behave in contexts other than interviews. As Silverman (1998) puts it, qualitative interview studies are 'fundamentally concerned with the environment around the phenomenon rather than the phenomenon itself'. He argues that the in-depth interview has perhaps been over-used in health research and that more observational methods (such as analysing what actually happens in a consultation, rather than merely patients' accounts of the interaction) would often provide more useful evidence.

However, if we remember that what we are accessing in interviews are *accounts*, rather than subjective beliefs, or objective reports of behaviour, interviews are an invaluable resource. Analysing interview accounts provides data on what people say and how they say it. Given that language is the primary way in which we make sense of the world, communicate that understanding to others and (from a constructionist perspective) shape the world, interview accounts can furnish data for many research questions.

Context and data

We have suggested that the interview is a format with which most people are familiar, in that they know the broad 'rules of engagement'. These include: the interview is a setting in which it is acceptable to ask relatively personal questions, the interviewee will respond to prompts provided by the interviewer, and the interviewer (usually) will provide less information about themselves. There is a 'social role' for the interviewee, just as much as for the interviewer, and qualitative interviewing relies on all parties understanding the conventions of an interview. However, these 'rules' about the meaning of an interview cannot be assumed. In some settings the format of an interview can carry threatening connotations, or simply not be a recognized format for 'normal' social interaction. Stone and Campbell (1984), for instance, report their study of the validity of information gained from surveys of family-planning knowledge in Nepal. Although they are concerned with interviews used for structured surveys, their comments are relevant to other research settings in which the interviewer would be a relative 'stranger' to the respondents. They note that many rural Nepalese people will be unfamiliar with the survey format of questions and answers, and with the notion of 'privacy' in providing answers. In some settings, particularly in rural areas, it may be impossible to interview people without others being present, and family-planning services may be one topic that is culturally inappropriate to discuss in public. One example of the interview providing misleading data was knowledge of abortion. In the survey, villagers had been asked if they 'had heard of abortion', and about a quarter said they had not. However, the researchers knew that villagers were all aware of abortions. Within the survey interview, interviewees had interpreted the question as one of knowing about the techniques, or knowing someone who had had one. This was how the topic of 'abortion' would have been framed within the relatively 'public' context of a survey interview. Although a more sensitive wording of the question could solve some problems of this nature, Stone and Campbell (1984) maintain that the very context of a questionnaire interview is 'socially and linguistically awkward' in this setting.

Even in cultures where there is an accepted interview format for generating information from individuals, cultural factors will shape the kinds of accounts particular kinds of people can legitimately generate within it. Those being interviewed will 'place' the interviewer in terms of their institutional allegiances, their presumptions about what they want to find out, and their social and cultural characteristics. There is a range of potential 'interviewee' social roles, and the placing of the interviewer will influence the one adopted. Institutional allegiances, such as whether the interviewer introduces themselves as a student, a researcher for a government department or from a university, will have an impact not only on willingness to be interviewed, but also the kind of person that the interviewee will present themselves as in the interview. Social, cultural and personal characteristics will inevitably shape the kind of relationship established, and how those involved frame the interaction. Characteristics such as age, gender and ethnicity cannot be eliminated, nor is it desirable that they are. Although there is some evidence that in some settings people are more willing to express less socially acceptable views to those of similar backgrounds, it should not be assumed that matching (for gender, ethnicity and so on) where possible is 'best' practice. There are likely to be advantages in terms of access and the establishment of rapport, but possibly disadvantages in terms of assumptions of shared meanings, and possibly (especially in relatively small sub-groups) a distrust of confidentiality. Instead, the researcher must reflexively account for the interplay between the social positions of the actors involved in the data generated, as this in itself is part of the data. Case Study 4.1 is a good example of this kind of analysis, looking at how attention to the gendered production of talk can provide insights into the topic. Here we discuss two particular contextual factors that need to be reflexively accounted for: the difference between 'private' and more public accounts, and social differences between interviewer and interviewee.

Private/public accounts

One aspect of the interview context is the relationship between interviewer and interviewee. In the one-off interview, however good the interviewer is at gaining rapport, the encounter is still one of strangers, and many researchers have contrasted the accounts provided in the first interview with those later on, when the researcher is more trusted, and treated as less of a stranger. Jocelyn Cornwell (1984), in her research on the health beliefs of people in East London, contrasted what she called the 'public' accounts given by her interviewees early on in the research with the more 'private' accounts she was given in follow-up interviews. In the 'public' accounts, people were more likely to provide 'socially acceptable' views, or those that reproduced the dominant moral meanings of health in wider society. These views were more likely to be provided when the researcher was less well known, and when she was asking more general questions about health beliefs. Private views were those that may be less acceptable, more 'deviant', and based on real experiences. These were more likely to be revealed once the interviewer was trusted as a confidante, rather than a researcher, and in telling stories about their own experiences of health and illness. These 'private' views are not necessarily more valid than the public ones (they may, for instance, be exaggerated for dramatic effect, or to present the interviewee in a sympathetic light), but there are different contexts in which each is likely to be expressed.

In his study of parents with children with a disability, Patrick West (1990) discusses these contextual differences as one explanation for differences in findings between his own and earlier studies on the same topic. In previous research, he notes, parents reported a relatively unproblematic process of diagnosis, a good relationship with medical personnel, and relatively little disruption of family life. In his own study, based on repeated interviews with families, and with his position as separate from the hospital and other agencies, he claims to have accessed more 'private' accounts from families. These interviews generated a very different picture of how families coped with a child with a disability, and stressed the 'troubles' of coping, rather than stoic acceptance, and negative or marginal views of professionals. The differences between his and earlier accounts from the literature, argues West, reflect the different types of interview undertaken. His were from the perspective of a 'family friend' who had gained the trust of parents over time, rather than from a one-off interview, in which parents may feel they have to present the 'acceptable' image of coping parents, grateful to the professionals caring for their child. West goes on to note that this, in itself, does not mean the 'private' accounts are necessarily more valid. People may tell negative stories about medical encounters for a variety of reasons, and we cannot assume that these accounts reflect any external 'reality' of the encounter.

Stimson and Webb's (1975) study of stories about consultations in general practice, for instance, demonstrates that interviews on this topic are useful for accessing the ways in which patients 'make sense' of the encounter, but may tell us very little about what actually went on. Stories about general practitioners are, they note, a common topic of everyday conversation, and ones that invoke empathy in listeners, and a desire to cast the teller in a more active role than might actually be possible in the real encounter. It could be argued that if we are interested in the phenomenon itself (i.e., the behaviour of medical professionals) rather than just the ways in which accounts of it are utilized in everyday conversation, then interviews alone would not suffice. In his study, Patrick West used observations of out-patient appointments to validate parents' accounts of issues such as delays in communicating diagnoses and reluctance to discuss medication or psychosocial consequences.

A qualitative methodology, then, foregrounds the subjective experience of the participants, but it cannot be presumed that the interviewer is simply a conduit for the expression of those experiences. Similarities and differences both in aspects of social identity and experience and in social power will clearly have a major impact on the social encounter that is 'the interview', and shape which particular experiences interviewees choose to discuss, and how they talk about them. Early discussions of the impact and ethical dilemmas produced by this were raised by sociologists exploring the implications of feminist methodology for research practice (Oakley 1981; Finch 1984; Smith 1988). Their resolution of the dilemma was that participants should be the subjects rather than the objects of the research, and that rather than pursuing the quantitative goal of eliminating difference (or bias), social differences in the interview relationship should be acknowledged and included in the analytical frame. This perspective has been influential in qualitative methodology more generally, with the acceptance that social differences and similarities between the researcher and those researched should be acknowledged, documented and accounted for in the analysis. Examining the salience of, for instance, differences and similarities with respect to ethnicity when talking about aspects of health is a useful way of identifying how ethnic identity may contribute to the ways in which people account for their health.

Social differences in interviews

Social differences between interviewer and interviewee can exist in relation to nationality, race, class, socio-economic status, age and gender. The impact of social 'difference' on the data produced in research is complex. As Rosalind Edwards (1990: 482) notes: 'race does not simply exist as an object of study or a variable in analysis, it enters into the research process itself ... and importantly influences the relationship with those we are researching'. This applies, of course, to other dimensions of social difference (and similarity).

From a feminist perspective, Rosalind Edwards (1990) notes that, as a white woman interviewing Afro-Caribbean women in Britain, race framed the whole process of her interviews, from gaining access to potential interviewees to the establishment of a trusting relationship in the interview itself. She found that, rather than assuming a commonality based on gender, interviewees were distrustful because of her different structural position in society. Many areas, such as details about family life, could only be addressed in interviews after she had acknowledged this different position, rather than assuming a similarity, as she did with interviewees of the same gender and ethnicity. However, Edwards did not see these factors as 'barriers' to be overcome in carrying out her research, but rather as data that helped her understand the ways in which gender and ethnic roles were experienced, and which aspects of identity are prioritized in different relationships. In contrast, Penelope Scott (1999), in her experience of researching white British and Caribbean people with diabetes, notes how her Caribbean background facilitated a level of trust and rapport, evidenced in the personal stories told, and the hospitality extended, with the Caribbean interviewees. This was not evident in most of the interviews with the white British participants, which were in general shorter and less likely to cover personal details. Scott suggests that a dichotomy of 'public' and 'private' views may not capture the diverse ways in which different groups will respond to the experience of being interviewed.

In more positivist research traditions, the problem of these differences is one of attempting to eliminate potential sources of bias. In qualitative research, though, there is more typically an acceptance that *any* interview account is situated and contextual, and that we therefore have to account explicitly for the ways in which social and cultural characteristics have an impact on the kind of data collected. For Edwards and Scott, who were interviewing people with both social similarities (of gender) and differences (of ethnicity), this was facilitated by an analytical awareness of the different kinds of data produced across their interviews. Other possibilities are using comparisons between the data collected by different interviewers within one project as an aid to thinking about the interplay of social identities and accounts of experience, or comparing your own findings with those of other researchers (as Patrick West did in his (1990) study of parents with children with disabilities, and the example in Case Study 4.1).

'Elite' interviewing

Much of the textbook advice on interviewing assumes that the researcher is in a relatively powerful position vis-à-vis the interviewee, and that methodological and ethical problems relate to offsetting this imbalance. However, many health research studies, especially those of policy development or implementation, involve interviews with those who are relatively more powerful than the interviewer. Interviewing senior civil servants, clinicians or health service managers presents somewhat different problems of 'cultural difference' if the interviewer is a student, or a less powerful health professional. First, many respondents in these 'elite' groups will be difficult to recruit to an interview study, if invited in their professional role, and may offer only brief appointments for the interview (see Case Study 4.2, below). Second, in brief interviews, managers or policy advisers will be speaking 'for their organization', and the public accounts you generate may have been more efficiently gathered from official documents or written replies. If the aim is to gather the less official accounts of, for instance, how policy is made or implemented, methods other than in-depth interviewing may be needed, such as the observation of meetings.

However, interviewing elite respondents may be the only method for accessing certain kinds of data. Renée Danziger, in her comparative (1998) study of HIV testing policies in Britain, Sweden and Hungary, characterized her interview method as 'elite interviewing' (Dexter 1970), as the data were gathered from civil servants, academics, directors of voluntary organizations and public health specialists. Her justification for using interview data is that in many countries (including Britain and Sweden) there was no official 'HIV testing policy' that could be identified in official documents. Such policies had to be pieced together from a variety of sources, including government and health service directives and the accounts of key informants. Danziger's interviews with policy makers and academics provided her with access to the kinds of cultural beliefs that underpinned HIV testing policies in the three countries, and contributed to her discussion of how different policies might be culturally appropriate in different settings.

Designing and doing interviews

Given the fact that the data generated from an interview are the product of the specific interaction of that interview, and that there is a need for sensitivity around social norms of 'interviewing' in particular localities, it is of course impossible to provide a general list of rules for 'good technique'. The key to developing research interview skills is to consider carefully the aims of the interview (is it to generate stories, to elucidate a broad range of views, to explore how people talk about an issue?), and to identify how these can be achieved within 'normal' interaction in the setting within which you are working and how they are likely to be achieved in an interview. The process of identifying the necessary skills is of course data in themselves, as you learn how to ask questions and what kinds of topics are discussed in particular settings, and how they are dealt with. A good way of developing skills is to look carefully at early transcripts with a critical eye on interview techniques and ask questions such as:

- Did you interrupt when the interviewee was still speaking?
- Could you have left longer gaps for them to continue speaking?
- Were there points at which you could have prompted for more information?
- Did your questions appear judgemental, or too inquisitive, or leading?

The following sections outline some of the practical considerations for planning and conducting interview studies to help you think through what might work best, given the aims of the study, the kind of data you hope to generate from the interviews, and the setting.

Access

How does a researcher get people to agree to be interviewed? Often 'key informants' are used as a means of gaining access to a more general population; thus a health care professional, the organizer of a pensioners' luncheon club, or the leader of a leisure club, may agree to ask (or to let you ask) other members to participate. The interview relationship depends on a certain amount of mutual trust and obligation. The most difficult interviews are those done with no introduction (cold calling), since the research and the interviewer have no external legitimacy to call on. For studies conducted as part of a research degree, being honest about the educative purpose of the study to the researcher may often be a good way to invite participation. In many parts of the world, people are generous with their time when it is for the purpose of assisting your education.

In settings with high rates of literacy, prepare an information sheet about your project, with your contact details, for potential interviewees. Given the particular problems of 'elite interviewing' outlined above, access to professionals can sometimes be particularly challenging. Chris Ntau's (2002) description of the process of accessing doctors in Botswana in Case Study 4.2 is perhaps typical of the experiences of many researchers.

Case Study 4.2   Problems of access in a study of doctors in Botswana

(Source: Ntau, C.G. (2002) 'Medical careers of Botswana doctors' (Report from the Phil Strong Prize), *Medical Sociology News*, 28(3): 9–12)

Chris Ntau carried out his PhD study on the medical careers of Botswana doctors. In Botswana, the migration of skilled health care workers out of the country has led to considerable pressures on the public system. His study aimed to explore the factors that influence doctors' decisions to leave by interviewing those in the public and private sectors. He discussed some of the challenges faced in getting permission to carry out the study and accessing interviewees:

> Interviewing doctors was a multistage process, involving a number of players before the interview could actually take place. The first stage started with the Office of the President, seeking a research permit. A quick response from the Office of the President gave me a false belief that things ahead would be smooth. Although obtaining the research permit was

---

quick, more hurdles lay ahead. More permissions were required to actually start interviewing the respondents. The second stage involved requesting permission from the participating hospitals. Delays were experienced at this stage as officials took their time to respond. In one case, a response came after three months, following a series of phone calls.

Once permission was granted by participating institutions, the next stage was to speak to doctors, and agree on the appointment date. A phone call to the hospital led to the hospital receptionist, who then put the researcher through to the doctor. On a bad day, it was normal to wait a long period before getting through to the doctors. On getting hold of the doctor, I quickly introduced myself, emphasizing that I was studying at a foreign university. Naming the university was helpful, in terms of getting some doctors' co-operation, as all of them had studied outside the country. The research purpose was explained and then an invitation extended to a doctor to participate. Guided by the doctor's schedule, an appointment date would then be agreed, which was by no means a guarantee that an interview would actually take place.

On the agreed day, if an interview was scheduled in the afternoon, a morning reminding call was important. If the interview was in the morning, one-day advance reminder was sufficient. Cancellations and postponements were the norm, especially with doctors employed in government institutions and government officials. Reasons ranged from 'I was "on call" last night, so, I wouldn't make it today', or 'he/she is in theatre', to 'still seeing patients'. Undoubtedly, interviewing doctors, especially in conditions where they are too few, or facilities are seriously understaffed, requires a lot of patience. However, once interviews were underway, doctors readily opened up, and 'told their stories' of the 'joys' and 'hurts' of the medical profession. (Ntau 2002: 10–11)

Setting

The setting of an interview, like the social and cultural context, has an impact on the kind of data generated (Green and Hart 1999). The same person may stress different aspects of their identity in an out-patient clinic, a private room in their home, or in their workplace. In general, in most developed country settings it is preferable to interview in a private space that the interviewee feels is 'theirs'. This ensures confidentiality, and a relaxed atmosphere to develop a rapport. Of course in many settings such privacy may be impossible, or may be viewed as a suspicious request. On a more practical level, interviewing someone in 'their' space, particularly at their home, can seem very intrusive. You are invited in but then cannot behave according to the social rules for guests, as you may have to ask to move furniture in order to be near enough to the microphone, or perhaps ask them to turn off the television in the room (some tape recorders pick up so much background noise that interviews can be impossible to transcribe if done in a noisy room), or ask others to leave. A quiet room away from other distractions is often suggested as ideal, but in practice it is not always possible. In settings where privacy is not so prized, requesting it can be interpreted as threatening: why is the interviewer so keen to get 'secrets'? When a request for privacy does cause disquiet, it might be worth thinking through, methodologically and ethically, whether it is necessary in order to collect the most appropriate data. It may be that the research can be done by using natural groups (see, for example, Case Study 5.1) or household interviews. However, even in settings where privacy is not a routine expectation, it might still be a necessary one for people to disclose confidential information. Catherine Riessman (2005) discusses the difficulties she had in finding a space to talk with Indian woman about childlessness (a stigmatized condition), but when she did manage to speak with one woman in a space where others could not overhear, it become clear that privacy was important:

> [her] account of discrimination and beatings in the context of the joint family, when she did not conceive ... could be told in the quiet space, overriding a cultural prohibition against talk with strangers about family problems ... as our interview was ending [she] said she felt 'relieved' to have talked about the violence she had endured. (Riessman 2005: 479)

Rapport

Building a sense of trust with the interviewee involves presenting yourself as both non-judgemental and interested. This involves avoiding questions, prompts and expressions that suggest disapproval or disagreement, and using prompts and body language to indicate an interest in what they are saying. Although these skills can be developed, at a deeper level, producing good quality qualitative data may well require a genuine and respectful interest in what people are saying, and an orientation towards actually attempting to understand their perspectives. This applies to whoever you are interviewing. Most people are more sympathetic to some types of respondents than others, but one hallmark of a good qualitative study is that there is a sense in which the researcher has genuinely attempted to understand the world view of those they were interviewing.

Building a rapport begins with an introduction that puts the interviewee at ease. This should include a repeat of your own name and the aims of the interview (which you will have already given at the point of recruitment), a reminder that the interviewee can stop at any time, and an opportunity for them to ask questions.

Phrasing questions

In-depth and **semi-structured interviews** give the interviewer flexibility in how to ask questions, but very careful preparation is needed to think about what to ask in order to generate useful information. Developing good **topic guides**, and identifying the 'right' question, can take a long time, because working out what to ask is in part an outcome of our growing understanding of how participants think about the topic. It is part of the analysis. There are, however, a number of rules of thumb that are generally helpful when considering how to ask questions in qualitative interviews, summarized below in Box 4.1.

Box 4.1   Some useful rules of thumb for phrasing qualitative interview questions

- Avoid asking respondents your research question.
- Avoid technical and professional vocabulary. (Ask about 'chest problems' not 'asthma'.)
- Avoid leading questions, which imply a preferred answer. (Ask 'For you, what is a healthy diet?' not 'Do you consider it important to eat fresh vegetables?')
- Avoid questions which suggest a judgement. (Ask 'Tell me about how you decided to feed your baby' not 'Could you tell me why you aren't breast feeding?')
- Use open questions in preference to closed ones.
- Ask about their experiences rather than abstract or theoretical questions. (Ask 'Think about the last time you went to the dentist – what did you like/not like about your experience?' not 'What do you like/not like about dentists?')

These rules of thumb do not always apply. There are of course points at which you might want to ask closed questions (about whether they have ever visited a particular hospital, for instance) or times when you want respondents' views on an abstract issue. However, they are useful pointers to some of the common problems researchers face when developing topic guides which must work well to generate the kind of data they were hoping for. To illustrate, suppose we are interviewing migrant nurses in a project on the problems they face adapting to a new working environment. Our research question is:

What problems do nurses face when coming to work in this country?

If we ask this question directly of our respondents we have several problems. First, this asks for their opinion about a generality that they may have no access to. To ask one person to speak on behalf of a whole group is asking for knowledge they may not have. It is our job, as researchers, to answer this question, and to answer it by analyzing the responses of all our participants.

It is not the job of the participant, who is being interviewed as an expert on their own experience, not as an expert on the topic in general.

We could specify the question as 'What problems did *you* face when you came to work here?', but this is still problematic as it is leading, in that it presupposes that the interviewee did face problems, or that he or she should have interpreted their experiences as problems. Instead, it would be more productive to start with open questions asking them to tell the story of how they arrived and started working, which will enable them to mention problems as they arose, if they did. We could start the interview with:

- Tell me about how you decided to come to this country to work.
- Tell me about when you first arrived to work in this hospital ... the first day, the rest of that week ... how did you feel at the end of your first week?

Once the interviewee has been asked to set the scene by describing their decision to seek a job in a different country and their first few weeks at work, and to frame this in their own way, we could ask more directed questions:

- On the hospital ward, tell me about what you've found to be different from [home country]?
- Is there anything easier/more difficult about nursing here than there?
- What has surprised you most about the differences?

In doing the study, we may well identify a range of relevant literature on adaptation processes for immigrants, which discusses concepts such as culture shock and acculturation. Although we may be interested in testing the usefulness of this theory for our study, again, this must be done at the point of analysis, not within the interview. So if we are interested in 'culture shock', asking 'Did you suffer from "culture shock" when you arrived?' is not likely to be useful. The phrase may well be familiar to the interviewee, but their understanding is unlikely to be the same as yours. Again, to produce information that will enable us to see if 'culture shock' is a useful way of thinking about early problems, we would need to take a few steps backwards. We would need to ask questions that would allow the respondent to give answers about their experiences and feelings that we could later analyse to see how they compared with the literature on culture shock.

There are a number of alternatives to straightforward questions asking about respondents' beliefs or practices. Some are listed in Box 4.2. The key issue is perhaps a flexible approach to the framing of questions, and close attention to the early interviews to assess what has worked well and what less well. It can take a long time to work out the 'right' question to generate the kind of data that will be useful, but if early interviews fail to generate anything useful, this can be a clue that the categories you are asking about do not reflect those of your interviewee, and your questions are not resonating at all with their experiences. If you are sure that you are asking the right people, this could be the point to rethink your interview strategy, and ensure that the topics or questions you have are not simply reflecting your own framing of the world, but are genuinely trying to prompt for theirs.

Body language

In many cultures, maintaining eye contact implies interest and active listening. However, interviewers do need to be careful about local cultural and social norms around body language. In most settings, for instance, it would be inappropriate to physically touch the interviewee except for shaking hands, but there are situations where not to do so would be unnecessarily cold. It is also important to retain an 'active listening posture', which usually involves sitting forward in one's chair, keeping your body turned towards the speaker, nodding for both agreement and encouragement, and not, of course, looking at your watch! This can, however, be enormously difficult to do as the interviewer is simultaneously having to worry about whether the tape is still running/ recording/about to run out, nod encouragingly and meet the interviewee's eye, not to mention planning the following question or link to another unexplored area of interest.

Box 4.2   Alternatives to direct questions for interviews

- *Verbal diaries*. Ask interviewees to describe a typical day, or hospital visit, or work shift. These kinds of questions are particularly useful for early data collection, or studies where the main aim is to understand the world-view of a group of respondents. Accounts of a 'day in the life' or a particular event provide some access to what respondents think is particularly important to report, and a general 'feel' for their world, as well as presenting opportunities to probe the areas of particular interest for the study.
- Asking about **'critical incidents'** such as worst or best experiences of care. This is a useful way of uncovering what the common features of, for instance, 'good' and 'bad' care might be from patients' perspectives. Equally, professionals can be asked which kinds of clients they most like/least like dealing with, or about the most satisfying or the most difficult work situations.
- Using *vignettes* based on case studies to access normative responses. This can be particularly useful for sensitive topics, as rather than asking interviewees to reflect on their own experiences, they are asked about fictional others. They are also useful for grounding discussion in concrete cases rather than abstract 'views'. Lindsay Prior and colleagues used vignettes to explore how Cantonese speakers in England referred to traditional and Western concepts of health and illness (Prior et al. 2000). These vignettes were summary descriptions such as 'Three month old baby with vomiting, diarrhoea and high temperature' and 'Man aged 45 with dizziness, headaches and blurred vision'. They were used to prompt discussion around what problems required help and what kind of help was appropriate.

(Continued)

- Using *visual cues*, such as photographs or objects, to aid discussion. Gillian Bendelow (1993), for instance, used a variety of visual images, such as paintings and photographs, to prompt her intervie-wees to talk about pain. On topics like this, which may be difficult for many people to verbalize, visual cues can be a useful way of generating data.
- Using *visual imagery* as an aid to data collection. Asking respondents to draw, for instance, a map of their neighbour-hood is a useful prompt for talking about the significance of local spaces and their health impacts. Many studies with younger children invite them to draw as well as talk, for exam-ple asking them to 'draw healthy food' or 'things that are bad for your health'.

Using prompts and probes

If the aim is to allow the interviewee to tell their story, or to provide detailed accounts of their experiences, the interviewer has to provide a facilitative audience for the story. This will usually entail:

- not interrupting
- allowing silences
- prompts, which include the noises we make to encourage people to continue ('uh-huh', 'mm') and the non-verbal cues such as head-nodding
- probes, to encourage elaboration, including questions such as 'Anything else?', 'And then what happened?' 'Tell me more about that'
- avoiding 'leading' questions that suggest a particular answer, or which frame the respondents' replies for them.

In summary, qualitative interviewing relies on skills most of us have as part of our repertoire of social skills, and they can be developed through practice and a sensitivity to the local norms of social interaction. However, interviews are a particular kind of interaction, and careful reflexive prac-tice is needed to ensure that the personal styles we bring to the interview are appropriate for the setting, likely to establish rapport, and likely to gen-erate the kind of data we need for the study. Like body language, this does differ across cultures: for instance, long silences may, in some cultures, be interpreted as aggressive, rather than facilitative (Simon Lewin, personal communication).

Improving reliability

Interacting and facilitating a research interview can be hard work, and it is gen-erally difficult to write down responses while maintaining eye contact, listening, providing encouragement and planning the prompt, probe or link to the next topic of interest. In addition, few interviewers have shorthand skills to take down exactly what is said. Ideally, then, interviews should be recorded on audiotape or with a digital recorder. It is a useful exercise to compare handwritten notes of an interview with a transcript of a tape of the same interview. Most researchers will find that they may have missed what could turn out to be the key issues, have quoted phrases that were never said, and have mistaken their own utterances for those of the interviewee in the notes taken by hand. An accurately transcribed recording is the most reliable record of an interview. It can also easily be reproduced if there are several researchers involved in the project, and archived (if there is permission from research participants and the data are suitably anonymized) for future analysis in other studies.

However, it is not always possible to record interviews. Some individuals will prefer not to be recorded, and in some cultures it can be a threatening request. Also, opportunistic interviews, done in the course of fieldwork, are unlikely to be recorded. It is also important, then, to improve both your skills in note-taking and your ability to write notes while listening actively.

If possible, it is worth investing in a good-quality tape or digital recorder and microphone, as poor-quality recordings are difficult to transcribe accurately. Transcription is time-consuming, typically taking six to eight hours to transcribe one hour of interview, and the time or cost must be considered in planning the study. Some researchers prefer to transcribe all their own tapes, as this is a useful way of beginning to familiarize yourself with the data. It is certainly good practice to transcribe at least the first few yourself, and to check the accuracy of those transcribed by others.

Transcribing interviews

Transcribing conversations is, of course, a translation process in itself. The choices of punctuation, spelling and detail of the transcript all affect how it is read by those analysing it. For those interested in conversation analysis, there are detailed conventions to record such nuances of talk as stress, pauses of various lengths, rising and falling intonation and non-verbal noises (see ten Have 1999). For most qualitative research, such detailed transcriptions are not needed, but it is important to reproduce reliably the precise words used by the interviewee, including slang words, stutters, hesitations and interruptions. Everyday conversation is rarely grammatical, or conducted in complete sentences, and transcriptions should reproduce the 'actual' talk rather than a tidied-up version. The important issue is that conventions used for transcription are agreed within the project team and whoever is transcribing the data. One possible set is suggested in Box 4.3. For ease of use when analysing, transcriptions should be printed with wide margins, numbered lines and each new speaker on a new line. To ensure confidentiality for respondents, remove any identifiers, such as names or specific locations, before these transcripts are used.

Box 4.3   Suggested transcript conventions

I	Start of each new utterance by interviewer
R	Start of each new utterance by respondent
?	Beginning of utterance by unidentified speaker
wo	Word interrupted by next utterance
(word)	Word(s) in round brackets indicate transcriber's guess at unclear word
CAPITALS	Words spoken more loudly than others
(...)	Indicate unclear material omitted by transcriber

In extracts reported in papers and reports:

[ ]	Square brackets enclose material added by author
...	Indicate material omitted by author

Sampling: how many and who to interview?

Perhaps the most common question from novice researchers is 'How many interviews do I need to do?' In quantitative work the answer can be calculated if you know something about the population, and the level of confidence you want in any differences found not being due to chance. The aim in quantitative studies is to produce a sample that is representative in a statistical way of the whole population of interest, and some kind of *probability sample*, in which each member of the population has an equal chance of being selected, is usually used. In qualitative work there are typically other considerations, and the sample size for an interview study depends on the aims – what you are expecting the data to do in terms of answering a question. As we have seen, in a case study such as a life history a sample size of one may be quite adequate, if the aim is to explore a deviant case or the subjective experience of one illustrative individual. For some studies, sampling decisions have to be made opportunistically, if there are few potential interviewees who may be willing to agree. In general, though, most qualitative research has the aim of *purposive* (sometimes called purposeful) *sampling*; that is, explicitly selecting interviewees who are likely to generate appropriate and useful data.

Patton suggests that the overall aim of purposive, as opposed to probability, sampling is to include 'information-rich cases for in-depth study' (1990: 182). To achieve this, a number of different sampling strategies are possible. These include: extreme or deviant case sampling, typical case sampling, and snowball sampling. Another interesting strategy proposed is 'political sampling', or taking into account the political considerations that apply to both the sample size and the selection. Patton (1990: 180) suggests that choosing politically important cases is one strategy for improving the chances of a project gaining attention and the findings being used. Thus, if evaluating a nation-wide health service reorganization, it may be possible to select case studies in high-profile hospitals to maximize the chance of media interest. Equally, such considerations will suggest not selecting high-profile cases if the findings are likely to be sensitive and such interest will be counterproductive. Less obvious political issues can also influence sampling strategies. For qualitative findings to be credible for those likely to be using the results, it may be important to choose respondents from a range that they would identify as 'representative'. Thus, if researching the views of cancer patients on information needs, it might be important to include patients from a range of social classes and localities and with different diagnoses so that oncologists are less likely to dismiss the findings as irrelevant to their practice, even if there is no theoretical justification for choosing these groups of patients. Thus one practical answer to 'How many people should I interview?' is 'However many will be credible to the users of your research'.

A more methodological answer to sample size is implied by a **grounded theory** approach (see Chapter 8). This approach advocates *theoretical sampling*, or including interviewees (or the 'events and incidents' that interviewees and other sources provide) in the sample on the basis of both an understanding of the field, emerging hypotheses from ongoing data analysis, and a deliberate attempt to 'test' such hypotheses. The intention is to keep sampling and analysing data until nothing new is being generated. This point is called '**saturation**' and the strategy is 'sampling to saturation'. Although initial decisions about sites and areas of interest have to be taken, and thought through very carefully, theoretical sampling involves a flexible approach that is to a large extent dependent on ongoing data analysis, which generates new conceptual ideas to test against the primary data. Strauss and Corbin (1990: 181–93) discuss a three-stage sampling strategy in which the early stages are relatively indiscriminate, because the researcher has little idea of which concepts are going to be theoretically relevant. A *convenience sample* would be sufficient at this point, and opportunistic interviews (for instance, informal interviews with those in the field) may be rich sources of data. As data analysis proceeds, the researcher deliberately seeks to include those who are likely to generate data of more relevance to the concepts that are emerging as important. Finally, in the later stages of a study, sampling will be more discriminating, and intended to test the emerging theories, by for instance deliberately seeking out **deviant cases** or testing how well hypotheses hold up in different settings.

In principle, the methodological justification for theoretical sampling is convincing and it offers a rigorous way of ensuring thorough data collection. However, there are a number of practical difficulties. First, in funded work few researchers have the kind of resources that allow the relatively open-ended commitment to data collection that theoretical sampling implies. We are likely to run out of time or money before 'saturation' has happened. Second, most sponsors of research will want a more or less detailed account of exactly who, and how many, will be interviewed within the protocol before research is funded. The same may apply to ethics committees (see Chapter 3), who may need to know precisely which population groups are being sampled. If each new category of interviewee has to be approved by an ethics committee as they are theoretically sampled, this becomes cumbersome to manage. Third, the point of 'saturation', in the sense intended by grounded theory, relates not merely to 'no new ideas coming out of the data' but to the notion of a conceptually dense theoretical account of the field of interest in which all categories are fully accounted for, the variations within them explained, and all relationships between the categories established, tested and validated for a range of settings. This process is potentially limitless, and the point at which 'saturation' has happened is perhaps more contentious than Strauss and Corbin imply. Certainly the phrase 'theoretical saturation was reached' has become rather a routine disclaimer in many journal articles of fairly thin analysis, with little evidence of the kind of density of theory intended by Strauss and Corbin.

If 'saturation' is not a practical answer to the question of sample size for most applied health researchers, it does perhaps suggest one. If addressing a fairly specific research question, the experience of most qualitative researchers is that in interview studies little that is 'new' comes out of transcripts after you have interviewed 20 or so people in one 'category'. To illustrate, in a study of bilingual children's experiences of interpreting for their families in health care settings (Green et al. 2002a), we were interested in including people from a range of more settled and more recently arrived communities, including both young men and young women and those who lived in areas where lots of other young people spoke the same language as well as those who were more isolated from others in the same community. The aims were both to sample a representative group of young people, in terms of the range of issues suggested in the literature as being important to how people perceive their language use, and to explore how social and cultural differences might shape experience. We thus proposed a sampling strategy that included 15 young people from *each* of four different language communities, and aimed to recruit both males and females within each group. We then identified established community groups (such as youth clubs and homework clubs) in areas that were socially mixed in terms of linguistic communities living there, and some that were more homo-geneous. The total sample size was therefore 60, but within that were various sub-samples, such as 30 young women, 15 Vietnamese speakers, 40 young people born outside the UK, and 20 who were the only people to speak their 'mother tongue' in their school class. This example illustrates the kinds of mixed sampling strategies that are used in practice to generate information-rich cases. Although 'theoretically sampled' in terms of the kinds of cultural variables likely to be important analytically, the sample was also a convenience sample to the extent that the actual young people invited to take part were those attending the community facilities sampled when we were doing field-work.

Conclusion

Interviews are the mainstay of much qualitative health research. The limita-tions of interviews as a source of data have been noted: they only provide access to what people say, not what they do; the accounts we collect are a pro-duction of the interview context, not any 'essential' truth about respondents' beliefs; the analysis of interview data relies on considerable local, cultural as well as linguistic knowledge. However, they are a relatively efficient way of generating data on almost all health topics. Their strengths lie in appropriate use: when the research question requires an analysis of accounts, and when the researcher is reflexive about how the research context impacts on the data collected. Good interviewing skills rely on sensitive use of the local cultural norms of social interaction. The development of appropriate interview protocols and techniques for a particular project is thus an essential element of good research practice, but is also part of the data analysis itself.

KEY POINTS

- The qualitative research interview is a particular kind of social interaction, which is recognized in most Western settings, but may be less familiar in other settings.
- The status of interview data depends on the epistemological underpinning of the study.
- Using interpreters in qualitative work is particularly problematic. When used, they should be an integral part of the research team.
- Qualitative research requires reflexivity about how the setting and social characteristics of the interviewer will affect the data produced.

EXERCISES

1   The best practice for in-depth interviewing is to carry one out. There is nothing quite like having first-hand experience of trying to juggle all the various social and environmental factors, thinking about the next question, and trying to decide how far to pursue a particular strand whilst still trying to keep focused on the actual spoken exchanges! If possible, identify a volunteer you do not know well to carry out a practice in-depth interview on a relatively neutral topic such as 'Experiences of dental care' or 'Preventing accidental injury'. Identify your aims for the interview (do you want to encourage narrative accounts of, say, experiences of accidental injury, or to identify health beliefs about dental hygiene?). Think of a number of prompts, and use some of the suggestions in Box 4.1 to frame some questions. After the interview, get your interviewee to give you feedback on whether you succeeded in putting them at ease, and whether they felt they covered the issues that were relevant to them on the topic.

2   If it is inappropriate or impossible to do your own interview, many insights can be gained from paying attention to the detail of interviews in other settings. Students may have access to

(Continued)

television, radio, newspaper or magazine interviews with a variety of 'respondents': these may be politicians, experts, lay campaigners, media celebrities or simply members of the general public. Select one or more of these interviews for analysis and then watch, listen to or read them with the following in mind:

• How does the setting influence the content or form of the interview?
• How does the 'world-view' of the interviewer or interviewee affect their questions or responses? Is their position implicit or explicit in what they say?
• How is the main topic of the interview approached?
• Do certain types or styles of question produce different answers?
• What particular aspects of replies are explored further? How is this done?
• In a political interview, for example, this may be by challenging the interviewee, which one would not normally expect in a social research interview. What effect does this have? How might it be approached differently?

Interviews of these types are in many ways very different from a social research interview. There are, however, many points of similarity. In the absence of the 'real thing', a great deal of insight and knowledge can be gained by the close observation of 'interview technique' more generally.

FURTHER READING

Kvale, S. and Brinkman, S. (2008) *InterViews: an introduction to qualitative research interviewing.* Thousand Oaks, CA: Sage. This takes an interesting approach to research interviewing as a method for finding out about people's experiences through an interchange of views. They discuss different kinds of interviews and approaches to analysis, leading from two metaphors of the interviewer as either a 'miner', digging for information about the world in a more positivist sense, or a 'traveller' on a journey which can change the researcher as well as generating knowledge about the world.

Wengraf, T. (2001) *Qualitative research interviewing: biographical narrative and semi-structured methods.* London: Sage. This may be a challenging read for those relatively new to qualitative methods as it does assume some familiarity with social science concepts, and it does use a large number of technical acronyms, but it is a mine of both theoretically-informed and useful, practical advice for designing, doing and analysing qualitative interviews.

5 Group Interviews

CHAPTER SUMMARY

Group interviews have the advantage over one-to-one interviews of providing access to interaction between participants, and thus some insight into how social knowledge is produced. In addition, they can be a useful way of researching some sensitive issues, such as dissatisfaction with services. In health research they have been used widely in health promotion, health services research and in needs assessment. Different types of group interview are discussed, including focus groups and natural groups, and the issues to consider when planning and conducting them.

Introduction

By 'group interviews' we mean any interview in which the researcher simultaneously gathers data from more than one participant. These range from opportunistic interviews held with small, naturally occurring groups during fieldwork to specially recruited focus groups gathered together purely for research purposes. In developed country settings, focus groups have become a widely used technique for gathering data to inform needs assessment, evaluate services and conduct research on group norms. In developing countries, community meetings are often used for data-gathering, as part of a participatory approach to set research agendas and in programme evaluation. What these various data collection formats have in common is that, unlike the one-to-one interview, they provide access to how people interact with each other as well as with a researcher.

Different kinds of group interview: an overview

The term 'focus group' is often used in the literature to describe any formal group interview. However, there are a number of more or less formal ways in which social researchers will use data collected from groups, rather than individuals, and it may be useful to begin by distinguishing different kinds of groups used in research. Jeannine Coreil (1995) has suggested a typology (outlined in Box 5.1) based on sampling strategy and aims. These are, of course, 'ideal types', and any particular interview might have elements of more than one type, but they are a helpful way of orientating us to the variety of aims researchers might have in conducting group interviews.

The type of group interview chosen will depend on the aim of the study and feasibility. If the aim is to generate 'naturalistic' data, then pre-existing 'natural' groups may be the format of choice, whereas selected focus groups would be more appropriate if a wide range of views across the population was needed. The setting will also influence the format. Coreil notes that in research in rural areas of developing countries, the lack of a meeting room means that in practice any group interview may involve a shifting group, as people (and even animals!) drift in and out of the room or space in which the interview is taking place. In many research settings privacy may not be possible, and group interviews may be used simply because it is not possible to talk to people individually. This chapter is concerned primarily with the methodological and practical issues raised by using focus groups or natural groups to gather data for qualitative health research, but as the other two formats in Coreil's typology (consensus panels and community interviews) are sometimes used in qualitative health research, we shall describe them briefly.

Box 5.1	Coreil's typology of group interviews	
Interview type	**Features**	**Typical uses**
Consensus panel	Often composed of key informants or experts Seeks group consensus or normative reactions More narrow, closed-ended stimulus material	Agreeing clinical protocols, resource prioritization

Focus group	Participants selected to meet sampling criteria Seeks broad range of ideas of open-ended topic Formal, controlled pre-arranged time and place Usually audio-taped and transcribed for analysis	Testing health promotion materials, exploring service users' views
Natural group	Group exists independent of the research study Format formal or informal Interview guide loosely followed Usually recorded by written notes	Ethnographic data collection (informal), social research (formal)
Community interview	Open to all or large segments of a community Usually recorded by written notes	Project planning, programme evaluation

Source: Adapted from Coreil (1995).

Consensus panels

Consensus panels are groups gathered to come to some agreement about an issue, such as priorities for health care spending, an agenda for health research, or guidelines for clinical practice (Murphy et al. 1998). Though not strictly an interview method, they are sometimes used in qualitative studies, and to help set research agendas (see, for instance, Bond and Bond 1982) as well as to inform planning. There are a number of different formal methods for reaching decisions, such as:

- *Delphi groups*. In Delphi groups the participants do not meet, but are mailed a questionnaire to garner views on the given topic. Summaries of the views of the group are then mailed back, with participants invited to change their responses in light of the views of the group. This can be repeated several times, until members of the group come to a consensus.
- *Nominal group technique*. This was developed to enable groups of people with an interest or expertise in an area to generate and rank ideas. The group is 'nominal' because it is a group only in name, and does not necessarily exist for other purposes. The structure is highly controlled to reduce the effects of dominating members. Each participant privately and independently writes their comments on the group's question. These are all then listed and discussed. Each participant now ranks their top ten ideas, with those with the most votes listed and discussed. Finally, points are awarded to the top ten ideas to rank them. Gallagher et al. (1993), for instance, used nominal groups to explore patient and professional views about diabetic care. Nominal groups of experts, generalist professionals, patients and carers were brought together to address the question 'What things are important in making people satisfied with diabetes care?' Qualitative analysis of the discussion

was used to explore the reasons for differences in how people ranked aspects of care, and Gallagher et al. claim that the technique is a useful research tool, especially in exploratory work.

- *Consensus conferences.* This is a generic term for workshops or discussion groups where participants come to some consensus through debate and interaction. Some aim to empower participants in addition to developing consensus (see Rowe and Frewer 2000 for a review). Citizens' juries are one such approach, where representative members of the public are invited to hear from experts, ask questions and discuss possible policy options. They are increasingly used, largely in developed country settings, as a way of including public views in policy development (see, for instance, Cosby et al. 1986; Lenaghan 1999). Consensus conferences are also used to involve professionals in such activities as guideline development (see Murphy et al. 1998).

Community interviews and participatory methods

Participatory methods aim to redress the unequal power relationships inherent in research such that researchers will share responsibility and knowledge with participants. Built on democratic principles, the intention is that communities will determine the research agenda, and participate in the process of research, action and development. Community interviews and workshops are a key plank in this kind of action research, as a route to developing participatory practice rather than merely gathering data. Development projects often rely on community meetings at the outset to generate interest in the project, answer questions from the community and include community priorities in the research agenda. As an example, look at the way in which workshops were used in the Stepping Stones project described in Case Study 2.2 to identify community priorities. Often these are not seen as part of the formal data collection process, although they may generate useful information. In other cases, community interviews are included as an essential element of gathering data and attempting a more democratic style of research. Rachel Baker and Rachel Hinton (1999), for instance, discussed their use of group interviews in their work on street children and refugee families in Nepal. Both were concerned to work with participants' own agendas for health and well-being. For them, group interviews were both 'an exploratory tool to illuminate issues of concern within the community' (Baker and Hinton 1999: 82) and 'to verify (or challenge) problems identified by the organizations, the community and the researchers' prior findings' (Baker and Hinton 1999: 82–83). They discuss the potential for group work to meet the needs of researchers and communities throughout the process of participatory work. One example was street children asking Baker to facilitate skills training to enable them to find employment, something that involved sharing knowledge and met the research aims. There are, though, limitations to how far participants' and researchers' agendas can both be met. Participants may have expectations of the researchers that cannot be fulfilled. In the work on street children, for instance, participants often asked if medical examinations would be carried out, something the research team could not provide.

Community groups are also vital in participatory studies towards the end of a project, to feed back findings to participants and their wider communities, and to maximize the possibilities of sustainability, if the project had development aims as well as research ones. One example comes from Eliana Lacerda's work with a *marisqueira* (women who harvested shellfish) community in Brazil (Lacerda 2008). This project was established as a participatory epidemiology, in which Lacerda worked with the local women to study the pollution risks they faced from working in an estuary, and used ethnographic methods to study the process of participation. At the close of the project, Lacerda organized a workshop to include local women as well as the community field workers who volunteered and collaborated in the project. She notes first that the workshop was welcomed broadly, and well attended, and that the women were delighted not to just be given a written report of the study. Second, she discusses the importance here of using appropriate methods of consulting:

> During the group discussions in the final workshop with the [Community Field Workers] and participating women, one of the groups concluded that our participatory experience 'valued' the women from the community ... their local knowledge was recognized and merged with academic knowledge. This was an empowering experience for them ... The use of visual devices and problem-orientated discussions helped me to establish a good interaction with the research participants ... [and] they reported an increased self-confidence and ... pride in our achievements. (Lacerda 2008: 145)

In participatory approaches, where working with participants, rather than extracting data from them, is the aim, it is productive to think carefully about the methods used in group processes, to ensure that they do enable participants to contribute fully. Lacerda used, for instance, mapping techniques, where women used coloured pens to describe their local community, and a cartoon figure of a *marisqueira*, which the women used to draw common health problems.

Focus groups

Until the 1970s, focus groups were largely a tool of market research, where they had been used to assess consumers' views of new products and publicity. In health research, they began to be used for similar purposes in evaluating health interventions, such as family-planning programmes. Basch (1987) suggests that their adoption by health education as a useful research tool relied on both the market research tradition and the history of group processes used in health education itself as a tool for behaviour change. Focus groups are now widely used (perhaps over-used) in a range of health research and evaluation settings. In essence, a focus group is a small (usually 6–12 people) group brought together to discuss a particular issue (such as local health services, or a particular health promotion campaign) under the direction of a facilitator, who has a list of topics to discuss. Typically, groups last between one and two hours and include a mixed group of participants from different social backgrounds who do not know each other. Each participant may also complete individual questionnaires to gather socio-demographic information and perhaps provide comparisons of what is said in public and private. These techniques are useful in social marketing, for instance in evaluating the suitability of health promotion materials for their intended audiences. They have also been widely used in studies looking at people's perceptions of health risks (Desvouges and Smith 1988). Focus groups have the potential for producing considerable information in a fairly short space of time on, for instance, how media messages are understood and talked about.

Natural groups

Participants in a traditional focus group will not have met before the discussion. However, in social research, rather than market research, the aim is often to access *how* social knowledge about a particular topic is generated, as well as what the content of that knowledge is. To achieve this, it is often useful to use 'natural groups' or groups of people who know each other already. This maximizes the interaction between participants, as well as between the facilitator and participants, and potentially provides the researcher with some access to a shared group culture. Natural groups can be informal or formal. Informal groups are those that occur fortuitously in the course of fieldwork – interviews with groups of workmates, for instance, or women gathered around a new mother, as in Case Study 5.1.

Household interviews are one kind of natural group that can be a useful source of information, as the household may be a key level of social organization that impacts on health. Interviewing all the members of a household together provides access to how household-level decisions may be made. These might include decisions about access to health care, or purchasing health-related goods and services. Household interviews have perhaps been under-used in developed country settings. In informal interviews, especially if opportunistic, there will not usually be a structured topic guide, and data will be recorded through field notes rather than tape recordings. Khan and Manderson (1992) suggest that, in practice, many interviews in developing country settings will be informal group interviews: as researchers start asking questions, more people will join in, and formal protocols will be adapted in practice, as the everyday demands of people coming and going or work being done interrupt a focused series of questions. As they note, this can be a real bonus, as such 'natural clusterings represent ... the resources upon which any of the group might draw ... a group that may weave or repair nets together [also] provides the scripting for the management of an illness event' (p. 60). The informal discussion groups formed either by design or opportunistically during fieldwork are exactly those in which health care decisions are typically made in everyday life.

Formal natural group interviews are those in which the group is invited to attend for the purposes of research. Usually, the researcher will book a private room and ask all participants to come for a specified time, and the discussion will be taped. Case Studies 5.1 and 5.2 both used natural groups for data collection. In the first, on Bedouin views of maternal child health services (Beckerleg et al. 1997), participants were interviewed in an informal setting, that of the homes of new mothers. The second, on understandings of HIV/AIDS, used more formal settings.

Advantages of using group interviews

In recent years, various kinds of group interviews have become popular in health research to offset some of the disadvantages of one-to-one interviews. In a group interview, the researcher ideally has access to the interaction between the participants, as well as between the interviewer and interviewed. This, in theory, provides a more 'naturalistic' setting, resembling in some ways the kinds of interaction people might have in their everyday lives. In terms of the discussion in Chapter 2 on research designs, the focus group can therefore be used in more observational designs. In health research this is a real advantage when we want to access not just how people talk to each other about health matters, but also how knowledge about health is produced and reproduced in 'natural' social situations. It can also be an advantage when researching workers in health service settings. For instance, interviewing ward staff in a group allows the researcher not just to observe who says what, but also who speaks most, which kinds of staff dominate, and whose comments are taken seriously. Case Study 5.2, from research by Jenny Kitzinger and colleagues on the effect of media messages about AIDS in the UK, illustrates how the interaction between participants was as important a part of the data as the content of what was said.

Case Study 5.1   Using natural groups to gather Bedouin views of maternal and child health services

(Source: Beckerleg, S., Lewando-Hundt, G.A., Borkan, J.M., Abu Saad, K.J. and Belmaker, I. (1997) 'Eliciting local voices using natural group interviews', *Anthropology and Medicine*, 4: 273–88)

Bedouin Arabs are a minority group of Israeli citizens, in socially disadvantaged circumstances. Although traditionally semi-nomadic, in recent years those living in Israel have largely been settled in towns, with many on low incomes and in poor housing conditions. Maternal and child health services are provided, for a fee, at clinics run by the Ministry of Health. As part of a larger study to improve maternal and child health care, this study aimed to consult with service users and non-users on the value and quality of the health clinics.

(Continued)

Previous research on child health had used structured questionnaires in home interviews with mothers. Susan Beckerleg and colleagues suggest that this approach may have been inappropriate in this cultural setting, as it is difficult to interview mothers on their own: if strangers come to the house, neighbours and family will gather to protect the mother and participate in the visit. Suspicion of outsiders might lead to inhibited discussion. Instead of attempting to interview mothers on their own, the researchers decided to talk to both women and men in groups with which they were familiar, and in which they could freely express opinions. Natural groups of men and women who would interact in everyday life were chosen to elicit views. In this setting, the most appropriate groups were family-based. To talk to women, the researchers invited women giving birth in local hospitals to take part in the study and consent to a group interview in their home during the 40-day post-partum period. Traditionally, women are secluded during this time, and are visited by related women who come to drink tea and eat lunch. These visitors form an ideal natural group for interviews about maternal and child health services, as this is a time when women would talk to each other about family news and childbirth experiences. Each extended family or sub-tribe has a guest house in which men regularly meet to enjoy conversation, tea or coffee and entertain guests. To include men's views, the researchers included groups in these guest houses. The research team recruited and trained Arab Israelis to conduct and record the group interviews in pairs, matched with the participants for gender. Key issues for the participants were confidentiality and full understanding of the aims of the study. As tape recorders inhibited open discussion, data were collected through detailed notes of the discussion. These notes were translated into English if necessary before analysis.

The findings suggested that preventative health services were important to both men and women in this community, but that several barriers to use existed, including financial barriers, distance to the clinics and problems in staff–patient interaction that resulted from cultural and linguistic differences between Bedouin users and nurses from other cultures. The methods of data collection worked well for the topic of maternal and child health, which was not one of a particularly sensitive or personal nature. For more private issues (such as family planning and household finances) the researchers identified women who could be interviewed in a private setting.

A further advantage is that some sensitive issues may be more readily discussed within group settings. One example is perhaps dissatisfaction with service provision. In a one-to-one interview, it may be more difficult for interviewees to disclose negative views (especially if the interviewer is a service provider), whereas in a meeting with other service users, it can be less threatening for participants if such views come from the group, rather than from one dissatisfied individual. Helen Schneider and Natasha Palmer (2002) provide a good example of this from a study of users' views of primary health care services in South Africa. They used both exit interviews (with users as they left the primary care facility) and focus groups in a study of the views of service provision at 19 sites across South Africa. Although in exit interviews users were generally satisfied with the services received, in focus groups many areas of dissatisfaction were discussed, including complaints about lack of privacy, rushed consultations, and dissatisfaction with communication and the treatments prescribed. Schneider and Palmer note that the focus group data are not necessarily more valid as a report of reality (indeed their transcripts contained many stories clearly told for dramatic effect, such as accounts of people dying through lack of care in the waiting rooms), but that the format does generate particular accounts that are not generated through interviews.

Clearly the kind of information that is easier to disclose in a group setting will depend on local cultural values, and the nature of the group. Asking for personal information in a 'natural' group that exists outside the research setting may not only be unproductive, but potentially unethical if the likely impact of disclosures on participants' everyday lives is not considered (see Case Study 3.1). This requires considerable sensitivity and local knowledge on the part of the research team. In their report of a study of young women's understanding of HIV transmission and their needs for AIDS prevention information in Zimbabwe, Davison Munodawafa and colleagues (1995) note the uneasiness of many of the groups in discussing their views of sexual behaviour and cultural norms. The groups they recruited were all 'natural' groups of women aged 15 to 22 who would work and socialize together after the research had finished, including self-help groups organized through the local mining company and church organizations. The research team used several methods to reduce the potential for embarrassment. First, they reassured the young women that men would not be allowed to come to the discussion, or to listen at a distance. They also assured them of confidentiality, by ensuring that no participant would identify themselves or others by name during the session. Young female group moderators were recruited, who were not only fluent in the local languages, but were also at ease talking with other women about AIDS and sexual issues. Group discussions were held in a relaxed atmosphere, with refreshments and dancing before and after the focus group. Finally, the disclosure of sensitive personal information during the discussion was discouraged by the moderator.

Case Study 5.2   Using focus groups to study the effects of media messages about AIDS

(Sources: Kitzinger, J. (1994) 'The methodology of focus groups: the importance of interaction between the research participants', *Sociology of Health and Illness*, 16: 103–21, and Kitzinger, J. (1990) 'Audience understandings of AIDS messages: a discussion of methods', *Sociology of Health and Illness*, 12: 319–35)

The AIDS Media Research Project studied the production, content and effect of media messages about AIDS in the UK. The researchers used group interviews to examine the effects of 'how media messages are processed by audiences and how understandings of AIDS are constructed' (Kitzinger 1994: 104). Focus group discussions were chosen for their potential to provide access not just to the content of people's views, but also to how those views were used and developed in everyday social interaction. For potentially sensitive subjects such as HIV/AIDS, the group setting may also encourage open discussion. The group participants were chosen to cover a wide range of different populations in the UK, including those who might be expected to have particular perspectives on the issue of AIDS. They were 'natural groups' in that they pre-existed the research, such as a group of women whose children went to the same playgroup, male workers on a gay helpline, a lesbian friendship group, a team of civil engineers who worked together, and members of a retirement club. That they were natural groups was important, as family, social and work settings are the ones in which we come to know about issues such as AIDS, and in which we develop our views. The intention was to maximize the interaction between participants in the groups to see how social knowledge was developed. As the participants knew each other already, there was also potential for access to what they did, as well as what they said they did, as other group members commented on how beliefs coexisted with everyday life. For these reasons, Kitzinger suggests that their use of natural groups is more 'naturalistic' than most research interview situations, but that it is of course an artificial research setting, in which the explicit aim is to explore often unarticulated views. Using natural groups 'allows for the collection of information both on group norms and the ways in which groups may mediate (relay, censor, selectively highlight and oppose) media messages' (Kitzinger 1990: 321).

To maximize interaction, facilitators used a number of techniques. First, group exercises allowed the participants to warm up and start to discuss the issues with physical prompts. These included cards with statements about who was 'at risk' from AIDS, which participants had to sort into groups of differing risk levels. This encouraged group participants to talk to each other, and to verbalize their reasoning. Another exercise was the 'News Game' in which the group was split into two teams, given a set of pictures and asked to construct a news report about AIDS. The pictures were taken from television news and documentary reports. The final exercise involved a health promotion advert from which the slogan ('How to recognize someone with HIV') had been removed. Participants were asked whether they recalled any adverts about HIV/AIDS, then asked to speculate on what the slogan was. Finally, the slogan was revealed and participants were asked to comment on the actual slogan and other parts of the text.

The second method for encouraging interaction was the use of the facilitator's skills in actively managing the discussion, pushing participants into accounting for their views, or exploring disagreements. Maximizing interaction allowed the researchers access not only to what people thought, but also to the cultural contexts in which views were held. Thus jokes, and the levels of agreement and disagreements between participants, suggested group norms, and the ways in which certain views are legitimate or not in the social settings in which they live and work. Even natural groups are not homogeneous, though, and Kitzinger notes the ways in which group participants were often surprised by differences in opinions among them. Disagreements forced participants to account for the views they held, and gave the researchers a chance to see what arguments are convincing in everyday interaction.

Exercises such as the card game were also useful sources of data on the assumptions participants made, where their knowledge came from, and for identifying areas of confusion and misinformation. The cards had descriptions of types of people taken from an opinion survey of the public, including 'people who donate blood at a blood donor centre'. In the discussion about how at risk this group was, it became clear that many participants assumed that the description referred to those who received donated blood, rather than the donors. This provides real insight into the meaning of survey results that suggest the public misunderstand risk activities. Participants' interpretations of the health education advert were also illuminating for showing how such images can be read in quite different ways from those intended by health educators. The advert was intended to persuade readers that there was no way of telling by looking at people whether they were HIV-positive or not – that they looked exactly like other people. In a minority of groups, participants read the image as meaning that there was a distinctive 'look' of someone who was HIV-positive or had AIDS.

What is and is not sensitive information is of course culturally specific. A discussion of knowledge about condoms, HIV risk and AIDS may be sensitive for young women in Zimbabwe, but not older women in London, whereas the latter might feel that a discussion of household income was too 'private' for a focus group.

Naturalism

The methodological strength of group interviews is that they supposedly approximate a more 'natural' interaction than individual interviews, thus providing the researcher with access to how people talk to each other about particular topics. The implication is that the researcher will capture some of the advantages of ethnographic research (see Chapter 6) in a focused way without the time-consuming and arduous business of actually carrying out fieldwork. A well-facilitated group has the feel of an everyday discussion, with participants interacting, joking and arguing with each other, rather than through the facilitator. However, it should be remembered that any specifically gathered or facilitated group is not a 'natural' setting, and that there are few situations in everyday life when peers will come together to discuss one topic for a lengthy period of time, and few in which they will be conscious of their utterances being treated as 'data'. In most group interviews, a facilitator also 'controls' the interaction to a greater or lesser extent, by deliberately canvassing views, controlling turn-taking, or asking for elaboration from participants. This facilitation obviously shapes to a greater or lesser extent the accounts participants give, and what they consider to be relevant to the researcher's needs.

It also has to be remembered that, for participants, the discussion itself is of course another source of both information and beliefs, in that it is one forum in which participants *come to know* particular things. The experience of taking part in a group interview may clarify, elaborate and even change participants' views. The following extract is taken from a study of how people with glaucoma cope with symptoms (Green et al. 2002b), and is part of a long exchange in which participants traded stories about the everyday difficulties caused by their eyesight problems. It is clear that taking part in the focus group had started to change the way in which one respondent (R4) thought about her difficulties, with her beginning to see the possibility of them being 'symptoms' rather than just problems of daily living:

> R1:   I can't follow things – and even, I go to church and, we've got large print hymn books and they are large print, you know – I can't even carry them!
>
> R2:   I have the same problem! And there's another problem ... putting your underwear on ... underslips you know, they have a seam down the side – I have to feel for the seam, otherwise often I come out with my underslip on inside out.
>
> R3:   Mm
>
> R1:   Oh yes!

R4:   ... I'm wondering, listening to you, because I have a job to recognize textures ... so maybe it's the glaucoma that does that.

In terms of generating more data about the impact of glaucoma on everyday life, the interaction in this group was an advantage, as other people's stories prompted group members both to remember, and to frame as significant, their own experiences. But the research setting itself has generated these data: there are clearly 'experiences of glaucoma' that are only recognized as such once other people help to frame them in this way. Similarly, in a focus group study of consumers' views of food safety, several participants mentioned during the discussion that taking part had made them think more about food safety, or that they had learnt about risks they hadn't known about beforehand from other participants (Green et al. 2003). The group interview does not just, then, 'collect' pre-existing ideas and viewpoints, but can also be part of the process by which these views are produced. Whether this constitutes a methodological problem or not depends on the aim of the study. If groups are used as part of a participatory design, in which developing the participants' understanding of a particular issue may be an explicit aim, it is clearly an advantage. It is also an advantage if research aims are to explore this process of knowledge production, rather than merely document the views of participants. For more positivist studies, in which group interviews are used as a tool for a survey of participants' views, this can look like 'contamination': the data produced reflect the opinions or beliefs that people develop during the process of the group discussion itself, rather than any pre-existing beliefs or opinions that they might have outside the research setting.

At a practical level, one disadvantage is that the more 'natural' a group discussion is, the harder it may be to analyse as data. The following extract comes from a focus group discussion with children from a study of children's views of accident risks. The participants were classmates who lived near each other in the same housing, which consisted of high-rise blocks of flats. The discussion was 'successful' in that there was considerable interaction between the children, who interrupted and spoke over each other in their eagerness to contribute, as can be seen in the passage transcribed here. The extract follows the children listing the risks for fire in their homes, and concerns a debate about what would happen in the event of a fire in the flats:

R1:   Would you jump out of the window or get burnt to pieces?
R2:   I'd jump out of the window
R1:   But if you lived on the fourth floor you'd be scared –
R3:   If you lived on the top floor ... and your house is on fire ... how you gonna get out? You can't jump out of the window because you'd be dead!
R4:   If you –
R1:   No, listen, if you could jump from the balcony –

?   You'd go splat on the floor and die
?   – no, you wouldn't die –

```
?      - you will die -
?      - jump carefully -
?      - you could land on your feet -
?      - your legs would break -
?      - how would your legs break?
R1:    - if your legs would break just like that, you wouldn't be able
       to walk for the rest of your life (Green and Hart 1999: 25)
```

Although this provides rich access to the kinds of discussion children might have without a facilitator present, it is perhaps limited as data, beyond telling us about the kinds of 'accident stories' that will be told spontaneously. The audio-tape of this section of the discussion was almost impossible to transcribe, as the number of unidentified speakers testifies, and as the participants all speak at once it is difficult to separate out particular points of view or how they are utilized in persuading others.

In other discussion groups held as part of this study of children's views of accidents, the young people themselves 'policed' the discussion to some extent, especially when the groups were held on school premises. In these more formal settings, children are used to calmer discussions, in which teachers or other adults will tightly control turn-taking so that only one child speaks at once, and everyone has a turn. When facilitating groups in school settings, we noticed that children would raise their hand before making a point, or insist that their peers took turns in speaking. In non-school settings, such as youth clubs, the discussions were less structured and there was more interaction between the children themselves (Green and Hart 1999). This illustrates the contextual nature of focus group data. Participants take on an appropriate social role, which is to some extent determined by the setting, and their contributions reflect this. What is appropriate to say in a youth club may not be appropriate to say in a school, even if away from the classroom and teachers. In other settings, of course, these contexts may have very different meanings. Baker and Hinton (1999), whose work in Nepal was referred to above, discuss the particular context of research with people living in refugee camps. Here, in contrast to the UK-based study, schools were a preferred location, as the researchers were seen as providers of services or material aid in other settings. Similarly, they argue that the home (with its lack of privacy) may be a less desirable setting than a relatively public space. The key point is that data from group interviews, like any other data, must be analysed with regard to the context in which they are produced, and the local meanings of that context. Care must be taken not merely to take particular utterances by individual participants as reified 'opinions' or 'views' without situating them within these structures of production.

Wilkinson and Kitzinger (2000) discuss a useful example of this in their work on the value of 'feeling positive' in studies of people with cancer. They suggest that much of the research that underpins the concept of 'feeling positive' is flawed because it takes little account of the ways in which people talk about 'feeling positive' in everyday settings. Using examples from their focus group study of women with breast cancer they show how, when participants talk about 'feeling positive', it would be a mistake to read this off as merely indicating some underlying mental state. Instead, they point to the ways in which the term is actually used interactively in the focus group talk. First, it is used as an idiom – an ordinary saying that is used in a formulaic way to summarize 'what everyone thinks' and to keep a conversation moving along. Phrases such as 'you've got to think positive' are ways of generating agreement in general in discussions. They are difficult to disagree with, and may be used at points where the speaker is seeking support and affirmation from others. Second, they note that if particular attention is paid to what participants are 'thinking positively' about, it is clear that it is not having cancer, but about other things in life or the possibility of recovery. Third, comments about 'thinking positive' are often made just after participants speak about difficult issues, such as feeling devastated by the diagnosis. The comment is thus used conversationally to enable participants to discuss emotional or difficult issues, which would be difficult to do in a group unless followed by a routine positive comment.

This kind of analysis clearly relies on cultural as well as linguistic knowledge to understand the ways in which particular phrases are used interactively, as well as what the content of them might mean. The issue of language was discussed in detail in Chapter 4, and the same principles apply to group interview data, which also require some attention to the *ways* in which talk is used in particular settings.

Limitations

The advantages of group interviews are also their limitations. Group settings may be ideal for accessing cultural norms, and how they are reproduced in everyday talk, but this means they are perhaps less useful for accessing in-depth accounts of socially deviant or marginal opinions. Group dynamics, with the dominance of particular group members, are a useful indicator of the hierarchy of opinions, and the ways in which marginal ones are 'silenced', but of course also limit the expression or elaboration of less acceptable opinions or the views of those who are lower in a status hierarchy. Thus, using ward-based natural groups to look at the views of health professionals in a hospital may be a useful way of accessing how various professionals talk to each other, but the more junior staff may feel too inhibited to speak out, or to disagree with senior staff. Again, the aims of the study will determine how far this is a problem. In the study on children's views of accident risks, referred to above, the aim was to capture how peer groups of young people interpret accident prevention messages and provide some useful information for planning health promotion materials for this age group. In many of the group discussions, young people discussed peers who were perceived as 'accident prone' in derogatory terms. These children were to some extent stigmatized for their clumsiness. If we had wanted to look at the experiences of these children specifically, the dynamics of a focus group would have been inappropriate – the most 'accident prone' children would have been unlikely to speak about their views within this dominant culture. Marginal or less socially acceptable views are unlikely to be explored in a group setting and may be best accessed in the more private setting of a one-to-one interview.

Local cultural and political considerations can also limit the range of views expressed in community interviews. Coreil (1995) discusses her experience of using community interviews in a participatory project designed to evaluate community management of a water system in Rwanda. Participants were recruited from users of standpipes in the locality, and although attendance at the meetings was good, with most turning into large community gatherings, women were under-represented. Not only did women have domestic responsibilities, which limited the time they had available to attend meetings, but also they traditionally had less involvement with public meetings. Those who did come did not speak much. 'Community interviews' may only access the views of particular (higher status) groups in the community, and in many settings may marginalize women's voices or the socially excluded.

Practical issues

The kind of group interview needed for the research, then, will depend on what kind of data you are aiming to produce. A focus group may well be appropriate for research that aims to gather a broad range of responses to, say, a proposed health promotion campaign, whereas interviews with less formal natural groups may be preferred if the aim is to gather more naturalistic data on how knowledge about a health topic is formed in social interaction. For any kind of organized group interview (as opposed to opportunistic ones carried out in the course of fieldwork), the practicalities of organizing group interviews need considering quite carefully for the method to work well. This will involve planning how participants will be sampled and recruited, what the topic guide will include (including ice-breaking and focusing prompts), how the groups will be run, where you will hold them, and how the data will be recorded.

Sampling

The previous chapter outlined some of the principles of sampling participants for interviews, and the same principles apply to focus groups. Essentially the aim of a sampling strategy is to maximize the opportunity of producing enough data to answer the research question. How this is achieved will depend on the research question, its feasibility and resources, and the setting. Convenience samples, based on networks of contacts, may be sufficient for exploratory or pilot studies. More systematic purposive sampling strategies will be needed for most studies in order to generate representative data that will be credible to users. One common strategy is to identify, from the literature and pilot work, the key demographic variables that are likely to have an impact on participants' views of the topic. These will then form a 'sampling grid', and groups can be recruited to reflect various combinations of variables. To take an example, in a European study of consumers' attitudes to the risk of BSE and other food risks (Draper et al. 2002), 'point in the life-cycle' was identified from the literature as a key influence on attitudes to food risk. Four important life-cycle groups were selected: adolescents, who are primarily reliant on others for choosing their food; 'young singles', who are responsible for their own food; 'family food purchasers', who choose food for their children as well as themselves; and 'older citizens', who may have memories of war-time food-rationing. In addition, in the UK it was known that geographical locality (whether urban and rural) and income (whether low income or more affluent) were likely to have an impact on attitudes to risk. Three other countries were involved in the study (Finland, Germany and Italy) and researchers there followed the same life-cycle segments and chose appropriate variables relevant to their own populations and what was known about differences in consumer behaviour. In Italy, for instance, the key difference was region, with sites selected in the north and south of the country. In the UK, 11 groups were selected to cover these key demographic differences (see Box 5.2).

The intention is both to represent the range of groups likely to have a different orientation to the topic, and also to provide some comparative data. Thus, the different life-cycle groups can be compared with each other, or with the different income groups. Using the same life-cycle groups in four countries also meant we could compare the views of, for instance, family food purchasers or older citizens cross-nationally. There are limits to using the same sampling frame in cross-national studies, as clearly demographic variables have different meanings in different settings. The groups of adolescents worked well in the UK study, as young people (aged 14-to-16) were already making some decisions about food choices, but less well in Italy where they reported merely that their mothers were the primary decision makers, and they had little to say on the issue. This sampling strategy also becomes unwieldy with a large number of population segments. Adding in, for instance, gender or ethnicity would have led to a very large number of cells.

Box 5.2	Sampling grid for UK groups in a study of public perceptions of BSE risk in Europe		
	Adolescents	Singles	Family food purchasers	Older citizens
Low income:				
rural	x		x	
urban	x	x	x	x
Affluent:				
rural			x	x
urban	x	x	x	

x = one group.
Source: Draper et al. (2002)

Recruitment

Recruiting participants can be time-consuming, and frustrating if attendance is poor. Many researchers have had the experience of booking rooms and sending reminders only to have few or no participants attending. Clearly the likely level of non-attendance will depend on how involved the researchers are with the participants' community, the interest of the community in the research topic, and the perceived benefits and gains of attending a group discussion. It is usually advisable to over-recruit by about 25 per cent, thus inviting 15 people if you are aiming to include 12 in the discussion, but in some settings higher over-recruitment will be needed. In other settings, of course, where it might be common to bring kin and neighbours, over-recruitment may be a problem, in which case some provision needs to be made to entertain 'extras' if there are too many participants arriving.

Once it has been decided which groups will be sampled, there are three potential strategies for recruiting participants. The first is opportunism. To recruit 'natural' groups, key 'gatekeepers' or contacts are invited to recruit their peers. Networks of personal contacts can be good gatekeepers for workplace and social groups, especially for pilot or exploratory studies. Nevertheless, however extensive the personal networks of the research team are, they are unlikely to generate a representative sample or to include all the population segments of interest. Advertising is one possibility, although most experience suggests it does not work well. Identifying community groups to work with is more productive. Community leaders can be asked to help contact key people to invite them. This may be the only way of including 'hard to reach' population groups. In a study of bilingual children's views of their experiences of interpreting for family members in health service settings, we contacted cultural centres, after-school activity groups and language schools to recruit bilingual young people. One disadvantage of working with established community groups is that it can be difficult to determine the sampling, and the researcher is reliant on community leaders to identify appropriate people to contact.

The second strategy is systematically inviting people, either as individuals, or as contacts for their peer groups, from a sampling frame, if there is one, for the population of interest. Such a sampling frame might be, for example, a list of all patients at a particular clinic, all nursing students in a college or all mothers giving birth in hospital (as in the example in Case Study 5.1). A sample of participants can then be drawn randomly from this list, or more purposively if you are aiming for a particular mix in each group. Unless the topic is of great interest to participants, this method may have low response rates. Using incentives, such as payments, refreshments or vouchers, can increase participation.

Third, commercial market research companies are one possibility for recruiting particular groups in short time scales and for groups that might be 'hard to reach'. Most commercial companies have large databases of potential participants, and can recruit the required number of people in each demographic group needed fairly quickly. They are of course relatively expensive, and pay higher fees to participants than is usual in social research. The groups constituted have other drawbacks. The main one is that participants can be, to some extent, professional 'focus groupees', who may be adept at adopting particular social roles for the purposes of research discussions. This may not matter, and indeed raises a question about how far the focus groups we recruit are adopting particular positions on the basis of how they were recruited. Most of us have a range of social roles (work-based, family-based, interest-based) and gathering a group of 'East African women with HIV' or 'elderly men with diabetes' to discuss issues of service use does presuppose that these identities shape the kinds of knowledge displayed.

Incentives

Following the example of market research companies, it can sometimes be beneficial to offer some incentive to participate, particularly for focus groups, in which the participants' stake in the research may be less than in more participatory studies. Incentives might include reimbursing travel and child care expenses, providing refreshments, or offering some kind of payment, or payment in kind, such as store vouchers. Offering incentives is more common than in one-to-one interview research simply because the researcher is often asking more of each group participant: they have to attend at a set time and place, rather than at one which is convenient for them, the time taken is often more burdensome, and out-of-pocket expenses such as child care and transport are needed. In countries with a tradition of market research, participants may well expect some kind of small payment, unless the study is one that is closely tied to their own interests. However, in academic health research the use of incentives is often rather contentious, with suggestions that we may be 'biasing' the response, and they may not be appropriate (or possible) in all settings.

The topic guide

A topic guide is a more or less structured interview schedule for the discussion, consisting of a small number of questions, with follow-up prompts to use to generate further discussion. The early prompts should be general, moving on to more specific issues. Box 5.3 shows the topic guide for the study of European consumers' attitudes to food risk, focusing on their views of BSE.

Ice-breaking tasks and focusing exercises

Ice-breaking exercises are primarily designed to generate discussion between the participants early on, so that everyone has a chance to speak and get to know each other enough to interact. Even when using natural groups, where people already know each other, an introductory exercise can establish preferred titles (whether participants want to use first names, or last names, or pseudonyms) and individual voices, so they can be identified on the tape. Focusing exercises are designed to get the group to orient themselves to the topic in hand, and sometimes to gather particular kinds of data. Case Study 5.2 has some examples of exercises used to explore how media messages about AIDS are interpreted and framed by groups, and the protocol for the European BSE study in Box 5.3 has examples of two group tasks. These examples are both exercises designed to generate data through facilitating members of the group talking to each other about the topic. The study by Munodawafa and colleagues (1995) on young women's understanding of HIV transmission in Zimbabwe, referred to above, used dancing to relax participants before the discussion. Ice-breaking activities need to be chosen with care. Not everyone feels comfortable with these kinds of 'games' and for some participants the embarrassment of joining in can cause considerable discomfort. Tasks requiring cards to be read are clearly unsuitable for any participants with limited literacy skills, and pictures or physical props could therefore be used instead.

Box 5.3   Protocol for a focus group discussion

Public perceptions of BSE in Europe

Protocol for focus group discussions
Groups to last 1–2 hours.

Group Task 1 (15 minutes):
'Order the following foods from the ones you feel most confident are safe to eat, to the ones you feel least confident are safe to eat'
Large cards with following words/pictures: Meat, Poultry, Fish, Eggs, Dairy Produce, Fruit & Vegetables

Group Task 2 (15 minutes):
'One food concern is BSE [check everyone has heard of this] – please sort the following foods in terms of how much of a risk you think they have of being contaminated with BSE'
Large cards with following words/pictures: Beef Steak, Ox Tail, Minced Meat, Dairy Foods

Prompts for general discussion (50 minutes):

1   Generally, do you think the food available is safe to eat?
2   Is it as safe as it used to be?
3   Whose responsibility is it to make food safe?
4   Who do you trust for information on food safety?
5   Do you worry about BSE? (Why? Why not?)
6   Why do you think BSE has happened?
7   Have you changed your/your family's consumption of beef because of BSE? (If so, what has replaced it?)

Conclusion/Debrief (5 minutes):
Ask each participant in turn if there is anything they want to add. Thank participants, ask them to complete the brief questionnaire, hand out travel expenses and ask if they have further questions about the study.

Source: Adapted from Draper et al. (2002).

Running a group

The role of the facilitator (sometimes called a 'moderator' in focus group studies) is vital. Like any interviewer, their job is to establish a relaxed atmosphere, enable participants to tell their stories, and listen actively. This involves greeting participants as they arrive, handing out refreshments, information sheets and consent forms if necessary, introducing any ice-breaking tasks and prompting each new topic. This is too much work for one person, and most groups will be run by a facilitator plus a note-taker, or assistant. The second person keeps written notes and ensures that tape recorders are working and switched on. If notes are the only form of data collected, they can also summarize at key points for the group, to check that views are being recorded reliably.

The skills needed to facilitate a discussion are similar to those needed for any interviewing, i.e., the ability to listen actively, be non-judgemental, and encourage others to speak (by not interrupting, adopting relaxed body language, making the right visual and verbal cues, not jumping in too quickly with the next question or prompt). Facilitators do not have to be an expert on the topic – in fact it is usually helpful if they are not, so that participants are not inhibited in discussing their views.

How far the facilitator actively manages the discussion depends on the aim of the group, and how tightly structured the topic guide is. If each group needs to cover all the topics on the guide, the facilitator will need to be careful to move the discussion on if it deviates too much from the guide. In more exploratory work, the 'deviations' can be left to run for a little longer, as topics that seem irrelevant at the time may be crucial at the analysis stage for making sense of people's understanding.

Setting

The physical setting is important. Ideally this should be a quiet, comfortable room where there will be no disturbances, although some trade-off may be necessary between accessibility and its suitability for research purposes. A local community centre room may be less quiet, but more accessible and familiar and less intimidating to the group than a university or hospital seminar room.

Recording data

Ideally, two good-quality tape or digital recorders are needed to record a group discussion, in addition to the services of a note-taker. In rural developing country settings tape recording may be impossible, or inappropriate. In this case, it is useful to summarize the views of the group as the discussion progresses so that the facilitator can check they have understood the key points. In literate communities, these summaries can be written on large sheets of paper throughout the discussion.

Sensitive issues

Great care must be taken in running discussions on sensitive topics, especially with natural groups who have to live, work or socialize together after the researchers have gone home. A good facilitator is likely to be skilled in getting participants to feel safe, and to reveal stories that they might not have shared in everyday settings, but this of course raises issues about how far the researchers need to protect participants from over-disclosure (see Case Study 3.1). However bland or non-controversial the topic appears to be, taking part in a group discussion may raise sensitive issues for some members of the group. As Michael Bloor and colleagues note in their book on focus groups (Bloor et al. 2001: 55–6), the research interview is not a therapeutic group, and if participants do get upset, or make disclosures that may be difficult for them later, researchers should not attempt to engage in 'therapy', but debrief quietly at the end of the session. For particularly sensitive topics, it is worth finding out the telephone numbers of appropriate service providers in case participants do ask for further help. Participants may also raise issues that are difficult for facilitators, if they express strong emotions or extreme views that are not those of the facilitator. In the research described in Case Study 5.2, Kitzinger reports some extreme homophobic views from some groups. On issues likely to generate this kind of data, it may be sensible to ensure that there is also scope for the facilitator to 'debrief' after the group. A formal arrangement with a trusted colleague or supervisor may be needed for the facilitator to talk through the experience of conducting the group interview and their feelings and reactions to it.

Developing appropriate methods for the setting

The key to running successful group interviews is to ensure that the methods used are appropriate for the setting, topic and participants. If working in unfamiliar settings, it is essential to work with partners who are sensitive to cultural norms about interaction, and what will be appropriate in terms of facilitation and structure. Bilkis Vissandjée and colleagues (2002) report their experiences of running focus groups in rural Gujarat in India, in which extensive local collaboration was necessary to develop appropriate protocols. The ethical implications of this were described in Case Study 3.1. Other issues they had to take into account included: when and what to offer in the way of refreshments, what characteristics the moderator would need, and how to introduce a tape recorder to groups who may be suspicious of being recorded. As described in Case Study 3.1, the rural setting had a number of implications for ethical methodology, including ensuring confidentiality, given that in small village communities the participants are well known to each other, and complex social relationships patterned what could be said in particular settings. Thus, whether groups included mothers-in-law or village elders had considerable impact on what women could say, and the researchers supplemented the group discussions with some individual interviews. In summary, they suggest a number of rules of thumb for what they call culturally competent focus groups: flexibility, taking time to understand local customs, consulting others with research experience in the area, engaging local communities in the research design, and being prepared to adapt protocols to make use of culturally appropriate techniques of data collection. Although Vissandjée and colleagues are reflecting on their experience in rural India, these rules of thumb are useful reminders for designing appropriate group interviews in all settings.

Conclusion

Group interviews are a flexible method for producing data on social interaction, and their key advantage is that they provide access to how people display, use and construct their social knowledge as well as access to what the content of that knowledge is. In this chapter we have concentrated on two kinds of group interview commonly used in health research, the focus group (with its traditions in market research) and the 'natural' group, which attempts to recreate naturalistic social interaction in a research setting. The key to using group interviews is to remember that, as with other methods of producing data, the researcher must be aware of the context of the data production, and account for how the particular setting produced data on views, or experiences, or beliefs. Utterances made in group interview transcripts cannot be stripped of their context and presented as the essential 'views' of the participants. The proper unit of analysis for a group interview study is therefore the group, rather than the individuals in that group, and group interviews are a particularly suitable method when this level of analysis is required.

KEY POINTS

- Group interviews have the key advantage of providing access to social interaction, and thus the process of how knowledge is acquired, shared and contested in quasi-naturalistic settings.
- However, it must be remembered that group interviews are not 'natural' settings, and the context of data collection must be taken into account in the analysis.
- The protocol for running a group discussion has to be appropriate for the topic, setting and population.

EXERCISE

Consider any professional or local community with which you are familiar. Design a protocol for a study using 'natural' groups from this community on one of the following topics:

(Continued)

1   Barriers to giving up smoking.
2   Dealing with stress at work.
3   Using dental services.

Include in your protocol some appropriate ice-breaking and focusing exercises and prompts to facilitate the discussion. What particular issues would working on this topic with this community raise in terms of: confidentiality, the impact of the research on participants after the group discussions had finished, sensitive issues, identifying an appropriate facilitator, recruitment?

FURTHER READING

Barbour, R. and Kitzinger, J. (eds) (1999) *Developing focus group research: politics, theory and practice*. London: Sage. A collection of chapters drawing on the authors' empirical experiences of focus group research that cover methodological issues including the impact of context, using focus groups in feminist and participatory research, using focus groups for sensitive topics, and approaches to analysis.

Bloor, M., Frankland, J., Thomas, M. and Robson, K. (2001) *Focus groups in social research*. London: Sage. Discusses the contribution of focus group methods to social research, including a chapter on the development of 'virtual' focus groups using email and Internet technology. Good discussions of the methodological weaknesses of focus group designs for many research questions.

Krueger, R. and Casey, M.A. (2000) *Focus groups: a practical guide for applied research* (3rd edn). Thousand Oaks, CA: Sage. A useful guidebook orientated towards the practical issues of planning, recruiting, running, analysing and reporting focus groups. The authors draw from their own experiences of running different kinds of focus groups, largely in North America.

6 Observational Methods

CHAPTER SUMMARY

The strength of observational methods is that they provide data on phenomena (such as behaviour), as well as on people's accounts of those phenomena. They can be divided into participant methods, where the researcher is present to some extent in the field studied, and non-participant methods, where researchers observe a field without involvement, through for instance analysing audio-tapes of encounters. Ethnographic accounts using participant observation have contributed detailed knowledge of how health beliefs are embedded in culture. The practical and methodological issues raised by ethnographic research, including doing ethnography close to home, rapid appraisal methods and pseudo-patient studies, are discussed, and this chapter briefly discusses the possibilities of utilizing non-participant methods by using analysis of naturally occurring data such as recordings of consultations in medical practice.

Introduction

If the aim of research is to understand a phenomenon, rather than people's accounts of it, then observational methods are often cited as the 'gold standard' of qualitative methods, given that they provide direct access to what people do, as well as what they say they do. As Becker and Geer put it:

> The most complete form of the sociological datum ... is the form in which the participant observer gathers it: An observation of some social event, the events which precede and follow it, and explanations of its meaning by participants and spectators, before, during and after its occurrence. Participant observation can thus provide a yardstick against which to measure the completeness of data gathered in other ways, a model which can serve to let us know what orders of information escape us when we use other methods. (Becker and Geer 1957: 28)

Interviews, in this 'classic' account of the strengths of observational methods, are flawed by only providing a partial account of a phenomenon. Observational methods allow the researcher to record the mundane and unremarkable (to participants) features of everyday life that interviewees might not feel were worth commenting on and the context within which they occur. Similarly, for Lofland (1971), participant observation is a route to 'knowing people' rather than 'knowing about them'. This perspective, that observational strategies somehow allow the researchers closer to some essential truth about social life, is implicit in much qualitative social research. The 'purest' form of data is that gathered directly from naturally occurring situations, in which behaviour and responses to it can be observed in situ. The idea of observational data being the 'gold standard' in terms of their validity is also a common theme in health research, with observations often provided as illustrating the truth about some event or process, in (often ironic) contrast to interview accounts, or statistical records. Certainly, there are a number of examples of observational studies on health topics that have demonstrated very nicely the limitations of other sources of data (such as official records) in terms of their reliability or validity.

Isobel Bowler (1995), for instance, draws on her observations of a maternity hospital in southern England to show how official statistics and 'facts' about women of south Asian descent result from particular bureaucratic processes, embedded in cultural practices, such as stereotypical assumptions made by staff. These particular social practices result in flawed records about women of south Asian descent. Examples include observations of record-making when women were booked onto the ward, when Bowler observed 'facts' such as nationality being recorded in line with what staff assumed about the women in front of them, rather than their actual answers, and details of their medical histories being missed because of difficulties in using standard forms with tick box answers. Another example was date of birth – for the staff, an unremarkable 'fact' that everyone would know, but for a few patients of south Asian descent, not a significant 'fact' about themselves, but one that they had learnt to respond to by estimating the year of birth and giving 1st January as the date. Bowler's observations thus provide essential information for anyone utilizing hospital records as a source of data on maternity patients, and point to some of the ways in which such records are likely to be incomplete or incorrect.

In a similar vein, Gillian Lewando-Hundt and her colleagues (Lewando-Hundt et al. 1999) looked at official statistics about birth in the Gaza Strip. Here, observational data explained why address data was missing from registrations, and also suggested that birth weight was often recorded erroneously (see discussion in Chapter 2). The findings from the observational study, suggest Lewando-Hundt and colleagues, demonstrate the unique contribution of qualitative methods:

> [Anthropology], as well as explaining how social systems function, can make explicit the ways in which people use documentation to cope. ... Anthropology can make its contribution to epidemiology. It is precisely here that qualitative methods can be used to *validate* health surveillance data and guide policy intervention. (Lewando-Hundt et al. 1999: 842, emphasis added)

Thus, observational data are widely assumed to be the archetypal qualitative method, producing the most valid data on social behaviour, and demonstrating the unique contribution qualitative methods can make to researching health. There is considerable merit to this claim, and the use of observational methods can add significantly to many qualitative studies, providing data on what participants do, as well as what they say they do. Shadowing staff over a shift at work, for instance, or attending organizational meetings, can be an invaluable way of not only seeing the organization through the eyes of those who work there, and providing some insight into what does go on in everyday settings, but can also provide a wealth of case study material for following up in interviews.

However, the argument that ethnographic methods are the 'gold standard' against which other sources of data could be compared is one that does make some rather positivist and empiricist assumptions, in which there is a rather idealistic view of the 'real', which can be reflected by a trained observer's eye, and perfectly recreated in the research write-up. It also assumes that all research questions relate to understanding phenomena directly, whereas in many cases the researcher is interested primarily in accounts, or narratives, for which interviews are an appropriate method. However, observational methods do have methodological advantages for many health research questions, and are perhaps under-used, especially in applied research, in part because of the time-consuming nature of many approaches.

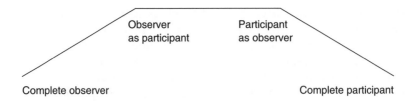

Figure 6.1   Gold's ideal types of research role

Participant and non-participant observation

A classic typology of observational methods was suggested by Gold (1958), who distinguished between potential roles the researcher can adopt in terms of how much they participate in the field being observed (Figure 6.1). At one end of Gold's scale, the complete participant is a researcher who is a 'native' in the field they are observing. Complete participation includes reflexive 'insider accounts', written by professionals or patients drawing on their own experiences as data for understanding a particular issue. There is a tradition of 'sociological autobiography' in which personal experiences are used to explore theoretical or conceptual issues. Christopher Adamson (1997), for instance, draws on a detailed diary he kept while ill with and being treated for inflammatory bowel disease and his medical notes to explore how 'existential and clinical uncertainty are mutually intermeshed properties of the medical encounter' (Adamson 1997: 138). Joel Richman (2000) used his experiences of time in intensive care as data for a paper on 'intensive care syndrome', which discussed how the environment of intensive care contributes to post-operative psychiatric disorder. In studies such as these, experiences only become 'data' in retrospect, and at the time there may be no intention to use them analytically. Less formally, many research studies begin as reflections on everyday experiences, and our own experiences as users of health services and professionals are an invaluable source of data and ideas for research questions.

However, in most studies the researcher is to some extent entering a field explicitly in order to research it. The next roles identified by Gold – the participant as observer and observer as participant roles – describe classic *ethnographic* studies, in which the researcher participates to a greater or lesser extent in the field that they are studying. Ethnography can be defined as a method of research in which the researcher 'participates, overtly or covertly, in people's daily lives for an extended period of time, watching what happens, listening to what is being said, asking questions; in fact collecting whatever data are available to throw light on the issues with which he or she is concerned' (Hammersley and Atkinson 1983: 2).

When describing research methods, the term 'ethnography' is often used interchangeably with 'participant observation'. In traditional anthropological studies, doing ethnography could entail many months or even years living in a small-scale community in order to understand the social structure and local culture. In these studies, the research design is primarily about the exposure to another culture, and the way in which the researcher comes to understand it, rather than a particular data collection method (such as 'observation'). Joseph Opala and François Boillot describe the aims of this kind of anthropology thus:

> The anthropologist can grasp a culture's world view only through long exposure. The researcher should ideally learn the language and live in the community for a year or more, spending as much time as possible interacting with people and absorbing their mode of reasoning. ... The anthropologist can also find clues through the careful observation of art, ritual and religion where ideas normally only hinted at are often brought to the surface. (Opala and Boillot 1996: 4)

Ethnography is, then, a holistic approach to research, involving interviews, observation and the interpretation of material culture. However, the *techniques* from this kind of ethnographic work, including the observation of 'naturally occurring interaction', have been used in health research both in studying the health beliefs of communities and in understanding health care organization.

Finally, at the other end of Gold's scale, the researcher can be a complete observer, and not participate in the field at all. Non-participant methods include the study of naturally occurring data, such as video-tapes of consultations in health care settings, in which the researcher is not even present in the field. They can also include studies in which the researcher is present to collect data, but does not interact with participants. This might include studies of patient behaviour in a clinic waiting room. These various roles generate rather different methodological problems. To start, we shall explore the contributions of ethnographic participant observation to health research.

Ethnography and participant observation

The term 'ethnography' refers to the methods of participant observation, but also to the *product* of ethnographic investigation; that is, the written report, often a monograph, is also called an ethnography. Classic anthropological monographs are the outcome of a considerable time spent living with a small-scale community, coming to understand in a holistic way their beliefs and social structure, including kinship structures, religious beliefs, political systems and material culture. Medical anthropology focuses on health beliefs and healing systems. Through living and working with the community, the anthropologist comes to see the world through their eyes and understand in detail how beliefs are embedded in local cultures. The first aim of an in-depth observational study in anthropology is, then, to produce an account of a social setting that is faithful to the perspectives of the participants.

What separates this from a common-sense account of the world is that it is not *merely* an 'insider' description, but also a theoretical description. Thus an empathetic and detailed description, although perhaps intrinsically interesting, is not enough. The 'insider' view must be related to the 'outsider' view, which brings in an analytical approach to social life. This entails a sensitivity to patterns in social behaviour, and regularities that indicate underlying 'rules' of social behaviour. Anthropologists distinguish **emic** and **etic** perspectives to label these activities. The emic perspective is that of 'insiders', or the explanation of a social world provided by a participant in it. The etic perspective is that of the analyst. In his account of analysing the ritual symbols used by the Ndembu of Zambia, Victor Turner discusses the role of the anthropologist in analysing meaning as well as merely recording the participants' own interpretations:

> How then, can an anthropologist justify his claim to be able to interpret a society's ritual symbols more deeply and comprehensively than the actors themselves? [F]irst ... he can place this ritual in its significant field setting and describe the structure and properties of that field ... the anthropologist has no particular bias and can observe the real interconnections and conflicts between groups and persons. (Turner 1967: 26–7)

The tension between an etic and an emic perspective is what drives an ethnographic analysis. It is also a tension that has practical implications, in terms of the roles adopted by the researcher engaged in any kind of participant observation. One way of describing this tension in fieldwork roles is to use the metaphors of the 'native' and the 'stranger from Mars' for potential stances the researcher can take. Thus, ideally, an ethnographer has to move between an understanding which resembles that of a 'native' participant, whether this is an urban slum dweller or an operating theatre nurse, and the complete alien, who is a naive outsider trying to make sense of the local culture: why things are done the way they are and how people account for them. The value of the 'native' perspective is that it allows an empathetic understanding of the motivations, priorities and rationality of those studied. Without seeing things 'through the eyes' of the insider, the researcher will never be able to understand fully their perspective. This is vital, particularly in applied work that seeks to intervene in health behaviour. An 'insider' perspective provides access to the logic and rationality of what might seem at first merely misguided or irrational beliefs. Thus, in reading Victor Turner's work on Ndembu rituals, we come to understand how the Ndembu attribute misfortunes such as illness to various kinds of ritual transgressions, spirits and witches. Female reproductive troubles, for instance, are believed to result from the actions of the spirits of dead relatives. Rather than being merely random superstitious beliefs, ideas about the causes of particular symptoms and the appropriate remedies tie into an overarching cosmology that 'makes sense' of the misfortunes that afflict individuals from time to time. Although Turner notes that the ritual therapies used by the Ndembu may not be effective in public health terms (Turner 1967: 356), his ethnographic account provides a rich account of how they work at the social level, through reintegrating the sick person into society, for instance, or dealing with conflicts within the community.

However, without the 'stranger from Mars' perspective, such accounts will be limited. In everyday life, most of us have experience of having to 'learn the culture' of a new setting and become an insider. Starting a new college, or moving to a new country, entails learning all kinds of everyday rules about social behaviour and we are usually anxious to do this as quickly as possible to reduce the embarrassment of being an obvious novice or newcomer. In a research setting this process of social learning has to be made explicit, and the researcher will then reflect on how the rules were learned and what their significance is. Michael Agar (1980) uses the phrase 'professional stranger' to describe this role. If the fieldwork is protracted, the researcher has to guard against 'going native' and being merely a participant in the field, rather than an active participant observer. The 'stranger' element of the role has to be consciously maintained, in order to be able to ask the naive question and analyse social life from a theoretical perspective.

Doing ethnography close to home

Early European anthropologists studied alien cultures, largely small-scale societies in colonized African and Asian countries, in which the key challenge was to make the unfamiliar familiar. More recently, anthropologists have turned their attention closer to home, with African and Asian researchers criticizing the misinterpretations of earlier generations (Fahim 1982) and those from the industrialized world focusing on the familiar as well as the 'other' with an ethnographic approach. Some examples of ethnographic methods used in industrialized settings include:

- *Studies of 'lay' health beliefs.* Cecil Helman (1978) looked at folk models of chills, fevers and colds in a North London suburb, and Charlie Davison and colleagues (1991) used ethnographic methods to look at lay epidemiological understandings of heart disease in South Wales.
- *Studies of health service organization and delivery.* Norman Fineman (1991) used observational and interview data to look at how clinicians, social workers and alcohol counsellors in a clinic constructed 'non-compliance' in the clients. Catherine Pope (1991) used observations and other methods to understand how waiting lists remain a problem for hospitals in the UK despite policy initiatives aimed at reducing them. David Hughes (1989) carried out a ten-month ethnographic study of an Accident and Emergency department, using the data to look at discretion in the work of reception and other non-clinical staff.
- *Cultural studies of biomedicine itself.* Deborah Lupton (1994) and Deborah Gordon (1988) have both used anthropological approaches to look at 'medicine as culture', and several anthropologists have analysed specific biomedical disease and epidemiological categories using the same approaches used for 'folk' categories.

Insider accounts

In these studies using participant observation methods in studying industrialized health care settings, health professionals are often in a position
of researching their own profession. Nurses, for instance, have carried out
many studies of nursing care based on ethnographic methods for data collection. This poses particular methodological problems for maintaining a
productive balance between insider and outsider perspectives and in making the familiar 'strange'. The advantages are clearly that access is much
easier, and the researcher is already familiar with the emic perspective.
Also, professional practice has provided a rich seam of potential research
questions, and a good understanding of the feasibility of researching
them. However, such 'insider' researchers face a far greater challenge in
gaining analytical distance from their data, and may have to work much
harder to treat the data theoretically. Jocelyn Lawler, in her work on the
body in nursing (1991), reflects on how this balance can be successfully
achieved. As a nurse, Lawler was interested in the 'invisibility' of nursing
work, and began thinking of how this could be related to the 'private'
nature of much of the work they did caring for patients' bodies. She notes
that although the physical body is taken for granted in everyday life, it
becomes the focus of nursing work, and yet there is a relative absence of
any 'talk' about it. She discusses the methodological challenges of
researching 'taken for granted knowledge' and getting nurses to discuss
explicitly what are not only taboo and sensitive issues, but ones that practitioners may have no adequate language to describe. Lawler argues that
her 'insider' status was an advantage, even essential, to carrying out
research on nursing:

> Because nursing is heavily influenced by experience, the
> researcher must share the same professional experience in order
> to decide what questions to ask nurses, if indeed the researcher
> wishes to get at the very essence of nursing practice. ... One
> persistent feature of research involving nurses' work is the
> extent to which researchers have asked the 'wrong' questions.
> (Lawler 1991: 6)

For Lawler, then, an adequate insider understanding is an essential precondition for valid analysis, and she claims that professional experience is necessary to develop this. However, this is not a sufficient condition. She also drew
on a combination of theoretical literatures to 'make sense' of the problem of
the body, and articulate the 'taken for granted' knowledge of practitioners.
This included a historical review of conceptualization of the body, literature
on nursing and 'surveillance' of the body, and feminist approaches to the
body and sexuality. This helps to maintain an analytical distance, but Lawler
(by suggesting that only nurses can ask the 'right' questions) is situating herself firmly on the 'emic' end of the continuum, where faithfulness to the participants' own priorities and frameworks is key to validity.

Ethnography in health care organizations

Doing ethnography close to home does not have to involve researching your own professional culture or organization. In complex modern health care systems, most researchers are only familiar with a few organizations, and most research fields will offer enough 'strangeness' to enable an attitude of ethnographic distance. Simon Carmel, for instance, in describing his role as an ethnographer researching Critical Care Units in the UK, a health care setting with which he was unfamiliar, notes that:

> The main disadvantage of being a 'complete observer' was that the setting was initially strange. However, this was advantageous as I kept a record of the ways in which the setting felt strange to me, and I entered the field with fewer pre-conceived ideas than someone more familiar with intensive care, thereby open to different ideas. (Carmel 2003: 95)

The advantages of observation over interviews in such a setting are that they enable the everyday routines of practice to be analysed from an 'etic' perspective. Although in principle we can ask clinicians or nurses about their activities and how their organization works, in practice these 'common sense' accounts are difficult for interviewees to access and make accountable: they become, after a while, taken for granted, and impossible to recount to an outsider. The ethnographer, as a stranger, can observe the minutiae of organizational life and, through analysis, offer an account of 'what is happening' in a setting that is rich, nuanced and based on a critical reading of insider accounts. Of course, it does not mean that insider accounts can be dismissed as biased or merely self-serving. Interviews, both formal and informal, are usually a key element of observational studies. Many studies of health care settings have used interview and observational data together to add depth, combining data on 'what goes on' with data on how insiders describe and understand what is happening. An example comes from Catherine Pope's (2002) work on surgery in the UK and the USA, in which she analyses the role of 'contingency' in surgery, suggesting that various sources of contingency can arise from variations in human bodies, the craft preferences of individual surgeons and the supporting technical and material assistance they can draw upon. The presence of contingency, she suggests, is one factor in the tensions apparent between the increasing reliance on 'evidence-based' guidelines in surgery and the practice of everyday surgical work. Had she just relied on interview accounts for this interpretation, there would be no way of accounting for the role of rhetorical over-statement by surgeons who may want to stress the 'art' of surgery. However, drawing on observations of operations, in which various kinds of contingency were seen to operate, provides useful evidence that this may be a useful way to characterize the *doing* of surgery, as well as to characterize surgeons' *accounts* of surgery. Similarly, relying just on observational work in a setting that is relatively unfamiliar would be not only more time-consuming, but also would make it difficult to identify, from the stream of activity and talk, what precisely would be useful to focus on. Interviews thus provide a framework and a space in which participants can explicitly make accountable the taken-for-granted knowledge and rules they draw upon in their practice, but which may not be note-worthy until the researcher asks about them.

Overt and covert roles

Overt roles are those in which the researcher is open about their role, whereas covert roles involve the researcher being 'under cover'. Most ethnographers are, to some extent, open about their role, but of course there are many potential ways to present your role in the field, and many interpretations people in the field will put on your account. Researchers working in areas where people are unfamiliar with the concept of research, or anthropology, are likely to be cast in more familiar roles by the host community – as spies or government officials, perhaps. One example comes from Richard Burghart's (1993) reflections on early fieldwork in his research on how people in Janakpur, in southeastern Nepal, used the wells that still supplied water for some residents, and how they kept the water pure. He discusses how one community, the Cobblers, who were using a hand-pump in a neighbouring community as their well water was no longer 'sweet', originally assumed he had a rather more powerful role than merely that of a visiting researcher. He explained to a gathering crowd that he was there to learn from them how the well had lost its 'sweetness' and what they proposed to do to cure it, but heard members of the crowd repeating a rather different account to each other:

> The Cobblers ... turned to explain to newcomers ... that the government had told the sahib to tour the country and see the condition of the common people, and that my government was going to help the Cobblers clean the well. ... I quickly corrected them, saying I had not come from Kathmandu [i.e., from the Nepalese government] ... rather I had come from London. ... The inner circle now explained to the outer that I had been sent by the London government to tour Nepal to report on the condition of common folk. Now the British government were going to help them clean their well. ... I attempted to explain my ethical neutrality, political impartiality, indeed the objectivity of scientific research. Again, confusion spread throughout the crowd. (Burghart 1993: 82–3)

Burghart realized that his attempt to stress his impartiality had misfired completely, as local residents then assumed he was, in the eyes of the villagers, the worst of all visitors – a political broker, whose only function could be to play the two governments off against each other. In the event, he settled for an identity of a minor 'Lord', who would help the residents to purify their well.

In an unfamiliar setting, it may be impossible to predict how the community will interpret the role of the researcher. Even when the research setting is in a familiar culture, the researcher has to consider assumptions that will be made about their position, and who they are while doing fieldwork. Professionals working in familiar settings may be assumed to be 'experts', and those funded by government departments may be assumed to be working to a political agenda.

If trying to explain the role of the researcher brings problems, covert research, in which the researcher does not tell the community what they are doing, brings even more. Lawler's 'insider' status as a nurse provided her 'cover' for much opportunistic observational work as she carried out normal duties, such as hospital-based teaching. However, she notes that these activities meant her role was more 'participant' than observer, and allowed little time for sustained observation. A longer-term period of observation was provided, also opportunistically, by the admission of a friend to hospital. Lawler thus had a legitimate role as a hospital visitor, allowing her to observe nursing work covertly. She notes:

> While I was aware of the ethical considerations inherent in using this situation for collecting data, I was also legitimately in the field as a visitor, and it was inevitable that I would find this time rich in ideas and data, and that it would contribute to my thinking on the ways in which nurses manage other people's bodies. I took advantage, opportunistically, of a naturally occurring event. (Lawler 1991: 13)

We discussed in Chapter 3 the ethical dilemmas involved in this kind of work, in which the role of the researcher is not disclosed to those in the field. Lawler's justification here is twofold: first, she wanted access to an 'undisturbed' natural environment in which the nurses' behaviour was not changed in response to a known observer (1991: 12). Second, as she notes above, it is very difficult to draw the line in long-term observational research between research and non-research activity. Health care is a diffuse activity, and we shall inevitably come across instances of our areas of interest in our everyday life. It would be impossible to discount all these stories and comments by friends and colleagues that might contribute to our eventual analysis, just because they weren't gained through a formal interview in which informed consent was sought. In addition, the meetings we have with potential gate-keepers, discussions with collaborators and observations made opportunistically while carrying out 'normal' activities such as visiting hospitals, all provide 'data' which cannot be forgotten just because it was not a formal part of the data set. Even if never quoted in a report, these encounters, at a time when we are explicitly reflecting on a particular issue, are bound to influence the development of ideas. They should be treated with exactly the same critical awareness as other, more formal data, and as a valuable aid to the 'sociological imagination'.

These opportunistic observations are, however, arguably rather different from extended periods of 'covert' research, in which data collection is the primary goal, but no attempt is made to secure informed consent from participants or be explicit about the research role. As Chapter 3 discussed, this kind of research cannot be undertaken lightly, and must be justified by the impossibility of gaining data in other ways and the likely 'public interest' value of any data gained. One covert observational strategy for data collection that has been widely used in health services research is the 'pseudo-patient study', deriving from market research's 'mystery shopping'.

'Mystery shopping' and pseudo-patient studies

Mystery shopping is a technique taken from market research, involving the testing of services by researchers pretending to be genuine consumers in order to find out how consumers really are treated by service providers in everyday, rather than research, situations. As a form of covert observation, it has been used in health research, although not often by this name. Martin Bulmer (1982) used the term '**pseudo-patient studies**' to cover research that involves researchers pretending to be patients in order to find out how services are 'really' provided. As he noted, such strategies are used by investigative journalists and consumer organizations to 'test' services, as well as by researchers. There are a number of examples of such studies. Rosenhan's (1973) study of psychiatric hospitals, described in Case Study 3.2, is a classic, and mental health institutions have attracted many covert studies. Other health service topics researched by pseudo-patients include homeless people's access to primary health care in a London borough (Hinton 1994), the differences between biomedical and Ayurvedic physicians in Sri Lanka (Waxler-Morrison 1988) and the routines of an acute hospital ward in Ghana (van der Geest and Sarkodie 1998).

Studies such as Rosenhan's are qualitative sociological studies of health care, in that they rely on ethnographic accounts from the pseudo-patients for their data. These covert methods are now not much used in sociological studies, largely because of the ethical problems involved. The need for informed consent from research participants in most settings means that many ethics committees would be unlikely to approve such a study. However, in health services research, there have been recent uses of pseudo-patients in evaluations of health care provision. Possibilities for securing consent include requesting consent retrospectively, and asking professional organizations to consent on behalf of their members. In these cases, the pseudo-patient is likely to have only had a brief encounter with a provider, rather than an extended period in, say, a mental hospital. Here, the method is used more quantitatively, and perhaps in an experimental design. Hinton's (1994) study of access to primary care, for instance, compared how often actors playing three different people (a homeless rough sleeper, a Kurdish refugee and a middle-class woman) successfully registered as patients in 30 primary care surgeries. In Waxler-Morrison's (1988) study comparing Ayurvedic and biomedical physicians, trained research assistants presented standard symptoms and recorded standard information about their visit and the medicines prescribed. In these experimental designs, the qualitative data on experiences of health care may contribute to the study, but the major aim is to generate comparative quantitative data.

Waxler-Morrison (1988), for instance, compared the number of times Ayurvedic and biomedical physicians carried out various investigations, volunteered particular information and prescribed Western or Ayurvedic medicines.

Madden et al. (1997) argue that these more quantitative pseudo-patient studies – or what they term *simulated client studies* – are a practical, feasible and economical method for researching health service provision in developing countries. For measuring actual practice, these methods provide better data than interviewing, as there are no problems with recall or social desirability bias, and better information than patient records, which may be inadequate. Reviewing studies that used simulated patients in developing countries, they note that they have been used to investigate a range of research questions, including evaluating training interventions, comparing pharmacy sales, and family-planning services. Although the main outcomes of these studies are quantitative, qualitative analysis might be used to examine issues such as communication in health care settings.

Following the ethical guidelines of the Council for International Organizations of Medical Sciences (CIOMS 1991), Madden et al. argue that provider consent may not be necessary if this would frustrate the purpose of the study. Despite noting that all researchers should be bound by the ethical norms of their own communities as well as those they study, they rather disconcertingly argue that weaker research governance is an advantage in developing countries, making pseudo-patient studies easier to conduct in these settings without consent: 'Government oversight tends to be weak, and there may be a general lack of labor/professional organizations, rights consciousness, and understanding of research. In many developing countries, social norms emphasize community rights over an individual's rights' (Madden et al. 1997: 1479).

Like all covert methods, pseudo-patient studies do raise particularly difficult ethical issues, particularly if (as Madden et al. are suggesting) the norms around consent may be different in the researcher's own institution and the fieldwork site. As we discussed in Chapter 3, a study to which participants cannot give informed consent is problematic. Justifications tend to focus on the high validity of data; the 'public interest' value of uncovering the real workings of health services, particularly in areas where patients may not be well served, such as mental health; and necessity – that such information can't be gathered in any other way. As the identity of the researcher is unknown to those in the field, the data gathered are uncontaminated by any researcher effects. Thus, if 'real' patient accounts are difficult to come by, or unlikely to be treated as 'valid', then the use of pseudo-patient studies may be the only way to generate convincing data on important topics such as discrimination in health service delivery. Aside from the substantial ethical problems, Martin Bulmer (1982) also argued that there are methodological problems. First, they encroach on the mutual trust and confidentiality of the 'real' doctor–patient relationship and involve deception. This can lead to a breakdown in trust between researchers and professionals. Second, there is the possibility of harm to the researcher if they are given unnecessary medical treatment, or are stressed by their experiences. Third, even the claim to greater validity might be flawed, as real patients (if not professionals!) may be adept at identifying 'pseudo-patients' and will presumably alter their behaviour in response.

Planning a participant observation study

So far, we have discussed in some detail the implications of various fieldwork roles (participant, participant-observer; stranger, insider; overt, covert) adopted by the researcher. Reflection on the methodological implications of the role is vital in thinking through the particular challenges of fieldwork (will it be learning the language? maintaining an analytical distance?), but there may be little leeway for choosing to adopt another role. Other decisions about participant observation studies will present choices, and these will need considerable thought before embarking on the project. Some of the practical methodological implications of participant observation studies that should be considered are identifying a site, gaining access, refining observational skills, and approaches to recording data. These are all affected by both the specific setting of the proposed research and the nature of the researcher's role within it. To some extent, decisions about, for instance, how best to take notes will be determined by those necessities of the field that can only be known once there, but they are issues that should be thought through at the outset to minimize potential problems.

Identifying a site

Traditionally, ethnographic work is based on an in-depth study of one site, and issues of generalizability are conceptual rather than empirical. In Chapter 4, we suggested that sampling in qualitative interview work is often orientated towards generating 'information-rich' (Patton 1990) cases. This is true when selecting a single or small number of sites, which may be chosen because they typify some larger population of sites (such as clinics, or villages) or perhaps because they are exceptional in some way. Often, site selection is in practice a pragmatic decision, based on existing networks of colleagues and contacts. Paul Atkinson (1995) discusses how he ended up researching haematology, despite intending to investigate the interface between clinical and laboratory issues in pathology. Following a meeting at a conference in which he outlined his research interests to a colleague, the colleague then negotiated for him access to a teaching hospital in the United States with an honorary hospital appointment – an opportunity too good to pass up. The pathologists he approached were less receptive than the haematologists, and in the end the study focused only on haematology. In health services research, though, participant observation methods may be used across multiple sites, and care should be taken to select ones that represent a range of typical settings. Here, the researcher may be responsible for 'cold calling' potential sites to collaborate, rather than relying on informal sponsors within organizations.

Gaining access: the role of gatekeepers

Gatekeepers are those people who control access to the site and the people within it. They include formal gatekeepers whose permission is needed before fieldwork can commence (such as hospital managers, government departments or consultants) and informal gatekeepers, without whose support fieldwork will be impossible in practice. The formal gatekeepers depend on the setting, and the appropriate people must be identified early on. For work in institutional settings (such as hospitals or health agencies) the formal gatekeepers will be fairly easily identifiable. Introducing yourself 'cold', for instance by writing to Chief Executives or senior managers in the prospective sites, can be a very difficult strategy, and it is often advisable to use personal and professional networks to smooth the way. If you can be introduced as a friend or colleague, prospective gatekeepers have some way of 'placing' you socially, and are likely to be more trusting. However, 'cold' calling can work. Van der Geest and Sarkodie, in their small-scale participant observation study of a Ghanaian hospital, wrote to the secretary of the nearest hospital, and were surprised by a very positive response: the hospital considered it an honour to be chosen. This was contrary to the previous experience of van der Geest in Western countries, where there may be more reluctance to letting unknown social scientists in to observe.

In community settings, it can be more difficult to identify the appropriate formal gatekeepers, and those with extensive knowledge of the setting should be consulted. Organizations for indigenous peoples now often have formal policies for collaborating with research, which outline the proper channels of communication and approval. As one example, the Hopi people in Arizona, North America, have a protocol for 'research, publications and recording' which requires proposals for studies to be sent to the Office of Historic and Cultural Preservation for review and approval, and for prospective researchers to outline how the Hopi tribe will benefit from the study, and how consent from participants will be addressed (HCPO 2001). In other settings the process may be less formal, but there are usually some gatekeepers who must give their permission before any fieldwork can commence.

Informal gatekeepers are just as important, in that the researcher is reliant on their goodwill to carry out the study, but can be harder to identify before setting out on fieldwork. Paul Atkinson (1995: 16) discusses an early problem in his study of haematologists. Although access had been negotiated with the hospital Chief of Staff and senior staff in the department, he had not had time to meet with more junior staff before commencing. One was initially hostile, and complained about his presence. Although Atkinson managed to resolve the problem by writing to all staff reiterating that he had no interest in evaluating their work or of intruding, these kinds of problems can completely undermine fieldwork.

Refining observational skills

Learning to 'observe' analytically is a skill that takes time to develop; it is not just a matter of looking and recording, but of knowing what to look for and how to reflect on what is seen. For William Foote Whyte, a foundational assumption is that 'human behaviour is not random ... but socially structured, and we need to discover the framework for such structuring' (Whyte 1984: 83–4). This is not, he suggests, a matter of looking at formal structures (such as organizational hierarchies or workplace divisions of labour) but looking at the regularities in social behaviour. Initial observations should be empirical: the idea is to describe what is going on, who is included, where it goes on and how, rather than one's 'impressions' or 'feelings' about the setting. This can be difficult to get started on, as any social field is a complex of many different activities and interactions. If it is an unfamiliar social setting, we may be tempted to impose our own assumptions of 'what is going on' from superficial similarities with those of our experiences. If the setting is a familiar one, it may be difficult to lose our professional frameworks for seeing what is happening. In Box 6.1 are John Lofland's (1971) suggestions for one way of dividing up 'the field' for observation.

Box 6.1   Lofland's headings for organizing observations

Acts:	brief occurrences of action
Activities:	of longer duration
Meanings:	verbal accounts that participants use to define what is going on
Participation:	holisitic involvement of participants in particular sets of acts and activities
Relationships:	who is involved, and with whom
Settings:	descriptions of whole sites

Source: Lofland (1971: 15)

Under each of the headings in Box 6.1, Lofland suggests that the researcher focuses on both static and 'phased' processes (that is, those that endure as features of a field, and those that change over time), either regularly or over the process of some change. One aim is to develop typologies for these different aspects of phenomena, by looking at how acts, activities and meanings are classified by those being studied. To take an example, if the fieldworker was beginning a period of observation of a community health clinic, they may begin by looking at the waiting room. Here, they might observe how patients wait (an *act*) for treatment, what they do while waiting in the waiting room (*activities*), who 'organizes' the queue for the doctor (*participation*), what communication there is between staff and patients in the waiting room (*relationships*), and what staff say their aim is in organizing the waiting area in a certain way (*meanings*). Putting together their observations of this and other phenomena, they can begin to build up a picture of the whole setting.

Note that 'observation' also includes, usually, talking to participants. 'Meanings' can only be elicited from asking people what acts or interactions mean to them. As well as people, the researcher observes space and material objects. How is the space of the clinic divided up, and how are these different spaces used? Who goes where, and when? Do people behave differently in different places, for instance taking off their uniforms when 'backstage' in the staff kitchen, or using formal titles to address each other when in public spaces?

Recording observations

Related to the issue of developing skills in observing is that of learning to record observations, and managing what can quickly become a large mass of data. The particular setting will determine to a large extent how observations are recorded, in terms of whether it is possible to make notes while observing (if on the less participant end of Gold's scale, or in an environment where writing notes will not seem 'odd') or whether the 'participant' role means that notes have to be written up at the end of each period of observation. But time to do this needs to be built into time in the field. One rule of thumb is to write up as soon as possible: at the end of the day, it is possible to remember most of the salient exchanges and decipher hurriedly scrawled notes; by the following day, these may be illegible and their salience forgotten. Tape recorders can be used to record opportunistic interviews, or a dictaphone to record observations for later transcription. It is good practice to keep separate empirical observational notes and your own initial interpretations, analytic comments and views, by using different notebooks, or colours. A fieldwork diary is essential for recording all aspects of the project, from early attempts to gain entry to the field and negotiations with gatekeepers to later reflections on the process.

Rapid ethnographic methods

As the examples so far in this chapter suggest, a key limitation of ethnographic work is that it is very time-consuming, taking many months for a researcher to gain access to a field, and to live or work there until their presence goes largely unnoticed. Agar reports that it usually takes about three months until he feels 'a functioning, accepted member of the community' (1980: 108). Meyer (1993) reports that her action research study of lay participation in care took six months to arrange access, one year of fieldwork and then six months of follow-up work, as she felt she could not withdraw from the field without consolidating the project. Turner's (1967) study of rituals in Ndembu society was based on two and a half years' fieldwork. This kind of extended study is typical of PhD studies in anthropology, but few researchers have the time to devote to such long-term participant observation later in a career. Additionally, few funding agencies are willing to take the risk of supporting a study that may have few clear aims at the beginning, and no guarantee of answering the research question first identified.

One attempt to preserve the advantages of observational work with feasibility in terms of resources is the development of so-called 'rapid' ethnographic methods, such as Rapid Rural Appraisal, Rapid Assessment Procedures and

Participatory Rural Appraisal (Rifkin 1996). These are controversial, with some claiming that brief incursions into a field are likely to collect superficial or even misleading information (Lambert 1998). Agar (1980), for instance, discusses his experience of carrying out a survey during the early stages of fieldwork in Pakistan. Only later in his research did he realize how unreliable the early data were. People had assumed he was either a spy or a government agent, and had under-reported both young males in the household and their land holdings. In their study of beliefs about leprosy among the Limba of Sierra Leone, Opala and Boillot (1996) also doubt that less intensive methods would have identified what the causes of leprosy were from the perspective of the Limba. Reporting how the Limba avoid discussing witchcraft openly, they note how in interviews respondents feign ignorance completely, or make oblique references that would only be recognized by other Limba. In interviews, early responses to questions about the causes of leprosy included 'God's will', insect vectors and infected water. Only careful questioning from an interviewer with a grasp of Limba world-views unearthed deeply held, but rarely voiced, beliefs that leprosy was caused by witchcraft or as retribution for the evil done by a family member. More importantly, from a public health perspective, the researchers found that although most Limba saw modern medicines as effective against leprosy, few saw the early signs (red patches on the skin) as signs of leprosy, but rather saw these as a different disease, with different causes, and thus delayed seeking treatment until late in the disease's progression. From a detailed anthropological understanding of Limba world-views, Opala and Boillot were able to work with health educators to shape public health messages about leprosy in ways that would mesh with the community's health beliefs. They suggest that programmes should employ a local anthropologist, even if they are not experts in medical anthropology, wherever possible to maximize the opportunities for an in-depth understanding of how ideas about health and illness are embedded in local world-views.

These examples suggest that rapid appraisal may do more harm than good, through identifying 'public' accounts of health beliefs that are given to strangers, rather than more deeply held beliefs that are more likely to impact on health behaviour. However, rapid methods have proved useful in informing many public health interventions, and when carried out with care can generate useful data to aid specific projects. Susan Rifkin (1996) points to the advantages: relatively quick and cheap data collection and data that are addressed to designing practical interventions rather than academic findings. She reviews the origins of Rapid Rural Appraisal in the field of agriculture and rural development as a method for improving on existing surveys and other fact-finding techniques that were inadequate for decision making. More recent approaches have incorporated a participatory element, with communities involved in the information collection and analysis. The resulting techniques of Rapid Participatory Appraisal have been widely used for health needs assessment both in developing and industrialized countries, and the World Health Organization publishes a guidebook on how to carry them out (Annett and Rifkin 1995).

Only data directly related to the project are collected, and the data collection methods come from a 'toolbox' of qualitative techniques, including interviews and various kinds of 'visualizations'. Visual representations are important not only when working in non-literate communities, but also because they are a good basis for discussion, and can generate information that does not come from an interview. Some of the data collection techniques in the 'toolbox' are illustrated in Box 6.2.

Care must be taken when choosing key informants to interview, to ensure that they can represent the interests of the whole community, and not just sectional interests. In the rapid appraisal approach, **triangulation** between these different sources of data aids validation.

The kind of data that this kind of 'rapid' ethnographic study produces, then, can, if done carefully, improve the effectiveness of public health interventions. Carl Kendall and colleagues discuss an attempt to widen access to oral rehydration therapy in Honduras through informing local people about the appropriate use of packets of oral rehydration salts (Kendall et al. 1984). Ethnographic studies suggested that one form of diarrhoea, called *empacho*, was seen as caused by eating the wrong kinds of foods, and treatable by massage and purgatives. However, this information was not taken up in the campaign to inform people about oral rehydration salts. The campaign did not mention *empacho*, because programme staff did not see it as a 'real' disease entity in the way biomedical classifications are, and because they were uncomfortable with the idea of oral rehydration salts being promoted as a 'purgative'. Ignoring this folk classification meant that in the evaluation of the project, although local residents reported higher knowledge of oral rehydration therapy, they were unlikely to have used it in cases diagnosed as *empacho*. However, it is not enough for ethnographic information to exist, it must also be seen as reliable and relevant information by programme planners. Rapid appraisal is thus best conducted within a multi-disciplinary programme setting in which the findings can contribute to interventions. Case Study 6.1 is an example, from a programme designed to reduce the morbidity from diarrhoeal disease.

Box 6.2   Examples of techniques from the Rapid Appraisal Toolbox

- Interviews with key informants such as: government officials, teachers, traditional healers, community leaders, shop owners.
- Visualization such as:

    o Seasonal calendars. Participants use illustrations to describe seasonal changes. These can be used to map disease prevalence, or household income, over different parts of the year.
    o Mapping. Local materials (sand, pebbles) can be used by participants to create spatial maps of the locality, with access to resources marked, or changes over time illustrated.

- Observations: of the physical environment, transport access, sanitation facilities, housing.
- Reports and other documents.

Sources: Rifkin (1996), Annett and Rifkin (1995).

Rapid appraisal methods, then, offer a way of utilizing the insights of medical anthropology without the cost of in-depth ethnographic fieldwork. To be effective, however, these methods need using with care, and ideally with the help of local people who are fully conversant with the beliefs of the community. Such techniques are only 'rapid' in contrast with traditional ethnography; they are not a 'quick and dirty' way of doing social research for health.

Case Study 6.1   Applied anthropology in a diarrhoeal disease control project

(Source: Scrimshaw, S. and Hurtado, E. (1988) 'Anthropological involvement in the Central American diarrheal disease control project', *Social Science and Medicine*, 27: 97–105)

Susan Scrimshaw and Elena Hurtado note the importance of a detailed understanding of local health beliefs, culture and language for effective health interventions. In introducing oral rehydration therapy (ORT), for instance, it is vital to know local terms for different kinds of diarrhoea in order to target health promotion effectively, and to understand local health beliefs about both the causes and potential cures. Anthropologists have a large role to play in planning health interventions, through presenting data on folk health beliefs to public health specialists. As a contribution to a programme on reducing the morbidity from diarrhoeal disease in Central America, they collated ethnographic information on 'ethno-classifications' of diarrhoea in four communities in Guatemala and Costa Rica. These proved to be complex. One taxonomy, from a highland community in Guatemala, included eight main kinds of diarrhoea, based on the primary cause: the mother, food, tooth eruption, fallen fontanelle or stomach, evil eye, stomach worms, cold or dysentery. These primary classifications were further subdivided. Different therapies were appropriate for different causes. Thus, if diarrhoea is caused by the mother being overheated (from pregnancy or being out on a hot day) and her milk being spoilt, the remedy would be to abstain from breastfeeding or weaning the baby. The only type of diarrhoea that was seen as appropriate to take to the clinic was that of dysentery, which was the most serious form and distinguished by blood in the stools. Others were seen as amenable to home cures (such as herbal teas, baths and massages) and various traditional healers. The ethnoclassifications of other communities differed in detail, but all included multiple types of diarrhoea with their own symptoms and preferred remedies. Explanations and therapies often combined biomedical and folk beliefs.

The implications for project planners are: that ORT has to be available widely in the community, through pharmacies and other stores, rather than only from the health clinic; that any information has to stress both the different kinds of diarrhoea in the local folk classifications and terminology; and that the need for rehydration in less serious categories of diarrhoea must be stressed. There is also scope for testing the effectiveness of home remedies identified, so that effective ones can be recommended.

To inform public health interventions, Scrimshaw and Hurtado recommend training project workers to carry out rapid ethnographic assessments in local communities to aid understanding of local health beliefs. They stress the need to present anthropological findings in ways that workers from other disciplines can understand. So rather than producing monographs using anthropological language, they summarize ethnoclassifications briefly as taxonomies, with diagrams if possible.

Non-participant observational methods

At the 'complete observer' end of Gold's continuum are those methods in which the researcher does not have to be present in the field, or at least does not participate in the field. They are, perhaps, more associated with quantitative techniques in health research, in which observations are used to count and analyse behavioural phenomena. One example is a study of adverse events in hospitals (Andrews et al. 1997), which used trained ethnographers to observe ward rounds and meetings to identify all discussions of adverse events. The researchers did not ask questions, but just observed and collected standardized data on each event. However, non-participant observation offers great potential for qualitative analysis as well. Naturally occurring data are perhaps underused in health research, but can often be gathered fairly quickly, and with less disruption for the working life of a clinic or hospital. Audio, or even video, tape recordings of professional–client consultations are a useful source for research questions on communication in health care settings. Again, they have often been used in a more quantitative way, for instance by looking for the number of questions asked by each participant, or the length of time spent on aspects of the consultation, but there is also the potential for ethnomethodological analysis.

Developed by the sociologist Harold Garfinkel (1967), 'ethnomethodology' means 'folk methods' and refers to the rules and processes by which people give meaning to behaviour and interpret social interaction. Garfinkel's focus was on the micro-level of social life: how interaction gets accomplished, and what potentially disrupts it. Although this branch of sociology has been criticized for being overly concerned with the minutiae of interpersonal communication, rather than broader questions of social structure, it clearly has a valuable contribution to our understanding of health care, where interpersonal communication is a key element. Of particular interest in areas of health care such as primary care and counselling, one aspect of communication is how well professionals allow patients or clients to 'tell their story', both to allow access to diagnostic information and as a therapeutic device in itself (see Greenhalgh and Hurwitz 1998, for example, on the renewed interest in narratives in medicine). The research described in Case Study 6.2 takes an ethnomethodological approach to look at how storytelling does or does not get accomplished in clinical settings.

Detailed analysis of naturally occurring talk from settings such as hospital clinics provides a useful source of research on how health care communication happens in practice, as opposed to participants' accounts of it. Like other observational methods, the key strength is that it utilizes data about 'real' behaviour. Following Harvey Sacks (1989), David Silverman (1993: 51–5) argues that an ethnomethodological approach has advantages over other ethnographic approaches, as well as over interview data, potentially addressing methodological shortcomings such as the tendency to generalize from small extracts from a data set. The methodological advantages arise from a focus on empirical, observable detail (using, for instance, reproducible data from transcripts of naturally occurring talk, which can be studied by a number of analysts) and the 'topicalization' of common sense. The 'topicalization' of common sense means that the kinds of resources individuals in any setting draw on to make sense of their world (and that we, as researchers, use to make sense of what we see in that world) are subject to analysis to see exactly how these understandings are accomplished, through focusing on what can be observed, rather than making assumptions about how categories or concepts are utilized and what they mean.

Case Study 6.2   Non-participant observation: using video-tapes to examine storytelling in consultations

(Source: Clark, J. and Mishler, E. (1992) 'Attending to patients' stories: reframing the clinical task', *Sociology of Health and Illness*, 14: 344–72)

Patients' stories are an important topic in research in physician–patient communication. Jack Clark and Elliott Mishler are interested in how storytelling does or doesn't happen in a clinical encounter: what interactional skills are needed by the physician, and how does a story get 'accomplished' in a particular encounter? The study uses data from video-tapes that are routinely taken for evaluation and training purposes in an out-patient clinic of a large teaching hospital in the United States. The clinic encourages patient-centred consultations. Two tapes were chosen for analysis: one that clinic staff thought exemplified a patient-centred consultation, and one that didn't. The video-tapes were transcribed in detail, with intonation, pauses and interruptions all transcribed. The two transcripts were then compared to identify the differences between them in terms of interaction. Although both patients had chronic illnesses and were from similar social backgrounds, and both clinicians had similar training, analysis revealed differences in how the initial problem is presented, how symptoms are determined and how therapeutic decisions are discussed.

In the first transcript, a man with epilepsy succeeds in 'telling his story': presenting a seizure he experienced in the context of his work as a car mechanic. His story 'embeds an illness event in the context of his lifeworld, combining personal knowledge, identity claims and relevant features of the everyday working life in which his illness is experienced' (p. 350). While gathering the clinical details needed for the consultation, the physician collaborates in the storytelling by reiterating key points, pausing for continuation and acknowledging the relevant facts of the story. In contrast, the patient in the second video, a woman with diabetes, does not manage to 'tell her story', but instead presents a list of disconnected symptoms as the clinician shifts the focus throughout her account to prompt for 'relevant' details, and ignores the context of her story. Her attempts to maintain the narrative are interrupted, and the physician misses the point she makes about her concerns. These differences in style continue through to the end stages of the consultation. In the first case, the physician collaborates with the man with epilepsy to request a blood sample (saying 'If it's okay with you I would like to have a blood test taken today. Is that all right?'). In the second, the physician announces his intention to do tests: 'We ought to check your sugar in the lab since you're here.' For Clark and Mishler, the importance of being able to 'tell a story' within a consultation relates to the need for patients to make sense of the physiological aspects of their illness in terms of its impact on the social fabric of their lives. Chronic illness, in particular, requires managing complicated treatment regimes while maintaining personal control. A consultation in which what the authors call 'the voice of the lifeworld' is heard is likely to lead not only to better patient satisfaction, but also to better control of illness for patients.

From analysing transcripts of consultations, Clark and Mishler are able to identify different ways in which patients and physicians actually accomplish clinical work. A detailed look at how the clinical tasks of diagnosis, ordering tests and deciding on treatment are managed in practice allows them to focus on the skills of physicians, and the ways in which consultations can be carried out in a more 'patient-centred' way.

Thus, if studying, say, 'how doctors break bad news in a consultation', the researcher does not trawl the transcripts looking for examples of 'bad news' from a predetermined definition of what this would look like, or ask participants what they think about how 'bad news' is broken. Rather, detailed transcriptions are analysed to look for how both parties achieve the communication of news in the setting. How do patients register particular utterances as 'bad' or 'good'? How do the participants in the consultation use talk to achieve shared understanding of the meaning of a particular utterance? Geraldine Leydon (Leydon and Green 2001) used this approach to analyse how information was shared between cancer patients and their doctors in hospital out-patient clinics. By looking in detail at transcripts of consultations, she demonstrated how doctors skilfully lead up to 'breaking bad news' by first establishing what patients already know about their diagnosis, and by pairing 'good news/bad news' statements such as 'we completely removed the tumour [good] but found cancer cells in the lymph nodes [bad]'. Using conversation analysis, Leydon was able to focus in detail on what actually went on in the consultation, rather than relying on either patients' or doctors' accounts of information exchange.

Detailed analysis of naturally occurring data has been used productively in a number of health settings, largely in industrialized countries. Examples include:

- Douglas Maynard's (1991) study of consultations in paediatric clinics, which identified how doctors break bad news through careful monitoring of the parents' perspectives and knowledge first.
- Anssi Peräkylä and David Silverman (1991) looked at the organization of talk within HIV counselling interviews, examining the ways in which counsellors covered delicate topics, and used particular communication formats to achieve tasks such as delivering information about safer sex, advising the client and gaining consent for a test.
- Derrol Palmer (2000) analysed recorded interviews between hospital patients and clinicians to identify how 'delusional' talk was recognized in practice by professionals.

Conclusion

Qualitative observational methods include, then, traditional ethnographic approaches associated with anthropology, more recent developments of 'rapid' ethnographic methods, and detailed non-participant observational work on naturally occurring talk or behaviour. In health research, there has often been an assumption that observational data are 'better' and more valid than those produced by other methods (such as interviews, or official statistics). Although observational designs do have undoubted methodological strengths, they are not appropriate for all research questions, and may not be feasible for many research questions. However, some observational work is essential in most qualitative studies, even if only as 'background' to a particular research topic, or as a way of assessing the feasibility of other designs in the study context. Brief periods of observational work (for instance, shadowing members of staff for a shift, or sitting in a clinic reception area) can be very productive for sensitizing researchers to issues to ask about in interviews, or for learning about the constraints faced by research participants. The methods used by ethnographers have, for this reason, been adopted in a range of qualitative health studies, and most research designs will benefit from some observational work.

Research designs that draw extensively on observation data are required for some research questions. If the concern is with the detailed analysis of particular settings in which transcriptions of talk are possible, then conversation analysis has been suggested as a reliable and valid method for studying how people actually interact in health care settings, rather than what they say they do. If the aim of the research is to really understand 'what is going on' in a particular setting in a holistic way, a long-term participant observation study, in which the researcher integrates both emic and etic perspectives, is the design of choice.

KEY POINTS

- The major strength of observational methods is that they provide data on what people do, as well as what they say they do.
- In ethnography, long-term participation in the field enables the researcher to capitalize on both distance and familiarity to analyse social behaviour.
- Doing ethnography in familiar sites has benefits in terms of access and familiarity, but poses challenges for the researcher in achieving analytic distance.
- Rapid ethnographic techniques have been widely used in public health research, with some success, although there has been debate about the validity of data generated.
- Non-participant observational methods provide access to social interaction with minimal intervention in the field and are one way of producing empirical and reliable data for analysis.

EXERCISES

1 Jocelyn Lawler argues that her 'insider' status was an advantage when researching nursing work. Consider a setting with which you are familiar (such as a workplace, neighbourhood, college). List the practical and methodological advantages and disadvantages of you carrying out an ethnography of this setting.

2 Carry out an observation of a public setting (such as a fast food restaurant or train station). Make notes on how different people in that setting behave, using the headings in Box 6.1 as a guide. You could consider: who uses the facility, how do they interact and with whom, how do they use space? Compare your observations with those of colleagues or classmates.

FURTHER READING

Agar, M.H. (1996) *The professional stranger: an informal introduction to ethnography* (2nd edn). San Diego, CA: Academic Press. This is a readable account of the practical and methodological issues raised by doing traditional fieldwork.

Hammersley, M. (1992) *What's wrong with ethnography?* London: Routledge. A more theoretical discussion of the methodological assumptions of 'ethnography', in which Hammersley argues that it is not a separate methodology. Covers issues such as generalizability, realism and theory in ethnographic work.

Hammersley, M. and Atkinson, P. (2007) *Ethnography: principles in practice* (3rd edn). London: Routledge. A thorough discussion of all the stages of planning and conducting an ethnographic study, from sampling cases though to fieldwork roles, analysis and writing up.

7 Using Documentary Sources

CHAPTER SUMMARY

It is not always necessary to collect new primary data for research, and using existing documents can be an efficient use of resources for many qualitative questions. Potential documentary sources include public records, private documents, research publications, archived research data and mass media sources. These sources are increasingly available electronically. There is a growth in interest in the secondary analysis of qualitative research outputs through systematic reviews for informing health policy and practice. Like data produced by the researcher, documentary data can be analysed from a number of qualitative perspectives.

Introduction

We use the term 'documents' here to refer widely to the whole range of written sources that might be available relating to a topic, and by extension other artefacts that can be treated as documents, such as photographs or video recordings.

This is, of course, a rather disparate set of potential data sources. Those that have been used in qualitative health research studies include (among many others) newspapers, government reports, personal and work diaries, letters, research articles, primary data from other projects, job descriptions, organizational charts, manuals, medical records, films, photographs and medical instruments. Given both the range of documents that researchers could access, and the disparate perspectives that researchers bring to them, it would be impossible to deal comprehensively with the practical and methodological problems raised by 'documentary research' as if it were a particular research strategy. Here, we address the possibilities of using existing documents instead of generating new primary data, and highlight how some of the most accessible sources of documents can be used for health research questions.

Why use existing sources?

All research of course relies on some analysis of documentary sources. At a minimum we have to review the existing research outputs in the relevant area, and perhaps draw on policy reports to make a case for the timeliness or policy relevance of our own research. Most qualitative projects also draw on a variety of documents in the field for background context on the setting, population or health problem addressed in the research. Case studies and ethnographic research will often draw widely on a variety of documentary sources in addition to data from interviews and observations, including perhaps reports from the organizations studied, diaries of research participants, or material artefacts used and produced in the setting. For some research projects this will be 'background' information, used only to orientate the researcher in refining the research question and design. In other studies, these documents and artefacts will be part of the corpus of data that will be analysed to answer the research question. Many research questions can be addressed by exclusively using existing sources of data, rather than by producing new data. There are a number of advantages in relying on available documents as the primary data source for research.

A first incentive for using documentary sources is their abundance and availability. Modern societies produce vast amounts of data, from official statistics such as censuses and surveys, birth, marriage and death certificates, to private records such as diaries, photographs and personal archives. In most countries, government departments and agencies devote considerable resources to collecting data about the population, and have the advantage of far greater resources than the academic researcher can ever muster. In addition to this 'official' record of our lives, many of us also produce throughout our lifetimes informal 'private archives' – data sources that ordinarily remain in the household, including photograph albums, letters and, more recently, videos, email correspondence and website postings. These diverse sources are sometimes divided into *records*, which are produced to provide evidence of some transaction or event (such as marriage, or a hospital visit), and *documents*, which refers to those produced for personal rather than official purposes.

Another existing data source comes from previous research studies. Increasingly, qualitative data generated as primary data for one study are being archived for use by other researchers (Backhouse 2002). Secondary research outputs (the research reports and published articles) are also now increasingly easy to identify and access through bibliographic databases which collate information about peer-reviewed articles. These include:

Medline Produced by the US National Library of Medicine, this contains records from 1950 onwards of articles from journals in medicine, dentistry, nursing and disciplines related to health care.

Web of Science This includes three databases, Science Citation Index, the Social Sciences Citation Index and the Arts and Humanities Citation Index.

Cinahl This covers bibliographic information from the nursing and allied literature, from 1982, and full texts from selected journals.

Qualitative research output published in journals is now identifiable on these and similar databases, although fewer databases cover books and book chapters. Given the sheer volume of potential sources of data already in existence, researchers perhaps have to consider whether their study really justifies adding to this by producing yet more primary data.

A second reason to use documents is of course that for some research problems, documents will be the only source of data. For historical research, there may be no living people to interview, and we are reliant on witness accounts recorded at the time, and other contemporaneous records. In a study of nursing in Uganda, Pat Holden (1991), for instance, wanted to understand contemporary tensions in a Kampala hospital, in which working conditions and salaries for nurses were very poor, but in which nurses still turned up for work, often in 'beautifully laundered uniforms', despite water shortages and few obvious incentives. To explore the current situation, she traces the development of nursing during the colonial period, which she argues has left a legacy of nursing ideology that may be inadequate for the crisis conditions now faced by nurses in Uganda. In her research, Holden draws largely on documentary data, including the papers of the Overseas Nursing Association and reminiscences collected by another researcher as part of a project on public health services in Africa, as well as contemporary ethnographic data. Documents provide the data for exploring the history of nursing in Africa and the concerns of the nursing profession in the early part of the twentieth century.

Third, there are some not insignificant practical advantages in using documents to address research questions when possible. One relates to the preferences of the researcher. Some researchers may be far more comfortable with documents than people: not everyone has the aptitude or desire to develop the interactive skills needed for qualitative fieldwork or interviewing. Finally, projects based solely on publicly available sources may be less resource intensive. Costs of retrieving existing data will be lower than those of producing new data, and documentary studies, if using data in the public domain, are unlikely to require ethical approval to conduct.

This chapter discusses potential documentary sources for research under five broad headings: public records, personal documents, mass media outputs, research outputs and **systematic reviews.** Each of these can be utilized for health research studies from a number of theoretical perspectives, from positivist studies using research reports as data for an extended literature review to social constructionist studies using **discourse analysis** to analyse documents as texts. The type of document (whether mortality reports from the World Health Organization, or newspaper articles, or diaries) does not imply a particular methodological approach: like any other data source, the use to which they are put depends on the research question and the orientation of the researcher. The approaches given as examples under the headings of public records, personal documents, mass media outputs and research outputs are not, then, the only approaches that can be used with these types of data, but are intended as illustrations of the potential for using documents for health research.

Public records

Public records, or official statistics, are produced by international organizations (such as the World Health Organization and the World Bank), national governments and other national agencies, and local statutory organizations such as health authorities. These data provide a rich source for quantitative secondary analysis (see Hakim 1982 for a discussion), and of course are often the source of new research questions, both qualitative and quantitative. Most qualitative studies will make use of these public records in some way, even if only in the literature review as part of the 'evidence' for the usefulness of the study proposed, or to document the characteristics of the population of interest. However, there are also a number of ways in which public records can be used as the primary data for qualitative research, as the topic for analysis. Indeed, official reports based on official statistics offer a rich seam for qualitative analysis. Social constructionists have inevitably made most use of these sources, as they provide an important longitudinal record of 'official' classifications of the social world, including that of health and medicine. What is of interest here is not the numbers reported (how many people died of cancer in this or that year, how many births this or that region had), but how they are categorized: how disease categories change over time, or what kind of illness episodes are officially reported. A social constructionist analysis of published data sets can address questions about what organizations consider it important to record at particular points in time, how this changes over time and space, and how the classification systems have changed. Case Study 7.1 is an example of this approach.

This kind of analysis has been a fruitful one for medical sociology, with a number of studies drawing on official statistics and reports to uncover the social construction of classification systems; see, for instance, Green's (1999) work on how the prevention of accidental injury has been constructed in public health discourse, or Sarah Nettleton's (1992) work on how the mouth has come to be stabilized and understood through the practice of modern dentistry. More recently, there has been an interest in including artefacts as well as written documents in these analyses, and focusing on technologies of classification (computer programs, statistical tests) as well as the texts (such as the International Classification of Diseases, or public health reports) that result from classificatory activity. One example is from Geoffrey Bowker and Susan Star, who aimed to explore 'the creation and maintenance of complex classifications as a kind of work practice, with its attendant financial, skill and moral elements' (1999: 5). Looking in detail at the tenth revision of the International Classification of Diseases (ICD), which is the internationally used tool for classifying diseases for epidemiological work, they show how it is a pragmatic system, which has embedded in it a host of social factors. For instance, in looking at the detailed breakdown of categories for accidents there are a wide range of choices for various falls (from a cliff, from a wheelchair, from bed, from a commode, and so on) but very few for differentiating the kinds of accidents likely to happen in less industrialized areas of the world. Similarly, deaths from snake or spider bites can only be differentiated as those from venomous or non-venomous species. As Bowker and Star note:

> The ICD is richest in its description of ways of dying in developed countries at this moment in history: it is not that other accidents and diseases cannot be described, but they cannot be described in as much detail. ... So the ICD bears traces of its historical situation as a tool used by public health officials in developed countries. (Bowker and Star 1999: 76)

Case Study 7.1   The social construction of Sudden Infant Death Syndrome

(Source: Armstrong, D. (1986) 'The invention of infant mortality', *Sociology of Health and Illness*, 8: 211–32)

David Armstrong's (1986) exploration of the emergence of Sudden Infant Death Syndrome in Britain in the twentieth century is an example of the use of official statistics to answer a research question about the social construction of the categories we use routinely in epidemiology. Tracing the ways in which deaths of infants were classified, reported and analysed in official reports, such as those of the Registrar General, Armstrong noted that infant mortality rates were only reported from 1877 onwards. The statistical technology needed to calculate a mortality rate existed before then, but only

(Continued)

once infants had been recognized as a socially significant category
was a rate for their deaths reported. This illustrates well the kinds
of questions a social constructivist asks of the data: not 'How did the
rate of infant death change over the nineteenth century?' but rather
'When, and why, did it become possible to report on deaths of
infants in this way?'

In the early twentieth century, the 'problem' of infant deaths,
Armstrong argues, moves from being a biological one to a social
one with a growing interest in the use of infant mortality as an indicator of the health of communities. It continues, of course, to be
used in this way, particularly in international comparisons. The
period of infancy became demarcated, with the gradual establishment of 'neonatal' to mean the first four weeks of life, and later a
concentration on the first week of the neonatal period. There was
nothing inevitable about this: at various points in the nineteenth
century, periods of two months and three months were used. Like
other categories, they appear 'obvious' ones that we may be accus-
tomed to using, but an analysis of their emergence unpacks their
social construction.

For Armstrong, these historical shifts observable in public
records are not necessarily evidence of the development of medical understanding of infant deaths or the inevitable outcome of
epidemiological analysis of those deaths. Instead, the records
and documents also create an object (in this case, the infant)
and can be analysed to demonstrate how that object is constructed. He argued that 'analysis and object are mutually con-
stitutive: that the infant is as much a product of the analysis as
the analysis is a reflection of the infant' (Armstrong 1986: 227).
In terms of the debates we reviewed in Chapter 1 about the epistemological underpinnings of qualitative research, Armstrong is
explicitly placing himself in the social constructionist camp, and
rejecting the realist position that 'infants' have a pre-existing
stable reality.

Public records, then, as well as providing essential information from a positivist perspective, are also a rich source of data for those interested in
exploring the ways in which the categories used in health and medicine are
constructed. At a minimum, these kinds of studies remind health
researchers that the taken-for-granted categories used in epidemiological
research are socially constituted, rather than inevitable or natural ways of
dividing up the world. Beyond that, qualitative analysis of official statistics
can explore how political and social factors (such as the development of
ICD to meet the public health needs of developed countries) shape the kinds
of data that are collected and reported.

Personal documents

Historians have perhaps made the most use of personal documents, as resources such as diaries and letters are often the only available source of data to shed light on lived experience in anything other than the most recent history. However, personal documents are also a useful source of data for any project that addresses, or aims to include, a biographical perspective. Norman Denzin (1989a) argues that the biographical method (using autobiographical and biographical sources) has been seen in the social sciences as a way of incorporating the subjective experiences of individuals, and how they give meaning to their lives. He cautions against any simplistic notion that diaries and other autobiographical sources are in any way reflections of a 'real' self, as of course all biographies (even the most personal diary) are produced as stylized narratives, written for particular audiences using conventional structures. They are, he argues, essentially literary constructions, and must be analysed as such, with due regard to the symbolic use of language, the social functions the writing performed, and the acceptance that biographies represent partial identities and lives, not the whole truth about such lives.

Some classic studies widely cited in qualitative health research have drawn extensively on documentary sources. Erving Goffman's essay on *Stigma* (1963), for instance, used a range of sources such as autobiographies, published diaries, examples from published studies and fiction to develop a sociological understanding of 'stigma' and its impacts on everyday social interaction. Goffman was interested in how discrediting attributes (such as disability, physical marks, or particular ethnic identities) disrupt the taken-for-granted aspects of interaction, and lead to damaged self-identities for those stigmatized. Given the wealth of existing sources of data, Goffman had no need to interview people, or undertake any extended observations to meet his aims, which were to 'review some work on stigma ... to see what it can yield for sociology' (1963: 9).

More recently, personal documents available on the internet have provided a rich source of data for studies on health. As access to the internet grows, websites are becoming a significant source of health advice for many lay users, and online communities have emerged for many patient groups, health professionals and interest groups. The comments and stories posted on the message boards or discussion spaces on these sites are a potential source of data on how health and illness are being constructed in what, for many people, have become a key domain of everyday life. Although these sources are relatively accessible to any researcher with internet access, their use does raise some ethical and methodological problems. Even if posted on a 'public' space, comments on websites are not usually made with the intention that they will be analysed as research data. If registration to use a website is required, the researcher then has to consider the ethical dilemmas of appropriate disclosure, just as in any other kind of ethnographic study (see Chapter 6) such as how their presence, if announced, is likely to change the style and content of contributions, and what responsibilities they have to disclosure of personal information about themselves.

Internet sources of personal documents have proved particularly useful for studies addressing marginal or stigmatised groups, who may have few other opportunities to express their views in public. One example is an ethnographic study of a website created by young women with anorexia (Fox et al. 2005). The website explicitly described itself as 'pro-ana'. Rather than helping each other 'cure' anorexia, subscribers were committed to being anorexic, and the site contained advice on keeping healthy while resisting the dominant discourse of 'recovery'. The researcher subscribed to the site, explaining her research interest, and after a period of 'lurking' without participating in the forum, then used the message board to prompt discussion. The study was, then, a mix of using existing personal documents and generated data. In a similar vein, Anu Katainen (2006) analysed discussion threads from the website of a Finnish tabloid newspaper to explore how smokers in Finland justify their behaviour, given the problemalization of smoking and abundance of health promotion on its negative effects. Like young women resisting a biomedical model of anorexia, smokers could be seen as a stigmatized group, and websites may be the most accessible source of data on marginal or private discourses.

Mass media outputs

Media outputs such as newspaper reports, television programmes and film provide an accessible source of data for many health research questions. Contemporary sources are easily collated or observed, and in many countries there are good newspaper and film archives. As with personal documents, these archives are increasingly available via the internet. Like public records and personal documents, media outputs can be used to address questions about the social construction and representations of health and illness.

On the social construction of health topics, one example is Elina Oinas's (1998) work on menstruation, which used data from the medical advisory columns of ten Finnish magazines. She identified all the letters published in these columns, with the doctors' answers, that related to menstruation to explore how the issue of menstruation is medicalized. For this kind of topic, these kinds of documentary sources are an interesting data set – Oinas suggests that medical columns are one of the few public arenas in which menstruation is discussed. From her analysis of the letters and answers, she identifies the key concerns of (largely) young women: normality and dealing with the etiquette of menstruating. Through the letters and answers, Oinas suggests that the women writers and medical professionals construct a 'proper' role for medicine as the arbiter of normality, and the need for medical expertise to determine the nature of the body and to be responsible for its functioning.

A second perspective in studies of mass media output is analyses of how health issues are represented in the media. Given the importance of the media as an influence on public perceptions of health and illness, exploring these public images of health issues can shed light on how they are framed and what messages (intended and unintended) they convey. Often, studies of media representations combine quantitative and qualitative methods of analysis. A study by Lesley Henderson and colleagues (Henderson et al. 2000) of how infant feeding was represented in the British media, for instance, used quantitative content analysis of newspaper and television coverage to identify how often references were made to breast and bottle feeding and whether any problems were associated with the method. They found that breast feeding was rarely shown, and when it was it was often depicted as problematic. Newspaper coverage often commented on potential problems with breast feeding, but rarely on its health benefits. Combined with this was a qualitative analysis of the contexts in which images of infant feeding occurred. This suggested that breast feeding was commonly associated with humorous story-lines in fictional television programmes, and with middle-class or celebrity women. In contrast, bottle feeding was presented as largely invisible and associated with 'normal' families. Here, documentary sources (national newspapers, a sample of television programmes) enabled the researchers to explore media representations of an important health issue in the UK, which has one of the lowest rates of breast feeding in Europe. Analysing representations suggested some influences on this health behaviour, in that breast feeding is portrayed as problematic and likely to fail whereas bottle feeding is represented as the normal and obvious choice.

Research outputs

In many ways, existing research outputs, whether primary data collected by other researchers or secondary sources (such as research reports and peer-reviewed journal articles), are the ideal source of data for projects when resources are limited. Primary data (typically, interview transcripts or diaries collected in the course of previous research) can be analysed to address new research questions, or re-analysed from new perspectives. Analysis of secondary sources is an efficient strategy for topics on which there has already been considerable previous research, as much can be gleaned by synthesizing existing research evidence. With the growth in interest in evidence-based medicine and policy, there has been an increasing demand for these syntheses of existing research knowledge, and we discuss this in a separate section on systematic reviews.

Using existing primary data

The efficiency gains of re-analysis of primary data such as interview transcripts from other studies may be particularly important for small student projects where there is limited time or resources for new data collection. However, there has been encouragement for all researchers to consider this as a good strategy for exploiting previous research activity to the full. Increasingly, qualitative researchers are archiving their data for future re-analysis. In the UK, the Economic and Social Research Council requires all grant holders to archive their data if possible and funds a service (called Qualidata) for encouraging the archiving, dissemination and re-use of data, based at the University of Essex (www.qualidata.essex.ac.uk). These archives require data to be anonymized, and any identifying details to be removed.

Networks of supervisors and colleagues are another good source of readily available data. Most researchers feel that they have never exploited their own data fully, and may be happy for someone else to explore different themes in their data, or use it to address a new research question. The ethical implications of re-analysis for a different purpose need to be considered, particularly if consent was only sought from participants for one particular study.

Some data sources are specifically designed to be repeatedly 'mined' for further projects. One example is the British Mass-Observation Archive. This was originally commissioned in the 1930s as a project to gather everyday accounts of social life in Britain from volunteer observers. A new panel of observers was recruited in the 1980s, who were asked to write about aspects of their lives in response to 'directives' suggesting particular topics. Their accounts are anonymized, so that they can be archived for future research. Helen Busby (2000) argues that these autobiographical sources of data offer potentially rich and fruitful insights into health and illness topics, particularly when the researcher is interested in subjective accounts of the interrelationships of health and other aspects of everyday life. Using the replies to a series of directives on topics such as staying well, the pace of life and doing a job, Busby is able to follow the case studies of individuals and explore how work, family and leisure have an impact on their health, and how moral discourses of 'keeping going' are used to describe poor health that does not necessitate time off work. These archives provide, then, invaluable resources for future researchers, and there is a growing movement in many countries to ensure that newly generated and existing primary data are being archived in searchable ways for future researchers (Corti and Thompson 2004).

Secondary analysis of research reports

Even more readily available are secondary sources, particularly published articles. These can be a rich source of material for studies using *discourse analysis*. The term 'discourse analysis' is utilized in a number of ways across the qualitative research literature (Potter and Wetherell 1987), but here we are using it to refer to those analyses of texts (including spoken language or artefacts that can be analytically treated as texts) orientated towards broad-ranging ideological explorations of how particular texts achieve their effects. The aim is to reveal how language (and indeed any other sign system, such as the uniforms of staff or the architecture of a hospital) does its work, in conveying not just the superficial meaning, but also the less obvious social meanings.

One example is from Patricia Kaufert (1988), who was interested in how the menopause is constructed through medical research. She looked at research reports on the topic of menopause not to review the findings, but to explore how these texts did their work of creating the discrete medical category of 'menopause'. Her data set includes a 1985 review of current research, aimed at informing gynaecologists and general practitioners about the state of medical knowledge, published by two leading researchers in the field, plus the 122 original research publications included in their review. For each publication

Kaufert classified the kind of study, how 'menopause' was defined, and the characteristics and size of the study population. There were three main categories of paper: epidemiological studies, clinical research and clinical case studies. She then analysed how the reviewers used these different materials in constructing their analysis. This included examining which sources were and were not used at various points, how they contributed to the overall argument of the review, and how important information in the original papers (such as the inclusion of 'artificially menopausal women' in the study population) was often missing from the review. A key element not in evidence was any sense of women's own voices – the review included nothing on how women talked about experiencing the menopause. The research papers reviewed also had limited data on non-Caucasian populations, although patterns were reported as though universal. Kaufert's study is a good example of how this kind of secondary analysis can reveal the ways in which medical knowledge is produced, and how the 'facts' produced through specific methodological processes then come to have a life of their own as 'knowledge'.

Qualitative secondary analysis of research reports does not have to be in this social constructionist tradition. In Case Study 7.2, the data used for secondary analysis are also research reports, but they have been used in a rather more positivist way, to shed light on a health problem, that of post-partum depression in the USA (Stern and Kruckman 1983). The authors do not have a primary aim of exploring the *production* of these anthropological studies, or analysing them as texts, although they do of course take into account how they were produced, in pointing to the limitations of taking data collected for one purpose to address a new question. Rather, they are reviewing the findings reported to extend our understanding of post-partum depression.

Case Study 7.2   Using ethnographic studies to shed light on post-partum depression

(Source: Stern, G. and Kruckman, L. (1983) 'Multi-disciplinary perspectives on post-partum depression: an anthropological critique', *Social Science and Medicine*, 17: 1027–41)

Gwen Stern and Laurence Kruckman are interested in a common syndrome in the United States, that of 'post-partum depression'. This mild and transient form of depression in mothers after the birth of a baby is very common, affecting 60–80 per cent of new mothers in Western countries, and is characterized by feelings of sadness, weeping, irritability and fatigue. Stern and Kruckman note that most research on this syndrome has focused on biological and psychosocial correlates and that there has been little attention to possible cultural factors such as the structure of the family or the role

(Continued)

expectations of the new mother. To explore the issue of cultural factors, they reviewed the ethnographic literature on childbirth. They
found very little evidence of similar 'illnesses' affecting new mothers
in non-Western settings. Studies from settings as diverse as Nepal,
China, Nigeria and south-east Asia identified post-partum depression
as a rare or absent disorder, although childbirth is recognized in most
cultures as a significant life event.

They suggest that post-partum depression could be described as a
culture-bound syndrome – an illness that takes a particular form in
particular social settings. Turning to why it may be that so many
women in the USA suffer from the disorder, Stern and Kruckman
draw on ethnographic descriptions of other culture-bound illnesses to
suggest a relationship between perceptions of 'role helplessness' and
mental illness. Specifically, they propose a relationship between the
strategies available within a culture to support the new mother and
her mental health. Compared with what is known from ethnographic
studies of other settings, mothers in the United States face a relative
lack of social structuring of the post-partum period, little recognition
of their role transition and little practical help. In many cultures, the
post-partum period is typically a time of rest and vulnerability, in
which the mother has to be protected and often secluded. This seclu-
sion and rest is often facilitated by practical help from female kin in
carrying out the mother's normal duties such as cooking, helping out
with the household and looking after other children. Alongside the
practical help, many cultural traditions entail emotional support for
the mother. These might include washing her body or hair or the
giving of gifts, ceremonial foods or massage. These traditional
rituals mark the transition to a new role and act as a focus for social
support for the new mother.

Using published ethnographic studies, then, Stern and Kruckman
are able to demonstrate that post-partum depression is not a universal phenomenon. They are also able to suggest some cultural factors that may make women in Western countries particularly
vulnerable by pointing to the range of traditional practices that protect the new mother in many non-Western societies. However, they
also note some limitations in this approach. First, childbirth has only
recently come to the attention of anthropology, so many ethnographies have little information on post-partum practices. Of those that
do, few studies used formal diagnostic testing. Given the ambiguity
over definitions of post-partum depression, this would also be difficult to do cross-culturally, given that the behavioural indicators,
such as weeping, may well be culturally specific. They cannot, then,
use these secondary sources to 'prove' their hypothesis about the
cultural aetiology of post-partum depression in the USA, but can
suggest some very fruitful avenues for investigating the role of
social support to new mothers.

Systematic reviews

In health care, the idea of a *systematic review* of the literature as a way of synthesizing the findings from quantitative (especially RCT) studies has become
popular recently, as an element of the move towards evidence-based medicine
and health care (Petticrew 2001). Although originally a method to increase
our faith in the findings of quantitative evaluations of health care interventions, there is increasing interest in using systematic methods of review with
qualitative studies to inform health policy and practice. A systematic review
differs from a traditional 'narrative' review of the literature in that it utilizes
an explicit and pre-determined methodology, which allows the review to be
replicated and updated. Although there are a number of available methodologies for systematic reviews, they share these features:

- they are designed to address a specific empirical research question
- they have clear and predetermined strategies for searching for the literature
- studies identified in the review are included or excluded according to defined
  criteria
- within these inclusion and exclusion criteria, there is an attempt to be
  comprehensive.

The strategies for searching typically include a list of electronic databases
which contain abstracts of published literature, the search terms used, and the
limiters (such as language of publication, and publication date). Given that
qualitative research may not be abstracted in these databases in ways that are
easy to search for, additional hand searches of the most relevant journals are
also done. Reports of research in books or in grey literature may be more difficult to identify, but these outputs are also increasingly being indexed electronically. On the kinds of diffuse topics that are often the subject of
qualitative systematic reviews, the literature can be spread over a number of
disciplines, and may be particularly difficult to identify. For this reason, many
systematic reviews of qualitative research use a multidiscplinary team of
researchers to conduct the review, in order to maximize the comprehensiveness of what is included, as well as the depth of synthesis of the included outputs. Systematic reviews usually also include an appraisal of the quality of
the studies, using a standardized checklist of criteria (see Chapter 11), and an
attempt to synthesize the findings from the methodologically sound studies in
the review. Many of the published qualitative systematic reviews to date
address questions such as lay health beliefs, illness experiences and barriers to
health care. Examples include:

- A systematic review of parental beliefs as barriers to childhood vaccination, which identified 15 studies using semi-structured interviews or focus
  groups. Using content analysis of the reported findings, the authors identified themes common to most studies, including concerns about the risk
  of adverse effects; a lack of trust; a belief that vaccinations are not necessary and barriers related to access (Mills et al. 2005).

• A synthesis of studies of the subjective experience of living with fibromyalgia syndrome identified 23 studies, using a range of different data generation methods. Four key substantive themes across the studies were: the experience of illness; the search for diagnosis; coping; and legitimacy. In the analysis, the authors conceptually linked these themes, with the central experience of pain as ambiguous and invisible raising questions about the legitimacy of the illness (Sim and Madden 2008).

The strengths of systematic reviews of qualitative evidence lie first in their potential to increase the generalizability of qualitative findings. By including studies from a range of settings and populations the researcher can identify common themes across settings, and therefore strengthen the credibility of findings. Discussing a review of evidence on medicine taking, for instance, Pandora Pound and colleagues (Pound et al. 2005) note that there are widespread concerns about the safety of medicines. Such findings, they suggest, are easily dismissed in single studies as insufficient evidence of patient concern, but become more convincing if found across the majority of studies. There is also the possibility of examining the impact of method on data generation. In the study of parental beliefs and childhood vaccination referred to above (Mills et al. 2000), for instance, the authors note that the focus group studies generated more issues related to access barriers than did those using semi-structured interviews.

Synthesizing studies

The description above suggests a rather empirical view of reviews, where the emphasis is on 'findings', as if they could be aggregated in similar ways to the quantitative findings from RCTs. To go beyond these rather positivist notions inherent in the process of simply 'adding together' empirical findings, a more analytical synthesis of the studies included can be done. In their study of fibromyalgia syndrome, Sim and Madden (2008) aggregated the empirical findings from the studies they had included into broader themes, informed by sociological concepts and theories, including theories about the legitimacy of illness and on illness careers. They use the term 'metasynthesis' to describe this process, and suggest that this can compensate for the methodological shortcomings in individual studies. The most common methodological weakness they identified in the primary literature was that of under-analysed, or descriptive, accounts of the data. Integrating findings across a set of studies enabled even the more descriptive studies to contribute to the development of deeper insights into the understanding of the experience of fibromyalgia syndrome.

Nicky Britten and colleagues (Britten et al. 2002) argue that there are good grounds for developing formal methods of meta-analysis for qualitative studies, as an alternative to traditional narrative reviews of existing literature, and suggest **meta-ethnography** as a way of doing this. Drawing on George Noblit and R. Dwight Hare's (1988) development of meta-ethnography, they conducted a meta-analysis of published papers on the lay meaning of medicines.

This approach entails going back if necessary to original data, and possibly to authors to check interpretations, so it may be difficult to include all the studies identified in a systematic review, but the primary aim of meta-ethnography is to 'synthesise understanding' (Noblit and Hare 1988: 10) rather than make comprehensive claims about a field of study. Noblit and Hare (1988) explicitly contrast their approach with positivist syntheses, which aim to accumulate findings, and stress that the guiding principle of a meta-ethnography is an interpretive one, rooted in an ethnographic approach.

Essentially, meta-ethnography entails a re-analysis of the concepts that are reported in published studies on similar topics. The first set of concepts included in the meta-ethnography are those reported from the participants in the primary studies: these are called 'first-order concepts'. In the meta-ethnography reported by Britten and colleagues, these were: adherence/compliance; self-regulation; aversion; alternative coping strategies; sanctions; and selective disclosure. Second-order constructs are social scientific concepts that are reported as outcomes of the original analysis. In the papers on the meanings of medications, these second-order concepts included the impact of cultural meanings, and 'cost-benefit analysis'. The second-order interpretations are the building blocks for the meta-analysis, in which the researcher develops an argument about how they are linked, and attempts to synthesize the insights from all papers included in the review. Britten and colleagues did this with the aid of a grid, in which all the first- and second-order concepts are listed. Thus, they can develop a generalizable theory about medicine-taking, from integrating the findings and analysis of a number of published empirical papers on the topic. These final 'third-order' interpretations that form the synthesis are then potentially testable hypotheses. Part of their synthesis is as follows:

> There are two distinct forms of medicine-taking: adherent medicine-taking and self-regulation. The latter reflects aversion to medicines. The use of alternative coping strategies is one expression of this aversion. In self-regulation, patients carry out their own cost-benefit analyses, informed by their own cultural meanings and resources ... . (Britten et al. 2002: 5)

The process of analysis is, then, very similar to that of analysing primary data, in that published findings are compared, contrasted, and integrated into a coherent argument. Meta-ethnography offers a qualitative approach to utilizing published research reports through synthesizing findings on topics where there has already been a considerable number of good-quality published studies.

Challenges of systematic reviews

A systematic review can be an efficient method for gaining an overview of the qualitative research on a particular topic, and reviews including qualitative literature are becoming increasingly important to research commissioners to inform policy and practice. There are, though, some methodological and practical challenges in undertaking systematic reviews of qualitative literature. For many topics and questions, such methods may simply be inappropriate. In a review of qualitative methods in health technology assessment, for instance, Elizabeth Murphy and colleagues note:

> The search tools often used for systematic reviews were not appropriate for this review as it would be necessary to cover the equivalents of MEDLINE in a range of disciplines and applied fields, many of which do not have databases of comparable coverage. In addition, important methodological writing in the field of social science started long before indexing for computer databases, and much of the most significant work has been published in books rather than journals. (Murphy et al. 1998: iii)

At the practical level, many published reviews note that identifying, accessing and abstracting data from articles can be more time consuming than predicted for qualitative research. Searches can generate large numbers of potentially relevant articles, and developing appropriate limits to the review can involve balancing the needs for comprehensiveness with those of having a manageable number of studies to appraise and synthesise. Not all journals provide abstracts for indexing services, and not all titles of qualitative papers reflect either the methodology or the topic. This can mean that large numbers of papers have to be retrieved and read in full before deciding whether they meet the inclusion and exclusion criteria. In a reflection on their meta-ethnography of adherence to tuberculosis (TB) treatment, Salla Atkins and colleagues (Atkins et al. 2008) note that reducing their scope to those studies addressing adherence only may have missed important insights from more general papers on the experience of TB, but that increasing the scope of the review would have been impossible to manage. They go on to note that the titles of many qualitative studies may not reflect the narrow empirical focus used in a review, so that some research that did address adherence, but did not include this as a word in the title, or key words, may have been missed. More generally, they suggest that the principles of an ethnographic interpretation may be difficult to apply to the kinds of reports most likely to end up in biomedical journals, which might lack the thick description and theoretical insight of more traditional ethnographic outputs.

This raises a more general methodological debate around systematic reviews, and the extent to which they are appropriate within a qualitative approach. Although there is now in general an acceptance of the usefulness of qualitative findings for informing practice and policy in health care, the style and terminology of systematic reviews is to a large extent taken from its origins as a way of integrating the findings from quantitative, particularly RCT, evidence. A stress on replicability, strict protocols for searching and abstracting, and checklists for quality, sit uneasily with the orientations of qualitative research. When the aim is merely to include all studies that used qualitative methods as if the findings could be simply aggregated without any attempt to take into account the context of data production, or the interpretation of the findings, this can result in rather thin and perhaps not particularly useful reviews. However, in practice, the methods and approaches of systematic reviews vary as much as those of any other kind of primary research, with researchers taking a range of positions, from the more positivist 'aggregations' of existing knowledge, through to explicitly qualitative approaches relying on narrative (see Jones 2004) or ethnographic interpretation (Noblit and Hare 1988).

Methodological issues in using documentary sources

Using existing sources if possible is, we have argued, often an efficient approach to research and one that can be used to address a wide range of qualitatively different research questions. It is not, though, always the method of choice, and a number of potential limitations need to be considered. First, the researcher is limited to what is available and accessible. Pat Holden, whose study of nursing in Uganda was discussed above, could draw on papers kept by the Overseas Nursing Association, but not all organizations keep their records, or would allow a researcher access to them. Second, data collected or generated for one purpose (even for research purposes) might be difficult to use to answer a different research question. It can be difficult to know before becoming immersed in the data what kind of research questions they will answer. This is a particular problem when designing research studies that need a clear research question at the outset (see Chapter 2). Third, the researcher has no control over, or often much knowledge of, how the data were collected. These issues will be more or less constraining on the feasibility of a study, largely depending on the methodological perspective employed.

Methodological perspectives

The illustrations used so far suggest that documents (like any data) can be read in a number of ways, depending on the perspective of the researcher. Within a positivist framework, we can see documents as representing some reality about the world, whether that is health care policies represented in written policy documents, or mortality rates represented by government reports of them, or women's experiences of the post-partum period. The same documents can also be read as giving us insight into the perspectives of those who produced them. So letters to magazines, or diaries, or official reports are a source of information for interpretative researchers in exploring the world-views of those who produce documents.

Bridget O'Laughlin (1998) takes this perspective in her discussion of the analysis of *grey literature*: unpublished reports from governmental and nongovernmental organizations. For O'Laughlin, grey literature is an important source of information not about the topic of the report, but about the political processes that produced it. Drawing on her experience of researching policy-orientated development issues, she argues that the report is 'the outcome of a process of negotiation between researchers and the commissioning institution' (1998: 107), and analysis of the document depends on locating it within the political processes and competing institutional discourses within which it was produced. To do this involves reading them with prior knowledge of the topic, and with a sensitivity to what has been omitted, what solutions are framed as possible, whose voices are present and absent, and what power relations exist between the subjects of the report, the writers and the commissioners. Grey literature is an essential clue in explorations of the political process:

> It tells us the ways in which important institutions in the politics of development, such as the World Bank, UNICEF, COSATU (the South African trade union federation) and national governments, view problems and solutions in the domain we are studying. When a poverty study on Mozambique informs us that the 'prospects for off-farm employment in Mozambique ... have never been very bright' (World Bank 1989) we learn that current World Bank thinking on Mozambique ignores the long history of migrant labour. (O'Laughlin 1998: 111)

For social constructionists, documents represent clues to the ways in which aspects of the world (diagnostic categories, management structures, policies) are socially produced. David Armstrong's (1986) work on infant mortality (Case Study 7.1, above) is one example. Another is Tom Shakespeare's (1999) analysis of medical and disability rights discourses in genetics. He explores the various narratives evident in public discourses about genetic technologies, identified by reviewing major journals and textbooks in the field. Medical writing about genetics, he argues, utilizes narratives of tragedy, in the metaphors about those with disabilities and the genes themselves (described as 'bad' or 'defective'), and of optimism in describing the potential role of medicine. Noting that the eugenic position is not presented in any clear-cut way in these accounts, he points to the methodological limitations of focusing purely on public documents as a source:

> ... [there is] a need to try and gather more unguarded statements or undertake qualitative research. Methodologically, this raises a problem for disabled researchers, because it suggests that clinicians and researchers would present different accounts of their views to a disabled researcher than they might to someone seen as less implicated in the new technologies. (Shakespeare 1999: 672)

Despite pointing to these limitations of 'public' documents as a source, Shakespeare does demonstrate their utility. In analysing the contrasting rhetorics of medical writers and disability activists, he identifies what is missing in the debate: a nuanced, balanced account of the embodied experiences of people with disabilities, and the challenges faced in developing an understanding of the potential and dangers of genetic research.

Whatever the orientation of the researcher, we have suggested that using existing sources of data has many advantages, including efficiency and the ready availability of many sources. However, there are some drawbacks to using documents as primary data, whether from public records, personal documents, media output or research products. In positivist approaches, some key considerations include threats to reliability and validity.

Threats to reliability

One major concern with reliability is the representativeness of records. Two sources of bias operate to potentially limit representativeness. First is *selective deposit*; that is, that not everything gets recorded (or published, or photographed) at the time. A second source of bias is *selective survival*, in that what survives of any data set is not necessarily representative of what is deposited (Webb et al. 1977). In Oinas's study of letters to Finnish magazines, for instance, she notes that we cannot assume that those who write letters are in any way representative of the wider population of Finnish young women, or even that those letters that get published are representative of all those who write. These limitations would be important from a positivist perspective, if we were, for instance, attempting to review the evidence to identify exactly what young women's concerns about menstruation were, but Oinas's study is not attempting to answer this question. From a more positivist perspective, we can see how in Case Study 7.2 one particular cause of selective deposit – publication bias – might be more problematic. It may be that reports of post-partum symptoms in non-Western cultures are simply less likely to get reported. In this study, the authors have to consider how to guard against conclusions based on a potentially biased set of data. Threats to reliability are, then, an issue for some research questions, but in others are better thought of as limitations on the kinds of questions we can ask of any particular data set, rather than limitations in the data themselves.

Threats to validity

A basic issue of the validity of a document is its authenticity: is the document genuinely what it purports to be? This may be a particular problem with historical sources such as diaries or letters, which may be deliberate 'fakes', such as the 'Hitler Diaries', or produced as fiction intended to imitate personal record. Again, from a positivist perspective, threats to validity have to be carefully considered. In more interpretative traditions, however, 'truth' is rather more complex, as Norman Denzin suggests:

> The problem involves facts, facticities and fiction. *Facts* refer to events that are believed to have occurred or will occur. ... *Facticities* describe how those facts were lived and experienced by interacting individuals. ... *Fiction* is a narrative which deals with real or imagined facts and facticities. *Truth* refers ... to statements that are in agreement with facts and facticities as they are known and commonly understood. ... A truthful fiction (narrative) is faithful to facticities and facts. It creates verisimilitude, or what are for the reader believable experiences. (Denzin 1989a: 23)

For Denzin, then, the essential question of validity (is this a true account?) is a rather inadequate one when faced with biographical sources from an interpretative perspective, as we are treating the text as essentially a literary artefact, and the aim is understanding the subjective experience of an individual, not merely accruing 'facts' about their life. For qualitative approaches outside the positivist traditions, threats to reliability and validity may be less relevant, as the object of research is what has been preserved, or cited, or is available, and the questions asked of documents relate to the social reality they represent or shape, rather than reflect.

A broader methodological drawback is that documents alone may furnish few clues about their production. If we are interested, for instance, in a policy process, documents may tell us little about the decision making that led to the policy, or the role of particular groups or individuals in its formation. In the study by Oinas of letters to magazines, described above, we know nothing about the motivations of the writers, how the letters were selected for publication or how they were edited by the magazine's staff. Of course, a research study can always include complementary components to address these questions of production, such as interviews with policy makers or journalists, and in practice many projects will use a number of methodological strategies in tandem.

Conclusion

This chapter has highlighted the potential uses of documentary evidence for health research. The key advantages of documentary sources, especially for unfunded student projects, lie in their efficiency, in that many documents (such as published research reports, official statistics, newspaper articles and published biographical sources) are usually freely available from libraries, reasonably easy to access, and it will take less time to assemble a data set than if producing primary data. Even data sources that take a little more effort (such as archived primary data, or mass media outputs) will require less time than fieldwork or a series of interviews. In addition to practical advantages, documents offer the potential for analysis from a number of qualitative perspectives. We have discussed in this chapter examples such as: positivist analysis of research outputs (Case Study 7.2); social constructionist analysis of public records (Case Study 7.1) and research outputs (Kaufert's study of papers on the menopause); interpretative studies of research outputs (Britten et al.'s meta-analysis of papers on medicine-taking); and critical approaches to grey literature (O'Laughlin's comments on reading reports from development institutions). But of course, this does not exhaust either the range of approaches or the potential sources that could be used. One source we haven't touched on, for instance, is artefacts. Qualitative sociology is perhaps most associated with language data, whether oral or from texts, but it has been argued that this has marginalized other material sources of documentary evidence, particularly visual documents such as photographs and art, which could also offer much for qualitative research questions (Harrison 1996). Anthropology has perhaps a stronger tradition of interest in the artefacts of material culture, but they are still perhaps underutilized as evidence on which we can draw in studies of health and related topics. The field of health has a rich material culture, including medical instruments, therapeutic and diagnostic artefacts, the material outcomes of therapy (such as x-rays, medical records), clothing (professional uniforms, safety wear), laboratory equipment and architecture, that has attracted some research, but is generally underdeveloped. Like any documents, or indeed any other data sources, these can be 'read' in a number of ways, depending on the orientations of the researcher and the research questions they are addressing.

KEY POINTS

- Using existing documents can be an efficient strategy for health research projects, usually requiring fewer resources than producing primary data.
- Accessible sources include public records, personal documents, mass media outputs, and research data and outputs.
- Documents can be analysed from a range of epistemological perspectives.
- There is a growing interest in methods for systematically reviewing and synthesizing qualitative literature.

EXERCISES

1 Suggest some potential research studies you could carry out using health promotion posters in a health clinic as your data source. What could these posters tell you about:

(a) The health problems considered important in this area?
(b) How messages about these health problems are framed?

What are the limits to posters as a data source to answer these questions?

2 What other sources of documentary data could be used in a study of health promotion policy? For each one you identify, consider the possible research questions you could address by using this data source, and its limitations.

FURTHER READING

Petticrew, M. and Roberts, H. (2005) *Systematic reviews in the social sciences*. London: Blackwell Publishing. This practical and accessible text describes how to plan, carry out and disseminate systematic reviews of qualitative and quantitative literature. Includes methods for assessing study quality and synthesizing findings.

Plummer, K. (1983) *Documents of life: an introduction to the problems and literature of a humanistic method*. London: Unwin Hyman. Ken Plummer's text is a plea for the serious consideration of sources such as life histories in the social sciences, as a way of accessing subjective meanings and lived experiences. He introduces some of the classic literature, the history of the method and how to go about doing a life history.

Prior, L. (2003) *Using documents in social research*. London: Sage. In one of the few textbooks devoted to the use of documents, Lindsay Prior starts from the assumption that documents are social products, and in using them as resources or data for research, we have to be aware of how and why they have been produced and how they are consumed. This text draws on many examples from the study of health to discuss the range of ways we can use documents in research.

8 Analysing Qualitative Data

CHAPTER SUMMARY

Analysis of qualitative data relies on both rigour and imagination. In health research, qualitative researchers are increasingly expected to report their methods of analysis in a transparent way, and this chapter focuses on methods to improve rigour and strategies for improving the reliability and validity of analysis. We introduce four approaches to analysis that is common in health research (thematic content analysis, grounded theory, framework analysis and narrative analysis) and discuss the potential for computer aided analysis.

Introduction

In disciplines such as sociology and anthropology, there has traditionally been little emphasis on techniques for the analysis of qualitative data. Many social science studies that have been influential in the health field report very little information about how the data were analysed, and indeed the most widely cited works in the field have been predominantly theoretical, with few empirical findings (Chard et al. 1997). Even classic research based on empirical research, such as Goffman's (1968) *Asylums*, on the social worlds of a mental hospital, rarely describes the *processes* of data analysis used. With the uptake of qualitative research designs in studies of health, rather than 'health' topics being coincidentally the subject of social science enquiry, and the growing market for peer reviewed journals as outlets for qualitative research findings, there has been increasing attention paid to the practice of analysis. This has addressed both the practical 'tools' or procedures researchers use to make sense of their data and the epistemological assumptions underpinning these techniques. In writing for audiences less familiar with social science writing, qualitative health researchers have had to be more explicit about what they *do* with data, and how their conclusions are built up from their interpretations. This has had benefits for relatively inexperienced researchers, who are often reassured by a set of steps that can be followed when faced with the task of making sense of data. It also, more arguably, has benefits for the non-social scientists who are the users of qualitative research in helping them judge whether the analysis was likely to have been done with due regard to issues of validity, rigour and comprehensiveness. However, it is impossible to reduce the task of analysing qualitative data to a set of tools that can be applied in a mechanistic way. Good analysis (in quantitative as well as qualitative work) draws widely on more general social science knowledge, and locates the particular findings of one study within a broader context. The American sociologist C. Wright Mills described this as a 'sociological imagination', an ability to 'shift from one perspective to another' (1959: 7), and to make the links between them. Thus it is rarely sufficient to focus purely on the data collected when doing analysis. Understanding the 'meaning' of data properly involves a broader perspective on history, social structures and comparative cases as well as an in-depth grasp of the particularities of the data set in question. To develop rules for integrating the more contextual and theoretical insights that contribute to analysing data is perhaps impossible: this constitutes the 'art' of qualitative analysis, utilizing imagination (the ability to make links) as well as a broad ranging knowledge base to draw upon. Norman Denzin (1994) argues that this art can only be learned by doing, and by thinking about interpretation as a kind of storytelling, in which practising the various conventions used develops an imaginative and theoretical approach.

To make claims for the importance of this 'imagination' is not the same as claiming that qualitative analysis is merely 'made up', and that the meanings inherent in data can be whatever the analyst wants them to be. Qualitative analysis should be rigorous as well as imaginative, and the requirements of thoroughness, reliability and attention to validity provide a necessary, if not sufficient, condition for conducting good and useful work in health research. The interpretations made by the researcher have to be credible, and the links between the empirical data and the claims made about them clear. This chapter concentrates on techniques for maximizing rigour, because these are the bedrock of good analysis. Outlining guidelines for the creative aspects of analysis is more difficult. For many people, this is an intuitive skill, but it is one that can be developed with experience and the cultivation of an enquiring approach.

Styles of analysis

There is a broad range of approaches to analysis in qualitative research, with the task of the researcher defined rather differently across that range. In the more humanistic traditions, the researcher may be conceptualized more as a 'conduit', through which other voices can be heard, than an analyst. If the aims of the study are to give voice to participants, and represent their individual subjective experiences, then talking of 'analysis' is perhaps inappropriate, and the task of presenting the raw data to a wider audience may be more akin to editing than analysis. If the researcher's aim is to allow participants to 'speak for themselves', their analytical task may be minimal, restricted to merely tidying up sections of transcript for publication. Ken Plummer's approach to life histories perhaps epitomizes the humanist tradition, in that he talks about a continuum of researcher 'contamination' (Plummer 1983: 113). At one end of his continuum is theoretical analysis that has taken no account of subjective experience, where empirical data are not really used. At the other end is simple editing of life history documents, where the researcher publishes accounts (from diaries, interviews or other sources) with no explicit interpretation, and the story is allowed to 'speak for itself'.

This chapter is concerned with the problem of studies in the middle of Plummer's continuum: those that utilize empirical data from the 'lifeworld' of everyday accounts, but that wish to go beyond merely reporting those accounts. Most approaches to analysing qualitative data attempt to 'intervene' at some level, to draw out the 'meaning' of the data that are not obvious at a descriptive reading. In health research, there are also usually requirements to be explicit about how the data were analysed, and how the 'stories' or other material are selected, interpreted and organized. Broadly, the aims of most qualitative analysis are to both reflect the complexity of the phenomena studied, and present the underlying structures which 'make sense' of that complexity. The task of the researcher is thus a dual and perhaps inherently contradictory one of simultaneously 'telling the story' from the point of view of the research participants, and unpacking that story in such a way that the broader meanings can be elicited. One way in which styles of analysis can be distinguished is in terms of the extent to which they maintain the integrity of the data, in aiming to reproduce for the reader a contextual, in-depth picture of a social setting, life story or experience. Description is of course a basic building block of all analysis styles, but in some a more holistic description is more central than in others, which focus more on 'unpacking' the data to reveal the underlying patterns.

Relating analysis to the aims of the study

The approach adopted for managing and analysing data from an empirical study is of course related to the aims of the study. One influence on the kind of analysis used will be what the findings are intended to do, whether it is to contribute to sociological theory, evaluate a health promotion intervention or inform the development of a survey questionnaire. These broad aims will influence the *style* of analysis: whether it attempts to merely report the views of the respondents, or a more detailed analysis that aims to explain how the accounts produced in the research illuminate a particular research question. Some common approaches are outlined below but, at a general level, analysis might aim for some of the following outcomes:

- developing conceptual definitions
- developing typologies and classifications
- exploring associations between attitudes, behaviours and experiences
- developing explanations of phenomena
- generating new ideas and theories.

If you look back at the study of asthma patients described in Case Study 1.1, some of these are illustrated. The researchers use a *conceptual definition* of 'stigma' that has been developed through other qualitative work (for instance, drawing on Goffman's classic (1963) study) to look at responses to asthma. From their own data, the authors identify a *typology* of three broad responses to asthma diagnosis: denial, acceptance and pragmatism. Within the data, they look at how attitudes (to, for instance, what kind of disease asthma is) are *associated with* experiences and behaviours such as taking medication, using the asthma clinic and disclosing the diagnosis to others. Finally, they were thus able to develop some *explanations* of phenomena such as the low 'compliance' with preventative medication.

In practice, most researchers probably use a pragmatic mixture of approaches to analysis within any particular study. The approaches taken may not be cited explicitly in written reports, especially if writing for a social science rather than a health audience. Those selected reflect both the needs of a particular project and the epistemological assumptions the researcher makes about what the data can tell them. Here, we outline four common approaches: thematic content analysis, grounded theory, **framework analysis** and **narrative analysis.** These have all been widely used in health research, and the differences between them illustrate the differences in emphasis across the range of qualitative research.

Thematic content analysis

The most basic type of qualitative analysis is an analysis of the content of the data to categorize the recurrent or common 'themes'. This is perhaps the most common approach used in qualitative research reported in health journals, and aims to present the key elements of respondents' accounts. It is a useful approach for answering questions about the salient issues for particular groups of respondents or identifying typical responses. In a study of community views about health needs, for instance, identifying the principle themes in interviewees' accounts might be the principle aim of the study.

Using data such as interview notes or transcripts, the researcher looks through them to categorize respondents' accounts in ways that can be summarized. This is essentially a comparative process, by which the various accounts gathered are compared with each other to classify those 'themes' that recur or are common in the data set. These themes emerge as the researcher looks in detail at transcripts, taking each segment of text asking, 'What is this segment *about*?' and 'How is it like, and not like, other segments?' The 'segments' you work with should be the size that pragmatically work in order to derive meaning, usually sentences, phrases or small groups of these. The easiest way to do this kind of analysis is using 'scissors and paste'. In the margins of each transcript or set of notes, go through to mark up the content of what is being said by labelling excerpts. Box 8.1 shows an example of a section of transcript marked up for some of the key themes. This is an extract from a focus group interview with people with glaucoma, and the aims of the analysis here were to look for triggers to referral and to describe the problems faced by people with this kind of eyesight problems. (There is more detail on the study from which this was taken in Case Study 8.1, below.)

Box 8.1   **Extract from focus group with five women with glaucoma, with themes marked.**

Transcript	Theme
1. **Ann**: The problem is that we all look, well, normal. It's not like	Symbols of
2. we're carrying white sticks or anything –	disability/passing
3. **Bertha**: No, and even if you're being guided, you could just be	Passing
4. with a friend or something	
5. **Connie**: I've got a white stick – but usually it's in my handbag!	
6. I hate using it – people stare at you, and you get offered seats on	Stigma
7. the bus – you get more attention, more than I want anyway	
8. **Ann**: Well, that's the problem – it's embarrassing. People,	Misunderstandings
9. people, who don't know, assume	

(Continued)

10. that if you're using a white stick, you can't see anything, so	
11. they look – quite openly, staring, thinking you can't see them	Embarrassment
12. starting.	
13. **Interviewer**: So do you prefer looking 'normal'?	
14. **Bertha**: Well, I feel pretty normal, mostly.	
15. **Connie**: With the white stick – it's meant for car drivers, really,	Aids for coping
16. so they see you in case you suddenly jump in the road – but I	
17. do feel very conscious when I'm carrying it. People jump out	
18. of the way like you've got the plague or something.	Stigma
19. **Donna**: I use one when I'm out on my own, when my sister's	
20. not with me, and it's mainly for dealing with stairs – I have	Aids for coping
21. real problems with steps, not being able to see, with depth	Problems
21. perception –	
23. **Ann**: Oh, me too!	
24. **Donna**: – and contrasts, you know, coming into a dark room	Problems
25. outside, can't see a thing	Impact of problems
26. **Bertha**: Oh, god, lifts are the worst! I just can't see anything	
27. when I step into a lift –	
28. **Connie**: because it's all dark! I know – you just have to hope	Strategies for
29. someone else comes in to press the buttons	coping
30. **Ann**: That's why I wear dark glasses outside – it makes the	Strategies for
31. contrast less	coping

There are a number of ways of laying out interview transcripts, but it is important to have some consistent format which leaves enough room for notes on the printed version. The extract in Box 8.1 uses typical conventions: each new speaker starts on a new line, line numbers are used to make the extracts easier to reference, and short lines leave the margins wide enough for **coding.** Note how codes might overlap: in lines 19–22, Donna's account of 'coping on her own' could be labelled as an example of both 'problems' faced, and as an example of 'strategies to cope' ('sister helping', using a white stick). For more detailed coding, it would be preferable to leave more space than in this extract.

Coding schemes (a list of code names to apply to the data) can be developed by looking through the early data to identify the key themes and how they will be labelled (the 'code'). If you are working as part of a team, you will need to discuss and agree on what the evidence for themes and codes is (that is, how particular utterances are 'indicators' of the concepts of interest) with your colleagues. If working alone, it is productive to consult with colleagues or a supervisor if possible during the early stages of data analysis. For instance, in Box 8.1, the extract starts with Ann's line 'We all look normal' (line 1) and Bertha's response (lines 3–4) about being with a guide looking like being with a friend. In discussion, it was agreed that these were examples of 'looking normal' as opposed to 'disabled'. This was in contrast to when they were carrying white sticks, when people could identify them as 'disabled'. We therefore labelled this code as 'Passing', to summarize a key theme: ways in which participants thought they looked 'normal' in everyday life, or 'passed' as normal. In qualitative work, it is more common to develop the coding scheme from the empirical data, but elements of it may be pre-determined by the research questions. In the example in Case Study 8.1, one aim of the study was to look at 'triggers for referral' – the signs and symptoms that people noticed, and which prompted them to seek help. This was therefore one element of the coding scheme, with a heading of 'Triggers for referral', although others were added as the data were analysed.

Copies of transcripts or notes can then literally be cut up and rearranged in piles or on large sheets of paper under the headings of the themes. In their focus group guidebook, Krueger and Casey (2000: 132–5) describe some practical suggestions for the 'scissor and paste' method of analysis:

- use a long table (or walls, or floor) covered with a flip chart or newspaper, with sections headed with themes (or interview questions)
- distinguish each of one set of transcript copies by printing each on different coloured paper, or using coloured lines down the margins so that the original source of the extracts cut out can be identified
- cut the transcripts up into separate extracts
- begin sorting extracts by assigning them to sections, and then compare each new extract with the growing pile: is it similar, or should you start a new pile or section?

These kinds of cut and paste techniques are 'low technology', but they work. They allow the researcher, or team of researchers, to compare, contrast, start to build up categories and typologies and to discuss the 'meaning' of their data. Word processors have made these processes a little easier, in that you can cut and paste transcripts on screen into new documents, with a separate document for each emerging theme. If there is a small number of interview transcripts, each can be identified with a different font, or colour. With larger data sets, you may have to type in a case identifier for the original transcript after each quote. At this point, the advantages of using computer software to help with managing the data will start emerging (see below).

This kind of thematic analysis can be as simple or sophisticated as is needed for the project in hand. If doing exploratory work in an area where not much is known, it may be enough to simply report the common issues mentioned in a community, and go no further than listing each issue, perhaps with some quoted excerpts to give 'colour'. If the qualitative study is a pilot for developing a questionnaire, you may want to pay more attention to how respondents discussed particular issues: what terminology they used, how difficult it was to talk about, and how often particular issues were mentioned.

Thematic analysis is also the basis of more sophisticated qualitative analysis, in which the researcher moves beyond simply categorizing and coding the data to thinking about how the codes relate to each other and asking more complex questions. The example in Box 8.1 for instance shows the 'first level' of thematic analysis of some focus group data. One outcome of this could be 'lists' of issues, such as a list of common problems faced by people with glaucoma in work, family life and leisure activities and a list of initial symptoms that alerted people to their eye problems. One of the aims of the study this is taken from was to inform health promotion activities for encouraging people to attend for eye tests, and this basic level of analysis is perhaps sufficient for this, as it provides some information from respondents about the kinds of information likely to be useful to the target population. However, to take this further, we might want to look at the *relationships* between the themes that emerged, and also at the context of particular codes. Questions an analyst could ask to facilitate this might include:

- Which kinds of respondents are more likely to report problems of daily living? Men, women, those who were relatively young when their glaucoma was diagnosed, those with little family support?
- Which kinds of respondents are more likely to report feelings of stigma, and is this related to their views of eye problems?
- How do respondents' accounts of their diagnosis relate to their accounts of current problems?

Thematic analysis is, then, enough for many health research projects, particularly if they are exploratory or the aim is to describe the key issues of concern to a particular group of people. However, many qualitative researchers will want to ask rather more of their data, and other techniques are needed if we are to move beyond the 'emic' summaries and typologies of participants' accounts that a thematic analysis provides. A good qualitative analysis should also say something about social life, as well as what participants say about it. It should provide a 'thick', rich description of the setting studied, link into theory and provide a satisfying and credible account of 'what is going on'. Two potential ways of developing a deeper analysis of qualitative data are grounded theory (sometimes called the **constant comparative method**) and framework analysis. They share many features, but are rather different in emphasis, so we describe them here separately.

Grounded theory

One approach to taking a more systematic view of qualitative data analysis was developed by two American sociologists, Barney Glaser and Anslem Strauss (Glaser and Strauss 1967; Strauss 1987). Their writings on what they called 'grounded theory' have been extremely influential on qualitative research. Glaser and Strauss attempted to operationalize the procedures they thought informed much qualitative analysis, but which were never written down. They argued that you could unpack the rules researchers use to, as they put it, 'discover theory from data' and that, with practice, most people could learn to use them. So it was in some ways an attempt to demystify the processes of qualitative analysis, and to provide a set of what they called 'rules of thumb' to help develop theory that was grounded in empirical data. Although this suggests an inductive method of research, in which theory is built up from empirical observations (rather than deductive, in which theories are 'tested' against the data), Glaser and Strauss argue that the strength of grounded theory approaches lies in the cyclical process of collecting data, analysing it, developing a provisional coding scheme, using this to suggest further sampling, more analysis, checking out emerging theory and so on, until a point of 'saturation' is reached, when no new constructs are emerging. At this point, you have a rich, dense theoretical account – but one that is completely grounded in empirical data. It is thus both inductive, and deductive, moving back and forward between emerging theory and data. The other key principle (and why this is also known as the 'constant comparative method') is 'constant comparison', and the notion that interpretation of data moves forward through comparing indicators (codes), cases and data sets.

A first step in a grounded theory analysis is the emphasis on intense coding of early data. This entails *open coding*, an intense line by line analysis of, say, a transcript, that attempts to open up or 'fracture' the data. This forces you to take a step back and open up all potential avenues of enquiry. In taking a small part of early data phrase by phrase, and asking the general question 'What's going on here?', the idea is to generate as many potential codes as possible. It doesn't matter if these are 'wrong' at this stage, as grounded theory involves going back to the data to check these emerging ideas, and refining the concepts and 'theories' about them throughout the research process. By 'codes' Glaser and Strauss do not mean merely descriptive summaries of the data, but more conceptual labels, which identify what general phenomenon is indicated by the instance, or extract of talk, being analysed.

To take an example from Box 8.1, we might start with lines 1–4, and interrogate these for the possible answers to 'What is going one here?' Some potential questions one might ask of these data are: how does Ann constitute 'looking normal?' Why does she say this is a problem? What signs of 'normality' are there in everyday appearances? Why would a white stick undermine this appearance of normality? Why would being guided undermine an appearance of normality? How is being guided different to being with a friend? Asking this barrage of questions intensively around a few lines of data helps generate some useful early ideas about the data, and lines of enquiry to follow. Even from these few lines, we might develop some initial concepts, including:

Constituting normality (how people behave normally, how they assess it in others)
Constituting disability (how disability is communicated)

Each of these initial concepts is subjected to further questions, in order to explore its *properties* and its *dimensions*. Properties are attributes, or characteristics. In the example above, the properties of 'constituting disability' might include behaving in remarkable ways, looking unusual, using mobility aids. Dimensions are the continua along which these properties can be arranged. For instance, one concept in the study of glaucoma was 'onset of sight problems'. The dimensions of this include: rate of onset (sudden, gradual) and expectedness (expected, unexpected). Open coding can quickly generate a long list of concepts, which can then be categorized into a more sophisticated scheme by gathering together those that appear to relate to similar phenomena.

One set of codes to look for are what Glaser and Strauss call *in vivo codes* – the kinds that participants use themselves to divide up the world. In the short extract in Box 8.1, there are a number of in vivo codes suggested. The idea of 'looking normal' is one, and we could look through the transcripts for what it categorizes: what examples are given of people who don't 'look normal'? Another is at line 8–9, of 'people who don't know', which could be contrasted with 'sister', and perhaps other examples of 'people who do know' in the transcripts. Examples of in vivo codes can be found in most data, and are useful first steps in exploring how respondents see their social worlds. A common one in many medical settings is the way in which professionals classify their patients or clients into categories such as 'good patients', 'interesting patients' and other, less complimentary categories. One example is from Roger Jeffrey's (1979) study of 'normal rubbish' as an in vivo category used by staff in an Accident and Emergency department to describe the patients they did not find interesting or deserving. These in vivo codes are useful as first steps in categorizing the data, though the analysis has to go further than simply noting them. In Jeffrey's study, he unpicked the criteria by which staff categorized patients, and linked these to normative ideas about legitimacy in sickness.

All codes should be labelled, at least provisionally, as the process of naming them is part of the work of thinking about what they are: what is the concept that this particular code relates to? What connects the different instances (extracts) that are coded in this way? This helps move the analysis from a rather descriptive level, where the researcher is merely summarizing what is in the data, to a more analytical level, which is focused on the phenomena in the data as examples of some more generalizable concepts.

Initial open coding is a first step, but can be returned to at any point when the data analysis becomes 'stuck'. However, it is obviously too intensive to apply to the whole data set. Once a provisional coding scheme has been developed, the analysis can move to the next stage: *axial coding*, in which the fractured data are 'put back together again'. Here, the analysis moves on to looking for relationships between categories. For the glaucoma study example, this might include looking at the following questions: How does suddenness of onset of symptoms relate to problems of daily living? Is there a relationship between 'passing' as normal and attitudes to eye disease? One strategy for axial coding is developing a coding paradigm, which entails a set of questions about each code. These are: what conditions give rise to the category? What is its context? What are the interactional strategies by which it is handled and what are the consequences of those strategies? For example, for the category 'passing as normal', we might therefore develop the following:

Conditions: Feeling that 'blindness' is stigmatizing
Context: Being in public, being with strangers
Interactional strategies: not using white sticks, not going out alone
Consequences: strain of managing, embarrassment

Finally, more *selective coding*, where the aim is to move towards more abstract and analytical and theoretically informed concepts is the stage at which the core categories emerge. These are essential in that they are related to most other categories, and explain most of what is going on.

Because grounded theory moves from inductive to deductive modes, and back and forward between theory and data, it ideally relies on what Glaser and Strauss call 'theoretical sampling'. The cases to include should be dictated by the emerging data, and data analysis will suggest further cases to investigate. In addition to advocating that data collection and analysis should continue simultaneously, rather than sequentially, grounded theory also encourages writing throughout the process. These ongoing written records are called 'memos', defined as 'the written forms of our abstract thinking about the data' (Strauss and Corbin 1990: 198). Writing memos is an essential part of the analysis, rather than something begun towards the end of a project. Memos will include operational notes about data collection, but also theoretical memos, which are an essential step in the development of analytical ideas. Theoretical memos include initial ideas about the data, emerging hypotheses about relationships between codes and the properties of codes, and detailed notes later in the analysis on how the axial and selective coding is developing.

Kathy Charmaz, discussing the importance of memos in her work (Charmaz 1999), describes them as a 'pivotal intermediate step between coding and writing', which allows the researcher to stop and think about the data and move beyond descriptive 'codes' to thinking about how codes can become categories for analysis, and alerts the researcher to gaps in the data and the point where comparisons can be made. Crucially, she suggests, memos keep the researcher writing, which is an essential element in the analysis itself (see Chapter 10).

Key to analysis in grounded theory is the constant attempt to challenge and develop theoretical insights. A close attention to *deviant cases* is crucial to this, in which the researcher both deliberately includes data with which to test the emerging theory (through theoretical sampling), and pays close attention to exceptions within the data set. The two case studies in this chapter have examples of the use of deviant cases.

Finally, it should be noted that 'grounded theory' is perhaps one of the most abused phrases in the qualitative health literature. Increasingly, researchers are making claims to have used a 'grounded theory' approach in what emerges as rather superficial thematic content analysis. An analysis that has used grounded theory should provide a detailed, saturated account of the data, rather than a list of 'key themes'. It should be possible to read the account to see how any variation within the data set has been used comparatively to develop the analysis, and how deviant cases have contributed to a credible and thorough account of the data.

To do 'grounded theory', and reach this point of theoretical saturation, is time consuming and much health research is constrained by practical issues of policy and funding. One constraint is on the flexibility sponsors will allow in collecting more data, or different data, as a result of early analysis. A second is of course timescale. Most projects are done to tight deadlines, and it is doubtful how often this saturation really happens. Nonetheless, the principles and some of the approaches of grounded theory have been invaluable to health researchers, and even if funding and resources do not allow the researchers to develop a saturated grounded theory, there are many elements of the grounded theory approach that are useful for any analysis. Open coding, for instance, can be an insightful way of bringing fresh ideas to your analysis, and ensuring that you have developed some 'analytical distance'. Case Study 8.1 uses elements of the grounded theory approach to analyse data.

Case Study 8.1   Using elements of the constant comparative method in a study of living with glaucoma

(Source: Green, J., Siddall, H. and Murdoch, I. (2002) 'Learning to live with glaucoma: a qualitative study of diagnosis and the impact of sight loss', *Social Science and Medicine* 55: 257–67)

This study used individual and group interviews to explore the experiences of people who had been diagnosed with glaucoma, an eye disease characterized by a gradual loss of visual acuity. The aims were to inform health promotion by identifying triggers and barriers to self-referral with eye problems, and to explore the relationship between 'medical' definitions of disability and people's experiences of sight problems.

Interviews took a narrative approach, asking interviewees to tell the story of how they first noticed eye problems, how they came to be referred for treatment and what impact the symptoms and treatment regimes had on their everyday lives. Interviews were tape recorded and transcribed, and some participants also provided written notes on their experiences. Although this was not a 'grounded theory' study, some of the elements of the grounded theory approach were used to aid data analysis. One was the use of 'open coding' of early data to generate categories. This enabled the range of concepts used by participants to be identified, and to extend the analysis so the research question could better be understood in terms of 'grounded' theory, that is, ideas from the data themselves. For instance, one research aim was to identify 'triggers for self-referral'. Although the data could be 'coded' for triggers (such as noticing blurred vision, noticing 'missing' patches in the field of vision), detailed analysis of the data, and of the contexts of these reported symptoms, suggested that these were 'post hoc' descriptions of triggers, and at the time the early 'signs' of glaucoma are indistinguishable from the everyday eye problems many expect as a result of tiredness or ageing.

A second element of grounded theory used was theoretical sampling. One emerging theory in the data analysis was that a worry about 'dependence' was a concern for some in the sample, but did not seem to be an issue for an older married man, who relied on his wife for extensive help in everyday tasks anyway. We then deliberately sampled older patients, and looked in detail at cases with a range of family support, to check emerging relationships between family support and concepts of dependence and independence.

Close attention to deviant cases helped develop the analysis. One example was the findings on attitudes to blindness. The majority of participants utilized one of two images of 'blind people' – either the 'victim' who was to be pitied, because they were dependant on others, or the 'hero', who manages to perform extraordinary feats despite their disability. Not surprisingly, neither was a very appealing image, and most respondents did

(Continued)

not identify themselves as 'blind'. Although (for them) this brought benefits such as passing as normal, and resisting the felt stigma of being labelled as blind, it had considerable costs as a strategy. For some, it meant they had no access to the material benefits to which they were entitled. A 'deviant case' was one man who had a less 'stigmatized' image of what blindness meant. He had diabetes, and because he already had come to terms with an identity including 'disease', could see that 'being blind' did not have to be incompatible with 'leading a normal life'.

Locating the empirical findings from this study within wider theoretical literature on disability and living with chronic illness helped make sense of the data. There is a large literature on issues such as 'independence' and 'stigma' and these were used to help make sense of the accounts of people with glaucoma.

The constant comparative approach, then, helped develop initial categories for coding, helped inform sampling, and provided a framework for looking at relationships between categories.

Framework analysis

The stated aim of grounded theory is the development of theory. Obviously this will generate policy-relevant findings, and much research from this tradition has developed our understanding of health and health services in ways that have had implications for practice. However, the aim of policy development is not at the forefront of grounded theory and, given that we can't say at the beginning what we will find out, or even who we are going to include in the sample, it can be a difficult approach to 'sell' to policy and practice minded funders. Framework analysis, on the other hand, developed by the National Centre for Social Research (www.natcen.ac.uk/) is explicitly geared towards generating policy and practice-orientated findings, and is popular with many health and social researchers for this reason (Ritchie and Spencer 1994). Described by the National Centre for Social Research as 'a content analysis method which involves summarising and classifying data within a thematic framework', the key difference between this and 'grounded theory' approaches is that the integrity of individual respondents' accounts is preserved throughout the analysis, in contrast to the deliberate attempt to 'fracture' the data in order to open up new avenues for analysis in grounded theory.

Reflecting this focus on maintaining the integrity of respondents' narratives, the first step in framework analysis is *familiarization* with the data. This involves listening to tapes and re-reading fieldnotes or transcripts until the researcher is closely familiar with them in their entirety. Following on, the second step is a *thematic analysis* to develop a coding scheme. The themes in the data become the labels for codes. In framework analysis, the process of applying codes to the whole data set in a systematic way is called *indexing*. Indexing is the third step. Like grounded theory, the analysis part of framework analysis entails comparison, both within and between cases. This is facilitated by the fourth step, called *charting*, which involves rearranging the data according to this thematic content, either case by case, or by theme. These charts contain only summaries of data, so the researcher can see across cases and under themes the range of data. Summary examples in the charts are referenced back to the original transcript. Case Study 8.2 includes an extract of a chart from a study by Geraldine Barrett and Kaye Wellings on how women use and define terms such as 'unplanned' when talking about pregnancy. Note how this organizes data under themes for each interviewee, and is annotated with page references to the interview transcript, so that the original data can be quickly retrieved. These charts can then be used to compare across each code, and see the whole range of phenomena, where they do and don't occur, and can also start to look at the relationships between codes.

Case Study 8.2   An example of framework analysis from a study of how women discuss pregnancy planning and intention

(Sources: Barrett, G. and Wellings, K. (2002) 'What is a "planned" pregnancy? Empirical data from a British study', *Social Science and Medicine* 55: 545–557, and Barrett, G., Personal communication)

In the family planning literature, terms such as 'planned/ unplanned', 'intended/unintended' and 'wanted/unwanted' to describe pregnancy are often used as if their meaning was obvious and unproblematic, but there has been little research on how women themselves understand them. Geraldine Barrett and Kaye Wellings aimed to develop a valid measure of pregnancy planning/ intention for use in quantitative surveys. A first step was a qualitative study with pregnant women that used in-depth interviews to collect data on a series of topics, including when they became aware that they were pregnant, their contraceptive use, feelings about being pregnant and decisions about the pregnancy. At the end of the interview, women were asked about their understanding of the terms planned, unplanned, intended, unintended, wanted and unwanted, and whether any of these terms applied to their own pregnancies.

(Continued)

When data collection was complete, framework analysis was used to analyse the data. The first four steps (familiarization, identifying a thematic framework and coding frame, indexing and charting) are described primarily as ways of managing the data. The table below shows this fourth stage of charting, in an extract from one of the charts.

Extract from chart produced for 'What is a planned pregnancy?' study

Interview No.	Partner's feelings about outcome	Partner's feelings about fatherhood	Definitions of planned/unplanned (introduced terms)	Definitions of intended/unintended (introduced terms)
105	Happy	Assumed would be father in future p.8. Enjoys fatherhood p.9	Planned – planned to have child, p.10. Unplanned is an accident, p.10	Intended – you intend to have the child, you wanted one p.10. Unintended – not planning to have a child and finding they are pregnant p.10, also accident
106	Happy	Says he probably wanted to be a father sooner than she wanted to be a mother p.11. Very positive about fatherhood p.11	Planned – same as intended pregnancy. Unplanned – not necessarily using contraception, had sex without contraception p.13	Intended – actively set out to create child, not using contraception, using fertile period etc p.13. Unintended – not intending to get pregnant, either using contraception or just get pregnant by mistake p.13 – moves towards seeing unintended as contraceptive failure p.13

107	Nervous p.4. Says he'll be at the birth p.13	Says he never actually wanted to have children, nervous about being a bad father p.12. He's acting as a father to her first child at the moment p.12	Planned – trying for a baby, find out best time to fall pregnant. Unplanned – fall pregnant without meaning to p.13	Intended and unintended – interchangeable with planned and unplanned p.13
108	Happy	Doesn't think he always wanted to be a father – wanted to find right partner, could have considered life without children p.12. Very happy as a father now p.12	Planned – something you want very much, you try and create it p.13. Planned and unplanned are similar to intended and unintended, but sound a bit more structured p.16, more focused p.17	Unintended – an accident, you didn't want or didn't consciously want. Intended – like planned p.16
109	Nervous about birth p.18	Doesn't really think of himself as a father yet p.13	Planned and unplanned – like intended and unintended p.20	Intended – you've planned for, actively tried to become pregnant. Unintended – pregnancy you weren't planning to have p.19 – doesn't include not using contraception p.20 (those are intended)

(Continued)

Charting involves rearranging the data within themes so that it can be compared across the interviews and within each interview. Barrett and Wellings describe the fifth step, mapping and interpretation, as the crucial one in developing their analysis of the data, involving:

> Drawing diagrams to clarify ideas ... looking for associations between the concepts and women's characteristics (e.g., age, marital/partnership status), and discussing the meanings of what we found. (Barrett and Wellings 2002: 547)

Framework analysis provided an appropriate approach in a study where some of the research questions were predetermined. Thus, in order to explore whether women did or did not use particular terms spontaneously, how these compared with definitions that were prompted, and how the use of terms varied across the sample, it was helpful to arrange the data across charts by themes. Diagrams were a useful way of graphically illustrating findings, for instance by drawing circles of various sizes to illustrate how many women used particular definitions. By looking across the interviews, they are able to show the criteria by which women judge a pregnancy to be, for instance, 'planned' or 'unintended'.

Barrett and Wellings use a number of strategies to increase the credibility of their findings and the reliability and validity of the analysis. First, quotes from the interview transcripts are used as examples of particular definitions, so the reader can see how the interpretation is built on the data. There is enough detail (such as the point in the interview at which the extract occurs) to judge the context of women's accounts. Second, they use numerical counts (of, for instance, how many women in the sample applied particular terms to their own pregnancies). Third, they report 'deviant cases' and demonstrate how they can be accounted for within their explanations of the data. For instance, the majority of women who applied both the terms 'unplanned' or 'unintended' to their pregnancies reported (not surprisingly) in their interviews that they had neither planned nor intended their pregnancy. One exception is discussed in detail: a woman who reports that she had intended to become pregnant, but that the pregnancy itself was unplanned. Looking through the whole transcript, it was possible to see that this woman did not meet the criteria other women used to describe a pregnancy as 'planned'. Although, like most, she and her partner had agreed to try to conceive, and she had deliberately stopped taking contraception, but unlike others who used both the terms 'unplanned' and 'unintended', they had not made wider preparations for a birth.

In summary, one key finding was the way in which the term 'planned' was used. To merely have *intended* to become pregnant and stopped using contraception was not sufficient; women also used two other criteria: agreeing this decision with a partner, and making wider life preparations for a pregnancy. This suggests that a survey question such as 'Was your pregnancy planned?' might only elicit a positive response from those who met all four criteria, and many women who 'wanted' and 'intended' the pregnancy might not answer 'Yes', if they did not also meet the conditions of agreement with partner and preparation.

What moves framework analysis beyond a sophisticated thematic analysis is the final stage of looking at relationships between the codes. This is what is known as *mapping and interpretation*, so a key tactic is to use diagrams and tables to physically explore the relationships between the concepts and typologies developed from them, and associations between the concepts. In Case Study 8.2, Barrett and Wellings are able to explore the use of different terms within their sample, and look at the relationships between characteristics such as contraceptive use and how pregnancy is discussed. Framework analysis in general has an overt policy orientation, with an end point of developing practical strategies on the basis of analysis. In this case study, the qualitative study is used to inform the design of a survey, through the development of a valid measure of pregnancy intention.

Narrative analysis

The final style we consider is narrative analysis. This term covers a number of approaches to data analysis, but what they share is a focus on the ways in which we make sense of the world through stories. Narratives have come to the fore over the last decade or so in both medicine (Greenhalgh and Hurwitz 1998; Charon 2006) and social science (Chamberlayne et al. 2000; Andrews et al. 2008; Riessman 2008), in part arising from a recognition of the role stories have in health and healing, as ways through which we understand illness in the context of our lives, and through which healers come to understand, and offer therapy for, their patients. Charon (2006) also suggests that a focus on narratives in health and medicine acts as a counterpoint to what many experience as the growing bureaucratization of health care in many countries. Accounting for the explosion of interest in narrative in the social sciences, Riessman suggests a number of contributing factors, including the legacy of 'identity politics' movements such as those of feminism, post-colonialism and gender identity, in which the personal experience was politicized and thus became a legitimate object of social scrutiny, and the cultural Western preoccupation with identity in modern times, which has prioritized the notion of a reflexive self that can account for his or her own biography. Broader cultural shifts mirror these developments, with, for instance, the rise of interest in such genres as personal memoirs. An example of the importance of stories to healing is suggested in Case Study 6.2, which focuses on a conversation analysis of medical consultations which suggested that those which enabled the patient to tell their story were more likely to lead to patient-centred care. Here, and in much research from narrative traditions, the story is the *topic* of the analysis. Riessman (2008) suggests this as one of three ways in which the term 'narrative' can be used in analysis. The first is that narrative can be considered the practice of storytelling, that is, of organizing events in an order that is intended to be meaningful for a given audience. Second there are narrative data that can be used as the topic for analysis. Third, narrative can refer to the methods for analysing those data.

In terms of narrative as data, biographical research, for instance, focuses on the stories people tell of their own lives, and the relationships between their life-histories (the experiences they have had) and their life-stories (how these are presented in the present). The study of chronic illness in particular has generated a large qualitative research output, much of it focusing on the ways in which a diagnosis of chronic illness can act as a 'biographical disruption' (Bury 1982), in that sufferers have to reassess the story they tell of their past, present and future in order to make sense of the misfortune that has happened. A first way of approaching narrative as method is to focus on the structure of stories. One structural method widely used in narrative analysis has its roots in early work from Labov and Waletzky (1967), which has been 'rediscovered' in recent years by narrative analysts (Riessman 2008). Labov and Waletzky suggested that narratives are stories told in chronological sequence that contain six elements:

1 An *abstract*, which summarizes the story
2 *Background* information setting the context, cast list and so on to orientate the listener
3 The *complicating action* (such as 'Then I collapsed' or 'I was completely lost') and subsequent events ('I called an ambulance')
4 The *resolution* of what happened at the end of the sequence of events
5 The *evaluation*, or moral, of the study
6 A *coda* finishing it off ('So that's my story').

(see, for example, Wengraf 2001: 115–6)

How far this structure does typify all stories told is hotly debated. If narrators miss out a section, should we still call it a narrative? Are we imposing structure on data if we look explicitly for these elements? And how are structures like this universal, in terms of describing how all stories are told, in all cultures? At a pragmatic level, Labov and Waletzky's elements do capture a form many listeners and readers will be familiar with, in that we recognize when we are being told a story, and when it has got to the end. Analytically, it can be useful to look at how stories get told in interviews and also at when they don't, or at least when interviewees have not used familiar structures to present their accounts, although there are clearly limits to how a focus on structural elements can account for issues such as the partial and contested ways in which stories get told in practice, and the ways in which storytelling might be socially patterned, in that different people tell different kinds of stories (Patterson 2008).

Exploring the types, or genres, of stories that get told can also be analytically fruitful. In a study of people who had self-harmed in the past, but have now stopped self-harming, for instance, Sinclair and Green (2005) used the kinds of stories interviewees told to help make sense of their data. They used Arthur Frank's (1997) typology of narratives to look at the different ways that people accounted for their past self-harm. Frank suggested there are three types of narrative that are typical of illness stories: 'quest' narratives, narratives of 'resolution' and 'chaotic' narratives. In the study of those who had self-harmed, younger interviewees, when talking about the time in their life when they were self-harming, told their stories in dislocated ways, with many pauses and disjointed chronologies. These sections of narrative did not easily fit the structure of a typical narrative, above, but rather reflected their chaotic lives at the time being remembered. When discussing their lives in the present, the narrative style shifted, with descriptions of a clear break (such as leaving the family home, or having a baby) followed by increasing steps to autonomy, and a sense of purpose to their lives. These were characterized as 'chaos' and 'quest' narratives, respectively. In health research, then, narratives can be the topic of analysis, but can also be an analytical device, used to help understand what is going on in the data. We can use narratives in this way because we assume that much of the *meaning* of a narrative lies in the unconscious structures, conventions and norms that speakers use to tell their stories. The ways in which accounts are given, in interviews or other settings, follow cultural rules of meaning-sharing, and paying close attention to *how* these are used provides us with some access to the narrative rules that pertain to our topic, as well as to just the style in which interviewees relate experiences.

One theme of this chapter is the tension in analysis between representing the world views of participants in the research, and analysing the accounts they provide in order to explain something more general about the phenomena we research. In narrative analysis, approaches vary between these representative and analytical goals. In life-history approaches, there is often an explicit aim of representation. Viney and Bousfield (1991), for instance, in a study of stories told by people affected by HIV/AIDS, begin by stating:

> We need ... to develop research methods which are both more respectful and more representative of our research participants ... narrative analysis may help us to achieve these goals. (Viney and Bousfield 1991: 757)

They conclude that the narrative analysis did enable them to treat accounts of their participants with respect, in 'undistorted' ways, but that in terms of detail, such as how much consistency different listeners had to what the core narrative themes were, or how to categorize elements of the narratives, the method lacked reliability. One implication of this is that structures such as Labov and

Waletzky's elements are a useful analytical device, but perhaps should not be seen as the output of an analysis.

At the other end of the representation–analysis spectrum, there are approaches to narrative analysis that draw more on traditions in literary theory, discourse analysis and semiotics (the study of signs). Here, the aim is not to preserve the narrative coherence of the account, but rather to analyse that account to explore what it can tell us about some other phenomena. Narrative analysis, then, does not describe a particular approach to qualitative analysis, but is usually used to suggest that the topic of interest is stories, and how they get told. These can be analysed from a number of epistemological traditions, from life-histories which stay close to the story as told by the narrator, through to more interpretative traditions (see Denzin 1989a) and those drawing on discourse analysis.

Using computer software to help manage data

Whatever approach, or mixture of approaches, is used, analysis requires considerable work, both mundane (transcribing and coding data) and more creative (thinking about categories). This can be very time consuming. We have already mentioned that word processors have made some tasks more efficient. The ability to 'cut and paste' electronically between documents, insert automatic line numbering and search for words or phrases are tasks that most word processors can do, and software available on most home computers can assist in the efficient management of qualitative research (Hahn 2008). Computer Assisted Qualitative Data Analysis, or **CAQDAS,** now covers a range of considerably more sophisticated packages specifically designed to assist those doing qualitative research (Bazeley 2007; Lewins and Silver 2007). Available packages and their capabilities change so rapidly that individual descriptions would quickly date, so it is advisable to use Internet sites to access details about available software. A good starting point is the CAQDAS networking project website at www.caqdas.soc.surrey.ac.uk/. This has links to websites for various packages, a useful bibliography of articles and other resources, and links to discussion groups. Early packages were of three main types (Fielding 1994):

- Those that retrieve particular kinds of text, such as searching for particular words or strings. These are useful for content analysis.
- Those that retrieve user defined codes. These take over some of the 'cutting and pasting' work of collecting together instances of particular codes.
- Those that are designed to aid with theory-building, which allow you to build links between codes and map emerging models of the relationships.

To some extent, these distinctions are blurring with every new version of each package, as the functions they perform become more sophisticated and extensive. However, there are still differences in how various packages work, reflecting the background disciplines and theoretical interests of their developers. Some, for instance, have been developed by those working in grounded theory traditions, with structures that reflect some of the elements of this approach, such as working with segments of text, connecting to memos and the ability to build up networks of codes. At the time of writing, some of the packages used by colleagues include The Ethnograph; ATLAS/ti; the QSR (Qualitative Solutions Research) stable of packages, including N7 (a development of NUD*IST) and NVivo; and QUALRUS. None of these are intrinsically 'better' than the others, and there is no answer to whether analysis is best done with the aid of CAQDAS. However, there are a number of issues to consider in deciding whether to use software to help, and if so, which package might suit the project needs.

Do I need to use CAQDAS?

The advantages of using these packages to assist with your analysis are:

- With large projects, having all the data and analysis in one place (or at least indexed in one place) aids management. Large numbers of paper transcripts and word-processor files can quickly become difficult to organize and manage.
- Analysis can be more *thorough* and systematic than if done by hand. If the whole data set has been coded, searches for segments relating to codes will produce all relevant data, rather than just those excerpts that the researcher has noticed.
- Your analysis will have greater *transparency*, as there is a record of how coding schemes were developed and theoretical concepts emerged through recorded memos.
- On large or multi-site projects, using (some) software can facilitate the transfer of data files, emerging coding schemes and research memos. This allows the whole team to contribute to analysis more easily, and in consistent ways.

However, there may be drawbacks. The first is the obvious one: none of these packages will do your analysis for you. They will help you to manage and retrieve data in more or less sophisticated ways, but the user still has to do the most difficult tasks of developing a coding scheme and coding the data. As Gibbs points out, 'code and attribute searching is only as good as your coding or assignment of attributes ...' (2007: 140). The advantage of 'thoroughness' clearly relies on the thoroughness of the original coding, and how useful this thoroughness is relies on the sophistication of the development of the coding scheme. There are also some practical disadvantages of using CAQDAS:

- It can be time intensive to prepare and code your data. Many packages have specific requirements for documents, and it is not always possible to directly import word processor files.
- It can take considerable time to learn a package for the first time, and it is expensive to buy licences for your own use.
- If your analysis will be reliant on looking at the minutiae of interaction, such as the pauses, stresses and tone of everyday talk, most packages will not be able to handle the transcribing requirements of conversation analysis. Formatting such as underlining or bold is often eliminated, and packages may require punctuation such as full stops to mark section breaks.

- Some researchers consider that CAQDAS loses the 'closeness' to the data they feel when working directly with transcripts or notes, although most packages now enable you to move more easily between original data and codes.

The final point relates to the type of analysis the research requires. Many of the available CAQDAS packages are built around a grounded theory approach, geared more towards the systematic analysis of segments of text. For those more comfortable with narrative styles of analysis, it may not be particularly useful to move away from an analysis based on the whole text. Deciding whether you are going to use CAQDAS is, then, a matter of considering your own needs and abilities (do you learn new technologies relatively quickly? Is this a skill that will be useful in future?), the needs of the particular project you are working on and the support you have (are there other researchers at your institution working with CAQDAS, who can help as you learn?).

Which package should I use?

All packages will do the basic tasks needed to help with your analysis. They enable you to code text, and retrieve segments coded, and search for words (and possibly words in particular positions relative to other words or codes). They all allow you to create 'attributes' for either your documents (such as gender, age or occupation for each respondent's transcript) or for coded sections of document, which enables more refined searching for codes. All work with a 'project' (called a 'hermeneutic unit' in Atlas.ti), which contains: either the documents as part of the database or links to documents which are stored elsewhere; coding, memos and any mappings created. Those packages which contain all the material within the 'project' (such as NVivo7), rather than linking to documents stored externally, make it easier to move an entire project to another computer. All will allow you to use plain text files (with no formatting), and some will work with documents in Rich Text Format (with minimal formatting) or some word processors. The Ethnograph will use any word processor files. Increasingly, packages also allow you to link to or directly code data in other formats, such as pictures or video, although some only offer minimal linking. HyperRESEARCH is a package designed particularly for use with different media, and this allows the coding of audio and visual data as well as text.

   Some of the things you may want to consider when choosing a package are: how the codes are displayed on screen (for instance, if you can see them in the margins); whether you can directly edit documents once they have been entered into the project; how much work it will take to prepare transcripts in a way that will work with the program; whether you can attach multiple codes to the same piece or overlapping pieces of text; whether you can include annotations or hyperlinks to your data and how the results of your searches are displayed. Once you have selected a particular package, try it out at the beginning of your project to make sure you produce the data (fieldnotes, or transcripts) in a compatible format, in terms of line lengths, line breaks between speakers or paragraphs, using consistent speaker identifiers, and the level of text formatting the packages can cope with.

The choice of package is made easier if you are working in an institution that already supports one. The advantages of an existing licence, other researchers who have experience with the package, and hopefully on-site training courses, will almost certainly make up for any differences in function between the one available and others. If, however, you have to choose a new package, it is worth exploring the links on the CAQDAS networking site to look at both the commercial manufacturers' descriptions of their products, test versions where they are available, and read the comments of other users on electronic noticeboards.

In summary, computer packages do not 'do analysis', but they can help both to manage data and allow you to retrieve these quickly. This can help facilitate rigorous, thorough analysis. They are particularly useful if you have a large amount of data to manage, and also perhaps if you are working with a team of people who will need to use the data set and need a high level of transparency about coding frames and the process of analysis. However, there are some costs in terms of the time needed to learn to use the software, and to prepare and code data.

Improving rigour in analysis

The different styles of analysis outlined above emphasize different elements of the process, but there are a number of general principles that apply to most qualitative research. These are the kinds of 'good practice' guidelines that will add credibility to your analysis, and increase faith in its reliability and validity. The criteria that typify rigorous analysis are summarized in Box 8.2.

Box 8.2	Some features of rigorous qualitative analysis	
Criteria	**Possible methods**	
Transparent	Provide a clear account of procedures used Keep an 'audit trail' that others could follow	
Maximizes validity	Provide evidence from the data for each interpretation you make Analysis of deviant cases and disconfirming data Including enough context for the reader to judge interpretation	
Maximizes reliability	Comprehensive analysis of the whole data set Using more than one analyst/coder Simple frequency counts of key themes	
Comparative	Compare data between and within cases in the data set Compare findings to other studies	
Reflexive	Account for the role of the researcher in the research	

Transparency

Transparency relates to the explicitness of the methods used, and how clearly they are outlined for the reader in research reports. This is perhaps a particularly important criterion when writing for audiences who may be unused to qualitative methods, such as biomedical journal readerships, or colleagues from other disciplines. The key is to provide an honest and clear account of the actual procedures used for analysing the data, rather than attempting to impress with jargon such as 'used a grounded theory approach' if it wasn't used. This might include a short description of how coding categories were developed, with perhaps examples of how debates around concepts led to labels for codes, how the sample was chosen (e.g., **purposive sample**? **theoretical sample**?), and how extracts used in the report were selected.

Maximizes validity

The validity of an interpretation is the 'truth' of that interpretation. In qualitative work, the notion of validity can be problematic, as in the interpretative and constructionist traditions we are working with 'truths' that are socially situated, and rejecting a positivist idea of one fixed and essential truth. However, this does not mean that qualitative researchers can dispense with all considerations of validity. There may be multiple readings of any particular data set, but the researcher does have to justify why their particular analysis should be considered a credible and legitimate one. Attempts to maximize validity are a way of answering the reader who asks 'Why should I believe this?' and 'How do I know this isn't just the researcher's subjective interpretation?' One common charge against qualitative work is anecdotalism – the idea that the researcher has merely reported anecdotes from the field that have struck a chord in some way but that are not rigorously and systematically supported by analysis. A similar charge is that of exoticism, with the suggestion that only the 'juicy quotes' or the most interesting or outlandish examples have been reported. In some of the social science traditions, presenting a subjective interpretation would be a legitimate exercise, but when working in health, especially if the research is aiming to influence policy or practice, it is usually necessary to demonstrate that the interpretation does have some validity: that the researcher has not focused only on the exotic, or drawn exclusively from the data that confirm their presumptions.

There are a number of approaches to increasing faith in validity. The key one is an approach that deliberately attempts to 'test' emerging theory. The aim should be to look for disconfirming evidence (such as deviant cases) and account for them, rather than just trawling through the data for examples that illustrate the points you want to make.

Simple counts can increase the reader's faith in the validity of your interpretations, and defend against anecdotalism, in that they give some perspective on how common particular kinds of views or experiences were. For instance, in this report of the problems faced by single handed GPs, based on an interview study, Green includes counts to indicate how common particular problems were:

Seven single handed general practitioners mentioned problems with finding locum cover: one claimed not to have had a holiday for nine years. There were practical problems in finding reliable locums and coping financially, but some of the single handed doctors also felt unhappy about leaving 'their' practice in the hands of someone else … five … reported providing 24 hour cover themselves every day … (Green 1993a: 608)

It is not always appropriate to 'count' in this way, but some indication should be given about the typicality of, for instance, observations or particular accounts and how they have been selected from the entire data set.

Providing enough context for the reader to judge interpretations is another way of increasing credibility. Depending on the nature of the study, this could include: the interviewer's prompts, details of the research setting, the history of the research project itself, or the interactions within which the 'quote' used was observed.

Respondent validation (sometimes called *member validation* or *member checking*) is one method sometimes suggested as a 'validity check'. This involves taking the findings back to the participants, and ensuring that they agree. Here, the assumption is perhaps that the aim of qualitative analysis is to achieve an 'emic' understanding (see Chapter 6), and that the ultimate mark of credibility is that the researchers' and the insiders' accounts tally. There are some good reasons to feed back findings to participants: it is good manners to inform those who contributed to the study what you found; there may be issues of confidentiality you need to check; participants may want to ensure that any reports are not going to damage their interests; participants may want to make corrections in, for instance, quoted material or examples (a reliability check); their comments on your analysis are an excellent source of further data. However, if the aims of the research are anything more than those of merely *reporting* participants' accounts of the world, respondent validation is a rather questionable exercise as a way of ensuring validity. First, the analysis might have to account for participants' views in the context of both contradictions and conflicts within a group of participants, and perhaps between them and others. More fundamentally, respondent validation presupposes a 'true' picture of the world, with which we can have more faith if two accounts (those of the researcher and the participants) coincide. Within qualitative traditions, this positivist position is rather untenable: there is no reason to suppose participants (or a group of them) are likely to analyse their own accounts in the same ways as a researcher.

Maximizes reliability

Reliability relates to the 'repeatability' of interpretation. In qualitative work, this is often interpreted as the likelihood that a similar piece of research would elicit similar kinds of themes. This kind of reliability is especially important if the research project has more than one person coding or analysing the data. However, one would not necessarily expect any two researchers to identify the same themes or codes in the data, as this depends to some extent on the analyst's interests, knowledge, theoretical approach and, ultimately, their epistemological framework. However, attention to reliability does ensure that whatever interpretation is followed through is credible, and the rationale for the codes and themes is identifiable. Ways of improving reliability include close attention to 'good practice' in fieldwork, including accurate note taking and transcriptions and discussing your coding with colleagues. In published papers, the credibility of your analysis is improved by including raw data, so the reader can assess how reliable your interpretations are, and demonstrating how data are linked to interpretation.

Comparative

Comparison is what drives qualitative analysis. Comparing cases within the same data set allows us to look for regularities in the data (key themes), exceptions to these and to build typologies. Comparing data within a case allows us explore the contextual meaning of accounts. For instance, in a study of people's accounts of accident risks, Green (1997) found that in many interview and focus group transcripts, respondents made very different claims about what an accident was in early responses to a direct question from the ones made later in the interviews when discussing their own experiences. Early in the interviews, respondents came up with 'ideal type' definitions of accidents (such as 'an injury no one meant to happen that wasn't anyone's fault') whereas in the context of discussing actual experiences of accidental injury they suggested definitions that utilized both intention and fault. Comparing instances across one case in the data set allowed an analysis of how such definitions were used in practice, and why.

Comparison also enables theoretical analysis to develop, as data are constantly compared with the emerging theory as they are generated. Comparing new analyses to the provisional theories and 'hunches' from preceding analyses allows the researcher to refine the emerging theory and amend it. Finally, good analysis also involves a comparison of the findings with other findings from the field. This does not necessarily just include findings related to the substantive topic of interest, but from the more general social science literature that relates theoretically to the issue.

Reflexive

Reflexivity was introduced in Chapter 1 as an essential orientation of qualitative research. It refers to the recognition that the researcher is part of the process of producing the data and their meanings, and to a conscious reflection on that process. In positivist approaches, the researcher is ideally invisible: the aim is to remove the potential biases that an individual brings to data collection and analysis, such that the data are 'pure' and untainted by social values. In most qualitative traditions, an alternative strategy is to account explicitly for subjectivity, in exploring how the context had an impact on the research and the data arising from it. In Chapters 4 and 5 we discussed in some detail how the researcher should account for the interplay between their presence, the research context and the data produced.

In practice, the term 'reflexivity' is used in a range of ways in reports of qualitative analysis. Perhaps least useful are routine statements of the sort 'As a white, European woman I was aware of how my status had an impact on my interviews with men in a Nigerian village'. Such statements tell us nothing about how the social roles of the interviewer and the participants were constructed within the research, or how these shaped the study. At the other end of the scale are intensely personal accounts of fieldwork in which the researcher is telling their story, rather than that of the research itself. Clive Seale (1999: 160–1) cautions against this more 'confessional' style of reflexivity, in which the researcher presents themselves as somehow, through a series of blunders and self-searching, achieving a true insider status. These are, he argues, more like rhetorical claims to authenticity rather than necessarily evidence of methodological awareness. He also notes (1999: 164) the limits of reflexivity, in that we cannot of course be aware of all the subconscious ways in which our assumptions shape our approaches to research.

Between the two extremes of routine triviality and research as self-exploration are, though, some 'good practice' approaches that demonstrate a reflexive awareness of the research process and increase the rigour of analysis. Some suggestions for developing a reflexive awareness might include:

- *Methodological openness.* Being explicit about the steps taken in the data production and analysis, the decisions made, and the alternatives not pursued.
- *Theoretical openness.* The theoretical starting points and assumptions made should be addressed, and the ways in which they shaped the study accounted for.
- *Awareness of the social setting of the research itself.* In interviews, or participatory fieldwork, the 'data' are largely the results of interactions between the researcher and the researched. Reflexivity requires a constant awareness of this, and the ways in which the data result from these particular interactions.
- *Awareness of the wider social context.* This might include awareness of how political and social values have both made possible the research (in whose interests is it funded?) and constrained it, and how the historical and policy contexts shape the data.

These are, at one level, a courtesy to the reader, who can then judge the findings presented in terms of the context for themselves. Beyond that, though, these are essential to thorough analysis, in that they are ways of taking seriously the elements of a qualitative approach outlined in Chapter 1.

Rigour is not enough ...

Addressing these elements of transparency, validity, reliability, comparison, and reflexivity will help produce credible analysis that is less likely to leave a sceptical reader asking 'How do I know this is not just your subjective interpretation?'

However, to return to the initial discussion about imagination as well as technical skills, rigour is not enough. To begin with, the data have to support detailed analysis. However thorough and rigorous the analysis, if the data consist of nothing more than notes of brief interviews, or comments on a questionnaire, it will be difficult to generate much of explanatory power. From her perspective as a journal editor, Janice Morse (2002) complains of the dangers of 'thin' data, such as those derived from semi-structured interviews or notes written under the 'Any other comments?' section of a questionnaire, which are then categorized as 'themes' and reported with no links to theory. The resulting analysis, Morse suggests, is inevitably 'shallow and trivial', with none of the rich descriptive narrative that would characterize good qualitative analysis. So, a precondition of good analysis is, inevitably, good data.

Second, however thorough the analysis, if it remains at the level of superficially attaching 'codes' derived from interviewees' own accounts, with little attempt to integrate these into existing theory, or to look for connections within the data, the result will look 'under-analysed' and rather trivial. This may suffice if working in a new field, or with participants whose voices are rarely heard, in which case simply reporting views is the aim in itself. However, this does not quite count as 'qualitative analysis'. The key to producing insightful, satisfying accounts of 'what is going on' in your data is to bring a social science imagination to bear: to identify connections both within the data and between them and the world outside. This is far harder to achieve than simply analysing in a rigorous and systematic way, and it is perhaps impossible to be prescriptive about how to achieve satisfying as well as rigorous analysis. However, there are ways of increasing the depth of your data analysis, and some suggestions for developing an imaginative approach are:

• Read and discuss widely – not just within your own topic and discipline, but from other disciplines, to look for connections and transferable concepts.
• Ask constantly about the context of the data: think about them in terms of historical, political, social and cultural contexts.
• Return frequently to the theoretical assumptions embedded in your research question (see Chapter 2): challenge them, think about how different assumptions might provide a fresh look at what is going on.
• Interrogate your data with colleagues: other people will have a different reading of your data, and may challenge your common-sense accounts of what is going on. Equally, helping others with their data analysis can help encourage a more imaginative approach to your own.

Generalizability and transferability

A final issue in qualitative analysis is that of generalizability. Generalizability refers to the extent to which findings from a study apply to a wider population or to different contexts. In a sample survey, random sampling allows generalizability through the principle that the study sample is likely to be statistically representative of the larger population of interest, so findings can be extrapolated to that population. In qualitative work, study participants are rarely randomly sampled in this way, and the logic of generalizability is rather different. Some argue that it is not an issue in qualitative work, which properly aims to provide 'thick' description, or to address particularities, rather than to provide 'typical' accounts or generalizable findings. There are, however, two reasons why researchers in the field of health do have to address this issue. First, if researchers are to make claims to their findings being useful, at whatever level, to health practice, they do have to consider the theoretical import of their findings: the extent to which they refer to some setting or population wider than that of the research itself. Second, and more pragmatically, the credibility of qualitative findings in non-social science fields is often fragile, and qualitative research is easily marginalized as 'interesting, but not research evidence' because the generalizablity is questionable. Addressing these concerns does not mean adopting, or even adapting, the procedures of quantitative approaches and attempting to imitate the kinds of random samples drawn, or comparing the study population to wider ones. Instead, it involves thinking through what *kind of relationship* the study findings have to other populations and settings, and unpacking exactly what inferences can be drawn from the data analysis.

Essentially, though, these all refer to the same question that generalizabiltity addresses in quantitative work, namely, how far can the findings of this particular study be extrapolated? There are various ways in which findings from qualitative work can be supported as more widely relevant. These include the following.

Sensitizing concepts

If researching relatively under-researched topics, or respondents, the issue of generalizability may be less salient that that of 'sensitizing' readers to new ways of thinking, or the potential views of respondents. In Case Study 1.1, in Chapter 1, for instance, the researchers found that many of the 'asthma' patients they interviewed did not believe they had asthma. At one level, it doesn't matter how representative their sample was of the whole population: the key point is that practitioners are sensitized to the fact that *some* patients may not accept the diagnosis. At a more theoretical level, qualitative studies may generate concepts that are 'good to think with', and thus will have a utility beyond their immediate research setting in sensitizing other researchers to useful concepts. Case Study 1.1 made use of the concept of 'stigma', from Erving Goffman's (1963) work on the impact of stigmatizing attributes on social interaction. In Goffman's original study, it perhaps matters little how far his data are representative of the population, or whether the findings can be generalized in an empirical sense: what matters is the theoretical usefulness of the concepts (such as stigma) he developed, which have been used widely in qualitative research. This suggests that the most appropriate way of thinking about generalizability in qualitative work is in terms of *conceptual generalizability*.

Conceptual generalizability

The key elements that are generalizable from qualitative analysis may not be the narrow findings, but the concepts, that is, the ways of thinking about or 'making sense' of the world. These concepts, whether at macro or 'middle' level (see Chapter 2) might inform our understanding of similar contexts or issues. Goffman's work on stigma is an obvious example from the 'classic' literature in medical sociology, but this also applies to more recent and more applied work. For example, in Chapter 1, one of the examples of qualitative research studies cited in Box 1.1 was Joseph Opala and Francois Boillot's ethnographic study of traditional beliefs about leprosy among the Limba. Here, the question of generalizability is not 'How far are the beliefs they identified typical of other groups, or the whole population of Sierra Leone?' but rather, 'How far do these findings help us understand what is going on when in situations where biomedicine meets traditional beliefs?' As Opala and Boillot (1996) note, workers in the field of leprosy are interested in studies of traditional beliefs, as they recognize that effective health care can only be provided when the user's perspective is taken into account. The 'generalizable' findings of Opala and Boillot are that to do this adequately relies on a detailed understanding of not just beliefs about leprosy, but also an understanding of the world view of which these beliefs form a part. In their study, which explored why different groups of Limba had different attitudes to the stigma of leprosy, they found that there were considerable variations in terms of views of traditional and biomedical treatments and when to take medicines. The specifics of beliefs about medications are not generalizable, but the *concept* that there are local variations – and these are important for health care workers to identify – is. Similarly, they found a number of misconceptions that medical workers held about local beliefs. These included the idea that local people believed leprosy was caused by eating one's totem, or that the majority used traditional medicines. Neither of these beliefs were supported by the research evidence, and 'counter' non-existent beliefs in health promotion messages might well be counter-productive. Again, these specific misconceptions may not be generalizable, but the general point (that we should focus on medical workers' ideas of lay health beliefs, as well as the health beliefs themselves), is.

Transferability

Here, the question is, 'To what extent are these findings transferable to other settings?' This is what the practitioner or policy maker reading your report is going to want to know: is this something I can apply to my clinic, or my patients, or my country? Answering this question relies on thinking through what is context specific and what might be more widely applicable within the findings. To return to Opala and Boillot's (1996) study, they also discuss the **transferability** of their recommendations. Opala and Boillot are able to draw out a transferable strategy for shaping health promotion messages, involving identifying medical workers' misconceptions about local beliefs; focusing on the differences between local and medical beliefs and using indigenous knowledge to provide analogies to use in health promotion.

Conclusion

Qualitative researchers working in the field of health have to pay rather more attention to the mechanics of data analysis than has perhaps been traditional in mainstream social science disciplines. This has had some benefits, not least in generating discussion around how we demonstrate the credibility of our interpretations, and ensure that analysis is done rigorously and thoroughly. However, we have also suggested that the application of practical techniques is not sufficient for producing insightful and useful qualitative findings. Researchers also have to ground their analyses in a broad ranging understanding of theoretical and other empirical work in their discipline in order to bring a 'social science' imagination to their own data.

KEY POINTS

- To provide credible findings for health, qualitative researchers need to address questions of reliability, validity and generalizability.
- There are a number of approaches to analysis, and in practice most researchers will use a pragmatic mix of techniques.
- Whatever style of analysis is adopted, it is important to be explicit about the methods used and rigorous in their application.
- Moving beyond merely descriptive accounts of data entails an imaginative as well as a rigorous approach to data analysis.

EXERCISES

1   Take an example of published qualitative work, and consider whether you found the report credible and interesting. Then identify what techniques the authors have used in their analysis that contributed to your answer: did they provide context, were they transparent about the methods used, were they reflexive?

2   The only way to develop skills in analysis is to practise doing it. This exercise requires a short extract from an interview transcript. If you don't have any data of your own, ask colleagues for an extract (suitably anonymized) to use. Take two or three pages, and first identify any 'themes' that might summarize what the interviewee is reporting. Code the text by 'marking it up' in the margins, with each theme labelled as a code.
    Next, try 'open coding' the extract, using the techniques of grounded theory introduced in this chapter.

(Continued)

Ask a series of questions about each line of the data: what is going on here? How can we label that as a provisional concept? Are there any in vivo codes? What are the properties and dimensions of the concepts that are emerging? Draw on your experience and reading to provide comparisons for each provisional concept, to aid this process. If possible, do this exercise in a group with colleagues. Compare your original list of themes with the provisional list of concepts generated by the open coding exercise.

FURTHER READING

Miles, M.B. and Huberman, A.M. (1994) *Qualitative data analysis: an expanded sourcebook* (2nd edn). Thousand Oaks, CA: Sage. Full of practical suggestions for organizing, analysing and presenting qualitative data. Miles and Huberman have a pragmatic approach which uses a range of methods for coding, comparing cases and thinking about the relationships in your data. Many of these are graphic, using data matrices to sort and display data.

Silverman, D. (2001) *Interpreting qualitative data: methods of analysing talk, text and interaction* (2nd edn). London: Sage. Silverman situates his introduction to methods for analysing various types of qualitative data within a theoretical discussion of the logic of qualitative enquiry, but this is a very accessible text for students, which addresses the detailed analysis of observational data such as consultations, texts and visual data as well as interview transcripts.

Strauss, A. (1987) *Qualitative analysis for social scientists*. Cambridge: Cambridge University Press. Detailed account of the principles of grounded theory, quoting extensively from Glaser and Strauss's (1967) book *The discovery of grounded theory*. This has extended examples taken from student and research team seminars on coding and analysis, taking the reader through common problems faced by researchers. Essential reading for anyone planning on developing skills in the grounded theory approach.

Part 3

Doing Qualitative Work for Health

Qualitative Research in Practice: Settings and Contexts

9

CHAPTER SUMMARY

Qualitative health research is conducted across a range of settings, from the small stand-alone study carried out as a student project, through to large international programmes conducted alongside health care trials. Qualitative methods are increasingly used in applied health research, where utilizing qualitative methodology does raise some challenges. We suggest these challenges necessitate close attention to the nature of collaboration, and that good communication with colleagues from other disciplines, from health care practice and policy and from the communities participating in the research, is essential. The aims and approaches of these various stakeholders may be very different. This chapter considers the opportunities and challenges of doing qualitative research in the context of these collaborations, particularly in applied settings.

Introduction

The methods of data generation and analysis discussed in Part 2 of this book are those typically considered part of the 'tool box' of qualitative methodology. We suggested in Chapter 1 that the principles of using these methods apply whatever the context of the study. However, the practicalities of actually doing qualitative research will vary, depending on whether the qualitative work is a stand-alone project or part of a larger programme, and on such issues as how much control the researcher has over the aims and conduct of the study. This chapter is concerned with using qualitative methods in applied settings, when the methods of data generation and analysis may be qualitative, but there may be constraints on how far the orientations of qualitative methodology introduced in Chapter 1 (naturalism, a focus on meaning, flexible research strategies) can be adopted. One focus of this chapter is on collaboration, because in practice actually *doing* qualitative research usually entails working with others, including research commissioners, participants, those from other disciplines and professionals who may be properly focused on other goals than those of the researcher. In general, the focus in applied studies may be on the *findings* of qualitative methods, rather than on the insights that a qualitative methodology might bring to the project.

'Pure' and applied research

A distinction is often made between 'pure' and 'applied' research. 'Pure' research, or basic research, is usually considered to be orientated towards a researcher's own interests, or problems that are generated from within a discipline. Research in anthropology or sociology that is focused on understanding health behaviour or beliefs, but with no explicit aim of improving practice or changing behaviour, could be considered 'pure' research. Of course, many of these studies do later contribute to improvements in health care, but their initial aim is one of 'understanding' rather than making a contribution to practice. In contrast, 'applied' research begins with a problem rooted in practice: how well something works, or what the needs for an intervention are, for instance.

Moira Kelly (2004) usefully outlines some of the issues of doing qualitative evaluations, as one example of applied research. The key distinction between basic and applied evaluation research for Kelly is its *context*: evaluations are instigated to address a practical problem, with the aim of 'appraising human activities in a formal, systematic way' (2004: 523). Although the methods used in evaluations may be the same as those used in basic research, the commissioners, or funders, are likely to have a greater interest in the study, with tighter control over how it is conducted. In terms of the orientations towards qualitative methodologies introduced in Chapter 1, there are clearly potential tensions. If the strengths of qualitative methodology include a flexibility of design and the ability to challenge common-sense understandings of the world, these may not be welcome in a tightly controlled evaluation, in which the funders, not unreasonably, would like a clear answer to a predetermined question or firm recommendations that focus on improving practice, rather than the rather more open and contingent reflections that might be typical of less applied research. Kelly (2004) notes that we can overstate the distinctions between pure and applied research. Increasingly, she argues, qualitative evaluations are theoretically informed, and many funders are keen to exploit the strengths of qualitative methodology (including a detailed understanding of context, and the contribution to 'asking the right question') as well as merely using qualitative methods of data collection. Similarly, funders of 'pure' research are increasingly asking for researchers to address the likely usefulness of that work for users, such as practitioners and the public. However, although the literature is full of examples of how qualitative methods contribute to applied programmes, there are also a number of published accounts of the tensions that arise in practice from the different imperatives that guide more applied work.

Sacrificing depth for speed

Applied research typically requires rather more condensed timeframes than those of pure research. In Chapter 6, we introduced the debate around rapid ethnographic methods, which is one illustration of the potential challenges that can arise in doing qualitative methods in applied health settings, particularly where there is a public health need for rapid results to inform practice. Examples might include the need to plan a condom distribution service, or the need to undertake rapid needs assessment in a disaster situation. The non-governmental organization *Medecins Sans Frontieres* (MSF), for instance, suggests that its staff might be using qualitative methods to look at people's beliefs and behaviours around hygiene before planning a hand-washing campaign in a refugee camp, or to collect narrative accounts from displaced persons to assist with planning or campaigning (Brikci and Green 2007). In these situations, the need is for empirical findings in the shortest possible time, rather than theoretical understanding. When the staff of organizations such as MSF are engaged in this kind of work, there may well be few challenges, methodologically, in using qualitative methods of data collection in relatively time-limited contexts. When anthropologists or sociologists are hired to conduct qualitative studies around similar issues, the trade-offs between the kind of depth usually prioritized in qualitative methodology and the needs for quick results may be more problematic. Helen Lambert (1998) notes that social scientists are often brought in to explain the failure of health projects and that, increasingly, medical anthropologists have been included in international health programmes around issues such as malaria, tuberculosis control, HIV/AIDS and diarrhoeal disease (see Case Studies 1.2, 2.2, 6.1 and 9.1 in this volume for examples). In developing methods for the rapid generation of focused data, in contrast to the more discursive and interpretative traditions of classic anthropology, argues Lambert, we have lost much of what was valuable about the anthropological approach. Often, anthropological studies will provide considerable insight into the contextual nature of health care decision making and therapeutic choices. In practice, people's decisions may well be shaped as much by local situational constraints as by the cultural models that can be generated through the focused interviews and mappings of rapid assessment. Lambert argues that what we lose through the rapidity of much applied anthropology, and its excessive focus on data collection methods, rather than an anthropological perspective, is any real understanding of how such choices are made, because such understandings can be impossible for people to articulate in the abstract. She concludes:

> The danger of 'rapid anthropological assessment' as currently practised is that it may produce findings which are quick, practical – and wrong. (Lambert 1998: 1009)

This conflict between the need for findings to inform practice in the shortest possible time and the risk that such findings are inadequate for informing policy because they are thin at best, and possibly misleading, is one familiar to many qualitative researchers working for practice and policy-orientated commissioners. Throughout this book we have stressed that applied work does need to be rigorous, thorough and informed by theory, but in practice, there may well be compromises in how far a properly qualitative approach can be adopted.

Research or development?

One potential strategy for dealing with the risk of thin (and possibly wrong) findings from rapid methods is the use of participatory approaches. Some have rejected the accusation that rapidly produced data are inevitably less valid, arguing that the foundation for producing findings of high quality is establishing a rapport and a good relationship with the community who are participating in the research. Robert Chambers (1994), for instance, provides several examples of participatory appraisals which have generated valid information, by which he means information which has not been contradicted by other research, or is of more depth than that previously gained. The first essential, he argues, is establishing good relationships between the 'outsiders' and the community at the start of the project:

> ... if the initial behavior and attitudes of the outsiders are relaxed and right, and if the process can start, the methods of [participatory rural appraisal] themselves foster further rapport. Early actions by outsiders can include transparent honesty about who they are and what they are doing; and participation in local activities ... Personal demeanor counts, showing humility, respect, patience and interest in what people have to say and show ... (Chambers 1994: 1256)

The second essential component is the use of what could be called a properly qualitative approach: asking open questions, which genuinely attempt to understand the perspectives of participants, and focusing on what local people do know about their area, its problems, and the potential solutions. Chambers' account of the gains of using participatory methods is one which will resonate with those who have had successes, in terms of the rapid learning that comes from opening up to others' knowledge for the 'outsiders' and the sense of empowerment for communities, when that knowledge is genuinely respected and used to stimulate change. For Chambers, what distinguishes participatory appraisal is the aim: that of empowerment, in contrast to traditional anthropology, where the aim is research. In situations where the primary aim, for the researcher, is research, this development setting may raise difficult issues of how far, realistically, the aims and needs of a community can be addressed within the scope of a project.

This raises a tension we alluded to in Chapter 3 on the ethical dilemmas of doing 'action' research, or participatory research. This is the challenge of ensuring that participatory projects are not compromized methodologically by the need to include the perspectives of all of those who participate in the project. Although in development projects, especially those from within a participatory approach, there is a focus on the knowledge and skills of participants and their lived experiences, it is unlikely that these skills are those of a professional researcher. If the primary aim is development, empowerment or an educational one of building skills in a community, shortcomings in the methodology may be unimportant. However, if the primary aim is to answer a research question, or provide knowledge that will be credible and convincing for policy makers, there may well be challenges.

An illustration comes from the work of Eliana Lacerda (2008), whose participatory epidemiology with shellfish harvesters was referred to in Chapter 5 as an example of community interviews in participatory work. Lacerda worked with the shellfish harvesters because they were concerned about the effect of polluted estuary water on their health. She needed a participatory design in order to work 'with' rather than 'on' the local women, but also wanted to conduct the best possible epidemiological study to answer the question about whether there were or were not effects on health from the pollution. In practice, she found the two aims in tension at a number of points. First, of course, the women's local knowledge was essential in designing a methodologically 'sound' study. Basic tasks such as defining both the population at risk (who counted as a shellfish harvester? Full-time workers, all those who ever went into the estuary?) and the outcome (the likely health effects of pollution) all required input from those who were experienced in the local economy and local health issues. Lacerda also found that the women who collaborated with her from the community had no problems understanding concepts such as bias and confounding, and indeed pre-empted various threats to the validity of her research. However, in designing a study – and conducting it in a way that collaborated with the women – she faced problems, with local women having different approaches to sampling and conducting the interviews than a more strictly 'scientific' study might have done. At one point, Lacerda notes (2008: 155) she became frustrated with the epidemiological component, considering that a more solid, traditional epidemiological design might have more clearly answered the question, perhaps using clinical examinations to record health outcomes rather than the more subjective survey interviews with local women. Such research would not only be more rigorous, it would also be more credible for agencies in a position to help the women, such as the local workers' associations or NGOs. These are perhaps inevitable problems in the politics of research with communities that have less power than the researcher. A traditional epidemiology study 'of' the women would have been impossible, for Lacerda would not have had their trust, or been able to learn from their experience. However, a participatory process inevitably had some costs in terms of methodological rigour.

The uncertain nature of qualitative findings

A final tension relates to the relatively open, and contingent, nature of the analysis and interpretations often generated by qualitative research. The strengths of qualitative research lie in their flexibility and in the potential for findings to unpack, or reframe, common-sense categories and assumptions. However, in many applied projects, there may be little interest in new ways of thinking about a topic, or in new questions, as there is an expectation that the researcher will stay tightly focused on the goals set out in the original protocol. Reflecting on 'doing ethnography' within a mixed method study of access to green space in the south-east of England, Ruth Pinder discusses her anxieties, as an anthropologist, at the end of a project that was rather more 'applied' than typical in anthropology.

> With a report in the offing and requests for soundbite recommendations in advance, it was clear that ... [the ethnographic findings] would not constitute proper research for policy-makers intent on wooing the Treasury with one-dimensional answers. I had introduced uncertainty – a more profound uncertainty than merely the lack of information – into the proceedings. (Pinder 2007: 113)

The ethnographer's aim is to produce a 'thick' description of social life, from the perspective of those in the field, whereas the commissioner's needs may be for clear answers to questions around the likely benefits of access to green space, or the barriers for people in accessing that space. The reflections and 'deep' descriptions produced by this kind of ethnography may not look like evaluation data that can easily be used by policy makers and practitioners.

Even when qualitative researchers do produce 'clear' findings, they may not mesh neatly with the needs of other parts of the project. Therese Riley and colleagues (Riley et al. 2005) discuss the contested nature of qualitative evidence within a community level intervention designed to provide support for mothers, in which the social science element was set up as a companion project to the original trial, with the intention that it would provide a theoretical input into the trial and describe the process of delivering the intervention. One area of contestation, they note, was around how to deal with qualitative data collected during the trial that could be used to improve its delivery, which was revealing a different picture to that gained by the trial organizers about how well the trial was progressing. They note that the 'status' of these data was questioned, given they were based on reports from those involved in running the trial, and seen as inferior evidence, and were therefore difficult to act on. This questioning of the validity and generalizability of qualitative findings is not uncommon when they conflict with those produced through other methods, and the difficulties of working across epistemological boundaries are discussed below.

These tensions are not insurmountable, and researchers on the whole will find ways of managing 'enough' depth, balancing the needs for development and research, or communicating as clearly as possible to commissioners the key implications of their findings. However, this does suggest that collaborative and communication skills are essential for doing applied work, given the need to work across what can be very different expectations of the research process and its likely outcomes. In practice, most research entails collaboration.

Collaboration

Academic research in all disciplines is increasingly likely to be a collaborative venture (Godin and Gingras 2000). Rather than working as a lone researcher, with sole responsibility for the research design, data collection, analysis and dissemination, qualitative researchers contributing to health research programmes will typically work as members of collaborative teams. These teams may be based in multidisciplinary departments, and many projects can span a number of collaborating institutions and perhaps countries. Researchers do not just collaborate with academics from other disciplines, but may also be developing partnerships with non-academics such as non-governmental organizations (NGOs) or health service providers. There are, in many countries, policies in place that actively promote various kinds of collaborative working, for instance those that encourage academic researchers to work with others in industrial and non-governmental sectors, and to work with the end-point users of the research findings, such as service providers and clients. There are certainly a number of incentives for researchers to work collaboratively. In a world of increasing information, and access to information, it is very difficult for the individual researcher to keep abreast even of developments in their own field, let alone those in related fields. Collaboration, in theory, increases the 'efficiency' of a research effort, through building information and dissemination networks. Working with users and those placed to implement findings can also increase the 'effectiveness' of a research, particularly for those working in policy- and practice-relevant areas. Planning research in collaboration with end-point users, rather than merely disseminating results to them at the end of a project, is perhaps more likely to ensure that research resonates with users' needs. There are also potential gains in terms of capacity-building, in that collaborations can help spread the skills and infrastructure needed to develop local research capacity, and can also raise wider awareness of and skills in qualitative methodologies.

However, collaboration of any kind brings a number of challenges. Most researchers will have learned their craft within a particular discipline, in a particular country, in which both formal and informal norms about research practice are acquired. Fundamental ideas about what research is for, and how we can produce valid knowledge, are closely tied to the kinds of epistemological orientations we introduced in Chapter 1, and those of qualitative research may not be shared by those trained in other traditions. The ways in which qualitative researchers address questions of research design, such as how to identify a credible sample, or what methods are appropriate for producing the data, may be unfamiliar to those more comfortable with more quantitative, positivist paradigms. The norms of 'good ethical practice', despite international guidelines, are to some extent locally specific, as we discussed in Chapter 3. Even expectations around how research protocols should be written are culturally shaped. There is some evidence, for instance, that deductive styles (in which the main point is introduced first, followed by information that supports it, or provides context) are preferred in Britain, whereas Asian writers feel more comfortable with inductive styles that lead up to the main point late in the protocol (Cortazzi and Jin 1997: 81).

Differences in research practice, epistemology or style are of course rarely neutral, and qualitative researchers can often face the challenge of having to 'defend' their approaches in institutions or programmes in which more positivist paradigms are the norm. Good working relationships across disciplinary, national or institutional boundaries cannot be assumed just because individual members of the team are enthusiastic about and committed to joint working. The experience of most researchers is that partnerships need considerable time and effort to develop. This is certainly true of large scale interventions, which are an increasingly common site of qualitative research, given the growing recognition of the importance of qualitative methods to evaluating the process of interventions as well as their effectiveness.

Qualitative research within interventions

In Chapter 2, we outlined some of the ways in which qualitative studies are used in conjunction with other research designs to build our understanding of health issues. In practice, much applied health research requires a number of different approaches to data collection within one study, especially if the study is supporting a public health intervention of some kind. If you look back at Case Study 1.2, for instance, quantitative methods were needed to address the *effectiveness* of the Kopana intervention (did it increase the number of TB treatments completed?) whereas qualitative methods were needed to explore *why* the intervention did or did not work. Typically, a mixed method approach to evaluating the intervention would involve using epidemiological methods to measure outcomes (such as disease incidence) and qualitative methods to explore the process and users' views of the intervention. The example in Case Study 9.1 illustrates this mixed methods approach in the context of a large programme of research on the effectiveness of microbicides, which are being developed to limit the spread of HIV.

This example of how qualitative methods are being used in one programme is perhaps typical of public health interventions that require both a range of data to support implementation, a flexibility in approaches to respond to the early stages of evaluation and qualitative data to provide detailed information on what might otherwise be the 'black box' of how the intervention actually works (or doesn't). The participatory evaluation of the Stepping Stones sexual health programme in The Gambia, described in Case Study 2.2, is another example of this kind of evaluation in a public health setting. These examples illustrate a model of interdisciplinary working in which different methods are used to address specific research questions raised by the study, and the skills of a multi-disciplinary team are brought in as 'experts' in the particular methodological approaches needed. Ideally, findings from each component of the programme inform each other as it progresses.

Using multiple methods within the same project is, then, common-sense good practice if the study addresses a number of distinct research questions, for which different methodological approaches are implicated. In some cases, the qualitative component may be to all practical purposes a 'stand-alone' project, with its own management and methods, and the process separate from other projects within the study. However, most multi-disciplinary projects aim to gain 'added value' from including a number of components, in the hope that the findings from each will feed into a broader understanding of the topic studied, or increase the validity of the findings from all contributing studies.

Case Study 9.1   Qualitative methods within large programmes: the example of the Microbicide Development Programme

(Sources: Montgomery, C.M., Lees, S., Stadler, J., Morar, N.S., Ssali, A., Mwanaza, B., Mntambo, M., Phillip, J., Watts, C. and Pool, R. (2008) 'The role of partnership dynamics in determining the acceptability of condoms and microbicides', *AIDS Care,* 20: 733–740.

Stadler, J. Delaney, S. and Mntambo, M. (2008) 'Women's perceptions and experiences of HIV prevention trials in Soweto, South Africa', *Social Science & Medicine,* 66: 189–200)

The Microbicide Development Programme is an international partnership set up to evaluate and test vaginal microbicides to prevent HIV transmission. MDP301 is a large, randomized, double-blind, placebo controlled trial of the microbicide gel PRO 2000/5, designed to prevent vaginally-acquired HIV infection. The trial intends to recruit around 9,000 participants from six sites located in South Africa, Zambia, Uganda and Tanzania, to test the efficacy and safety of the microbicide. This is a complex programme, involving several local teams of researchers, community mobilization teams (to lead recruitment) and workers and participants across different sites, all of which are multilingual. The trial design included social science research from the outset, to contribute to feasibility studies; collect more detailed data on key topics relating to sexual behaviour; assess the acceptability of the gel and its applicator; assess the validity of trial data through triangulation using qualitative methods; and also to study participants' own understandings of the study itself, including the consent procedures.

(Continued)

Qualitative data from feasibility studies for the trial generated evidence for understanding how women perceived participation in the research, which is essential for planning appropriate recruitment and information strategies. In a feasibility study in Soweto, South Africa, Jonathan Stadler and colleagues discuss the widespread fear and denial of AIDS in the community, and the negative connotations medical research might have in the South African context. Lack of community involvement can impede the successful roll out and completion of a trial, and understanding the social and cultural contexts in which products such as microbicides are being investigated is crucial to not only understanding trial findings, but also to the likely success of the trial. In the feasibility study, focus groups were first conducted within the community, before any trial recruitment began. These included a range of participants, including students, traditional healers and those from community health committees. The second phase involved interviews and focus groups with a random sample of women who were recruited for the trial feasibility study. This enabled the researchers to understand better how the participating women understand the consent procedures of the trial, and what effect their participation might have on them. For most of the women, participation was a positive experience. Not only did it provide health care services they might not otherwise receive (e.g., screening for sexually transmitted diseases), but the testing and counselling received as part of the trial were reported as empowering, in that they gave the women knowledge about their health, and an added confidence in discussing sexual health with their partners.

Catherine Montgomery and colleagues reported on interviews with 320 women and 45 male partners, as part of the pilot study for the trial in four of the participating countries. Women were asked about their attitudes to the gel, and about the involvement of their partners in deciding to take part in the trial. Analysis of interviews with women and their partners suggested that women used a process of persuasion to overcome the resistance their partners often had to their participation in the trial, and men reported using this resistance to gain more knowledge about their partners, and the new technology. Although the microbicide gel could be considered a 'female controlled' technology, in practice it might be difficult to use covertly in relationships because of the changes it produced in how the vagina felt. However, it emerged that the 'meaning' of microbicide gel within relationships was very different from that of condoms. Whereas condoms were associated with a lack of trust (and were therefore difficult to use in long term relationships), the gel was associated with sexual pleasure (in part, because using it involved intimacy) and with greater communication within relationships, thus making it suitable for long term relationships.

The roles of qualitative research in large trials such as the Microbicide Development Programme are complex. First, the research (in the examples here, from feasibility and pilot studies) generates useful data in its own right, addressing questions about how sexual health is experienced in the context of relationships and health care provision. Information about the different ways that microbicide gel and condoms are perceived in terms of 'trust' is extremely useful information that could be used, for instance, in planning roll-out campaigns for the product if the trial does show that microbicides are effective and safe. Second, such data also have to function as 'useful' for the primary purposes of a large quantitative trial, in which adequate recruitment and retention, and the reliability and validity of trial methods, are crucial. This potentially raises problems if the qualitative data are not consistent with data from other parts of the trial. Third, there are issues of integrating findings from the quantitative and qualitative components during the analysis.

In this case, qualitative interviews and focus groups helped in the design of the trial's quantitative instruments, especially in terms of clarifying key concepts and the range of ways in which they were understood locally. This included defining terms such as 'long term partner' or 'penetrative sex', which may be difficult to standardize across study settings. They also aided in designing recruitment strategies that maximized informed consent and ethical participation. Finally, interviews and focus groups provide essential information on the *process* of the trial, and on issues such as how women completed the diaries developed to monitor adherence through the trial and how their answers to study questionnaires may change over time as a result of their participation in the project.

Following on from the discussion of epistemological approaches in Chapter 1, there are two models of how this can happen. The first assumes that there is a range of (theoretically informed) questions raised by the consideration of any health problem, and that different research designs will be needed to address them. Here, the different methodological approaches are seen as 'adding depth', such that the whole research programme moves towards a richer understanding. If using multiple methods for adding depth is relatively straightforward (at least in principle – we will come to some problems below), a second model for using multiple methods within one study is perhaps rather more contentious. This is the idea of *triangulation*, or using more than one method to increase our faith in the validity of findings.

Triangulation

The notion of triangulation borrows a metaphor from navigation, with the idea that taking two readings will enable us to pinpoint the 'truth' more accurately than one. Thus, one method of data collection can be used to off-set the weakness of another, or to 'check out' the validity of findings. Examples might include the use of other data sources to 'validate' behavioural accounts from interview data: using sales figures for contraceptives, for instance, to compare with interview reports of contraceptive use, or medical records to check interviewees' accounts of medication prescriptions. However, there are of course limits to how far we can use different strategies for collecting data to improve the 'accuracy' of those data. Clearly, looking at sales of contraceptives and asking people about the use of contraceptives are generating data about two rather different phenomena. Less contentious is the use of triangulation to provide another perspective on a particular phenomenon, or 'fill in the gaps', for instance by using oral history interviews to complement historical documentary research. Norman Denzin (1989b) discusses the possibilities of triangulation from a more qualitative perspective; that is, that validity might refer to an improved understanding, rather than improved 'accuracy'. He argues that triangulation does not necessarily imply a naive positivist position, in which one can more accurately pin down some reality that is the object of research, but rather an approach that can bring the object more sharply into focus:

> ... each method implies a different line of action toward reality – and hence each will reveal different aspects of it, much as a kaleidoscope, depending on the angle at which it is held, will reveal different colours and configurations of objects to the viewer. Methods are like the kaleidoscope: depending on how they are approached, held, and acted toward, different observations will be revealed. (Denzin 1989b: 235)

Thus, the aim is not to produce a consistent version of the object of study, as that object is inevitably socially constituted, but to offset the particular weaknesses of each method, and challenge the biases that come from only one perspective. As an example, look again at Case Study 2.1, which described how Hilary Graham used both interviews and diaries in her study of women and smoking. Note that the diaries were not used to 'validate' women's interview accounts of the number of cigarettes smoked, but were used to generate slightly different information, and that these differences were what helped Graham unpack the meanings of smoking for the women in her study. Using qualitative data to 'validate' the more quantitative measures in a trial can, then, be problematic, as it is not always clear what should be done with different accounts. Neither could be considered the 'gold standard' if we are serious about treating the data as telling us about situated accounts, which need to be understood within the context of their creation, whether that was as answers to a questionnaire, or records made in a diary.

For Denzin, triangulation of methods is only one possible strategy. We can also use data triangulation (in utilizing as many diverse sources of data as possible), investigator triangulation (using different observers) and, most challenging, the idea of theoretical triangulation. This involves widening the theoretical frameworks utilized in a study as the research progresses, such that a range of models and theories is at the forefront when analysing the empirical data collected. It is with Denzin's idea of theoretical triangulation that researchers in multidisciplinary health studies are perhaps at a particular advantage. Most public health projects can draw on the theoretical traditions of a number of disciplines, widening the potential interpretative frameworks to be used in analysis. However, in practice, few health projects will utilize the possibilities of theoretical triangulation.

Combining methods

In considering the implications of 'mixing methods' in health promotion research, for instance, Kathryn Milburn and colleagues (Milburn et al. 1995) argue that in much health promotion research methods are combined uncritically, with little consideration of exactly what was to be achieved by using them together. This applies, perhaps, to health research more generally. Combining methods is assumed to be 'a good thing', an end in itself, and there is often insufficient attention paid to the relationships between the various components:

> ... are the researchers concerned about ... choosing methods for their appropriateness to the topic and the purpose of the research? Or are they concerned with 'illumination', and therefore with using different methods sequentially, the one to inform the other? Alternatively, are they concerned with 'saturation', with several methods being used simultaneously either to verify or augment the findings of each single approach? Or is there concern with 'diversification', so that several approaches are used in order to tap multiple realities in a particular setting? (Milburn et al. 1995: 348)

They advise clarity on exactly what is to be achieved in using a number of methodological approaches within one project. Given the varying expectations those from different disciplinary backgrounds can have about the relative contributions of different methodological strategies, the partners in any collaboration may well have to spend considerable time in exploring these differences to reduce the risk of frustration when outputs do not 'fit together' in the predicted way.

Trans-disciplinary research?

One approach to multidisciplinary work is, then, to be explicit about the epistemological differences within the team, and to highlight the range of expectations about the separate contributions of each of the partners. Another is to try to move towards a shared approach – a more 'trans-disciplinary' model.

Here, the aim is to integrate the different theoretical and methodological insights from each discipline throughout the project, rather than at the point of combining the findings. For some researchers, the division of labour between epidemiologists, anthropologists and clinicians is an artificial and unhelpful one that should be struggled against: they are, in this light, 'natural partners', and indeed the separation of health research into the camps of quantitative epidemiologists and qualitative social scientists is a relatively recent one (see for instance, Yach 1992; Inhorn 1995).

This vision of a coming together of social and health sciences is an appealing one, and 'breaking down barriers' is difficult to argue against without appearing elitist or protectionist about one's own discipline. However, it does perhaps ignore the 'political economy' of public health research, in which the research agenda tends to be set by those from particular health professions, and not social scientists, and it is perhaps naive about the epistemological (rather than merely methodological) differences between the contributing disciplines. Often, pleas for 'breaking down the barriers' appear to be little more than exasperated requests for anthropologists or sociologists to do the fieldwork that public health specialists want doing, rather than genuine collaborations around a research agenda, and research questions (see Pelto and Pelto's 1992 complaint about the paucity of trained social scientists for applied health research in developing countries for one example of this). As we have seen, the theoretical and epistemological starting points for research will shape the kinds of questions seen as legitimate, and what methods will produce valid answers to those research questions. In this light, anthropologists may well be reluctant to contribute to yet another 'rapid appraisal', considering the data collected are a poor guide to local beliefs.

There are of course many examples of such collaborations working well, and Case Study 6.1, on using ethnography in a diarrhoeal disease project, demonstrates the possibilities of informing public interventions on the basis of ethnographic work. But productive multi-disciplinary work does not just happen: it requires considerable planning. In their reports of the project described in Case Study 6.1, the authors discuss some of the reasons for anthropological perspectives being successfully integrated into practice (Scrimshaw and Hurtado 1988), including building on a field prepared by earlier anthropologists who had worked in Central America, the receptivity of project staff, and the care taken to prepare reports and findings in useful formats for nonspecialists, especially by using face-to-face meetings to explore how they could be used in the project. As Scrimshaw and Hurtado note, this is time-consuming and resource intensive. In many studies, researchers are too busy with the next project to consider appropriate dissemination formats, or to explore the implications of their findings for practice. Susan Rifkin (1996) also notes that there are unexpectedly time-consuming parts of the 'rapid' appraisal process, and she suggests it can take a long time to develop the research objectives if the team do not share a common language or approach, and a new shared one has to be developed. Rifkin suggests that visualizations are one way in which members of teams can share ideas more easily: using diagrams and rankings to get across key points in ways that are not tied to disciplinary ways of thinking. In the diarrhoeal disease project, Scrimshaw and Hurtado used typologies of ethno-classifications to introduce other members of the team to the basic concepts, rather than extensive written reports.

Communicating across disciplines

It is not only in rapid appraisals that problems of communication can be a barrier to productive working across disciplines. In Case Study 9.2, Gillian Lewando-Hundt (2000) describes the different expectations of various stake-holders in a project on maternal and child health around such issues as how to disseminate findings in appropriate ways. In this case, political sensitivities as well as disciplinary traditions created challenges. The political sensitivities of working in the Middle East meant that such difficulties were particularly acute in this project, but similar challenges face most multidisciplinary projects in the dissemination phase. Some typical areas of tension faced within many research teams include:

- *Publications.* Researchers from particular disciplines will be keen to publish in 'their' journals. Although most large projects will furnish enough findings for several publications, it is helpful to have discussions at the outset of the project about who will take the lead on which publications, who will contribute to particular papers (and have authorship) and where the project findings will be disseminated. (Authorship is discussed further in Chapter 10.)
- *Ownership of the data.* On a large, collaborative project, writing up will probably continue long after the project itself has finished. Again, it is essential to be clear at the outset who will have access to whatever data have been generated at the end of the project, and who will have 'rights' to exploit those data.
- *Outputs.* Given the flexibility of qualitative designs, the research 'answers' that come out may not be the ones expected. It is not uncommon for a key finding of qualitative studies to be that the original research question was the 'wrong' question. In a stand-alone project this is not a problem, but in collaborative projects, with research partners perhaps reliant on the qualitative phase to provide data for their contribution, colleagues can find this extremely frustrating. Writing up these unexpected findings (and explaining why the aims may not have been met in expected ways) can present dilemmas for the project team.
- *Language.* Even if teams are working in the same language, disciplines still have their own vocabularies, with terms that have specific meanings. 'Observational study' means something rather different to epidemiologists and sociologists, for instance. Further, the concepts used in health research may carry quite different connotations across different disciplines. Clinicians, for instance, may be comfortable with the concept of 'lay perceptions' to distinguish their patients' understanding of health from their professional, biomedical ideas. However, for many sociologists and anthropologists the term implies that lay and expert beliefs are distinct and that lay ones are somehow 'faulty', so terms such as 'public views' may be preferred. In collaborative projects, if all partners are expected to agree to the wording of all outputs, the time taken to reach a consensus around terminology can be considerable.

Case Study 9.2   Collaborations across disciplines and nations: problems of language and politics

(Source: Lewando-Hundt, G. (2000) 'Multiple scripts and con-tested discourse in disseminating research findings', *Social Policy and Administration*, 34: 419–33.

Gillian Lewando-Hundt reports on some of the challenges in dis-seminating research findings from a study of maternal and child health to Palestinians in Gaza and Bedouin in Israel. The study was funded by the European Commission as a collaboration between universities in the UK and Israel and a research centre in Palestine, and included researchers trained in epidemiology and public health – some of whom also had service responsibilities – and anthropologists. Lewando-Hundt argues that the different national, disciplinary and research orientations of the team led to different understandings throughout the project of issues around study design, interpretation of the results and dissemination. These can be a productive force for developing research ques-tions. In this study, the members of the team with responsibility for service provision and a public health perspective wanted to focus on non-attenders at pre-natal clinics, and find out whether they were informed about the service on offer and why they did not attend. From a more social science perspective, the anthro-pologists were more comfortable asking questions about profes-sional and client views and experiences, and focusing on what the women gained or did not gain by attending. These differences in focus were accommodated by dividing the research questions according to methodology, such that the epidemiologists led on designing a questionnaire survey to measure service utilization, and the anthropologists developed qualitative studies using focus groups and interviews to explore users' views and experiences (one of these studies is described in Case Study 5.1). By con-ducting both quantitative and qualitative studies as part of the same project, the two disciplines could see that using a combina-tion of methods provided answers to slightly different questions, but both contributed to understanding the issue of maternal and child health.

When it came to dissemination, there were also differences across the research team in terms of expectations about what was legiti-mate. As an EC-funded study, the coordinators had an obligation to disseminate widely, but this did not form part of the normal expec-tations of the local research teams in Gaza and Israel, where the accepted process was to move on to planning interventions, without a lengthy phase of dissemination. The challenges of disseminating the key findings included difficulties in addressing diverse audiences, and conflict over which languages to write it in. The Palestinians were keen to have Arabic translations to disseminate widely in an accessible format, whereas one member of the team wanted a more limited dissemination, and only in English. In the end the draft report was summarized and translated into both Arabic and Hebrew, with these as well as the English versions bound into one document.

Expectations around the format of dissemination also led to conflicts. When the researchers first presented some of the qualitative data from the focus groups, they included data on women's views of the issue of *wasta*, or using influence or connections to jump the queue. They had intended this to be a way of informing health centre managers and others about the key findings, and generating discussion about the implications. However, the sensitivities about the topic (*wasta*) and the lack of understanding of the methods (group interviews) meant that the findings were challenged by the audience, who commented that the methods were unscientific, and the data could not be believed. In another meeting, the researchers were advised to tone down some of the criticisms reported of the clinics, and to use the word 'social' rather than 'political'. Some of the particular difficulties faced were the result of political tensions in the Middle East, but Lewando-Hundt suggests that all dissemination strategies have to take account of the ethos of local health services, the sensitivities of the various groups involved, and their expectations about what data 'should' look like.

Political sensitivities also shaped how findings were disseminated in academic journals. For instance, although the context for the Gaza setting was health service provision by the Israeli Civil Administration, this was usually too contentious to note. Direct comment by the authors on the position of Palestinians was avoided, in case it appeared to be politically biased, and they instead quoted other authors. Choosing whether to use Hebrew or Arabic names for places, or whether to use the term 'Bedouin', 'Bedouin Arabs', 'Palestinian Israelis' or 'Israeli Arabs', was not just a matter of linguistic preference, but one that suggested particular political affiliations. For joint papers a compromise had to be reached on terminology, with drafts being discussed by members of the research team until a consensus was reached.

In this study, then, not only disciplinary differences but also political and institutional differences had to be negotiated throughout the research process. Although these issues might be particularly explicit in settings in transition, such as the Middle East, they are likely to shape research in most collaborative settings, and we have to pay attention not just to the technical aspects of research design, but also to the politics of research.

If we assume that the contribution of qualitative research is to bring methodological expertise to address particular research questions, these practical differences between disciplinary research cultures can be addressed, given adequate time for teamwork and debate. However, there are perhaps more fundamental differences in the epistemological starting points of many of the social sciences and the more biomedical sciences, which can potentially be more undermining of fruitful collaboration. Within health research programmes addressing a 'public health problem', the agenda is perhaps inevitably set in biomedical terms, and if bringing a social science approach, rather than just qualitative methods, many qualitative researchers will feel rather uncomfortable with an uncritical biomedical perspective. Robert Pool (1994), for instance, reflects on the tensions raised by the 'biomedical' framework he had to adopt in order to fund anthropological research on health and illness in Cameroon:

> The goal of my original research project was to discover the cultural factors related to infant nutrition and illness. ... These insights were to lead to recommendations for improving infant nutrition. ... [However] I was opposed to the idea that the anthropologist studying health related beliefs should adopt an evaluative attitude based on bio-medical assumptions. Rather, I preferred to explore people's ideas about illness and food and place them in a wider cultural context. However, grant-giving agencies desired a more applied approach. ... (Pool 1994: 27–9)

Pool was working in an area where local health workers considered kwashiorkor (protein-energy malnutrition) to be a major health problem. From a biomedical perspective, the 'causes' of this problem were perceived to be dysfunctional health beliefs and practices, which could be identified through anthropological methods. However, as Pool notes, this sits rather uneasily within a broader anthropological perspective, which would aim for holistic understanding of local culture without *a priori* assumptions about the validity of local health workers' ideas about causation.

In her critique of the 'natural collaboration' model for anthropology and epidemiology, Susan DiGiacomo (1999) is rather pessimistic about the possibilities of genuinely collaborative partnerships between the disciplines. She outlines a number of assumptions made by epidemiological science that led her to question whether there could ever be a 'cultural epidemiology'. First, she argues, epidemiology, with its 'web of causation' model, tends to reify culture as simply one more risk factor to be accounted for in models of epidemiological risk. Disease incidence is merely the sum of individual cases of disease, and culture reduced to a list of 'social' factors (age, sex, race) that are similarly individualized as attributes of particular people in particular places. A more holistic, anthropological notion of culture is difficult to maintain against this reductionist concept. She identifies five underlying assumptions in epidemiology which are at odds with anthropological practice:

1 It is possible to isolate cultural concepts from their context.
2 Culture can be reified as 'value', 'attitudes' and 'beliefs' and these can be attached to particular social groups.

3   Culture is a 'risk factor', even if a protective one.
4   Culture is an attribute of 'others', defined in terms of ethnicity, or social class.
5   The beliefs of these 'others' tend to be unreasonable, irrational and in need of explanation.

DiGiacomo argues that the stress on methods, rather than theory, in the intersection of anthropology and epidemiology has reduced anthropologists to mere data-gatherers, with the focus on collecting information on these cultural 'beliefs' rather than producing 'thick descriptions' that can provide the context and holistic understanding needed to interpret the meaning of beliefs. She also notes that it is not just epistemological differences that constrain the role of anthropology within epidemiology, but also institutional pressures. Spain, where she was based, like many other countries, puts pressure on its academic departments to publish in high-impact journals in a narrow range, and not more imaginative pieces in social science journals. As she concludes:

> The requirements ... of genuinely collaborative work go well beyond matters of epistemology to include the politics of scientific research, and demand some degree of courage from all concerned, but especially from epidemiologists in pursuing lines of research that do not necessarily promise fast returns with high bibliographic impact value. (DiGiacomo 1999: 451)

Projects involving partners from a number of disciplinary backgrounds involve, then, at a minimum, challenges in terms of working across varying communication and research cultures. They can also raise more fundamental challenges of addressing epistemological differences, and developing research agendas that can accommodate social science as well as biomedical or epidemiological perspectives.

International collaborations

International projects can range from studies based in one country that use data from another, through to major international collaborations with research management spanning several continents. Jessica Ogden and John Porter (2000) point to the rhetoric of collaboration for international public health, and criticize a simplistic notion of 'partnership' to describe international collaborations, given the inequalities of power between research institutes in the north and south. In their examples, from collaborations between institutions in the UK and India, they argue that it is important to separate out relationships between institutions and those between individual researchers or research teams, and to distinguish both from short-term 'consultancy' relationships, in which researchers will spend time in other countries as technical experts, working to the agenda of the host institution. Institutions may have a formal collaborative agreement, but this only becomes a partnership in practice if individuals within the research team can develop a collaborative working relationship. Individual power differences between members of the research teams, in terms of seniority or the relative status of their discipline, can undermine collaborative working. Ogden and Porter also point to structural barriers to collaboration. The costs of research can vary considerably between countries, with those in the UK five to ten times higher than those of the Indian institutions. This creates an image of the northern partners being 'worth more', which is hardly conducive to partnership.

Even when there are no structural inequalities between the international partners to manage, there will still be cultural differences. Cultures of communication vary across national boundaries, as well as across disciplines. Martin Cortazzi and Lixian Jin (1997) discuss the impact of different communication cultures on teaching and learning for students, but many of their points apply equally well to research collaborations. First, there are different academic cultures that frame our expectations of what 'good' research and academic activity look like. Experienced research practitioners come to think of these as obvious and universal, but they do vary from country to country. Thus, our expectations of whether team relationships should be hierarchical, 'master–disciple' or collegial, or whether persuasive rhetoric is an essential element of professional skills, will depend on our cultural background. How far junior members of a team are expected to show originality, creativity or critical skills also varies across cultures, as do expectations of how far disagreement, rather than consensus, is tolerated within teams. Second, styles of written and oral communication used in academic settings reflect broader cultural patterns. The length of pauses we are comfortable with in discussion, whether interrupting other speakers is legitimate and how animated speakers can be all vary cross-culturally, and differences in discussion styles can be misinterpreted as rudeness or lack of understanding. In written communication, different styles are also favoured in different cultures. One example is the use of citations to other work. In British reports, there is an expectation that the literature and previous research will be reviewed to put findings in context, whereas Chinese scientific reports, for instance, typically focus on the contribution, rather than the background, with the aim of minimizing the 'irrelevant' material for the reader (Cortazzi and Jin 1997: 83). Over long-term collaborations, partners can develop their understanding of these cultural styles, but the time taken to establish good international working relationships is often underestimated.

Opportunities

This chapter has focused on the challenges of doing qualitative health research in practice, particularly in applied settings. We have pointed to some of the issues that may arise in working with those from other disciplines, particularly from the epidemiological perspectives that may dominate health research, and working in projects that may have development or other aims. However, while these challenges need to be considered, this discussion has perhaps ignored the opportunities and privileges that working in applied settings can bring. First is of course the satisfaction from doing research that does inform practice or policy.

Health is one arena where social scientists can, and do, have a contribution to make in improving health service provision, and for many qualitative researchers, the opportunity to 'make a difference', even if on a modest scale, is a real attraction of working in applied fields.

Second, there are often enhanced opportunities from applied work to contribute at a more theoretical level. Case Study 9.1 illustrates this. Although the qualitative research summarized here was conducted as part of a larger programme, and primarily to inform a randomized controlled trial, the social scientists have used the wealth of data from interviews and focus groups to not only help understand local behaviour, but to also make a wider contribution to our understanding of issues such as the role of health knowledge in empowerment, or how the use of contraceptives relates to trust in relationships. We have touched on the problems of the rapid timescales of much applied work, which can leave insufficient time to fully analyse the data generated from a project. To find the time for this kind of analysis might be difficult in short-term projects. One solution is to try to attract extra funding to carry out further work on the data after the project is complete, given that some research funders may be enthusiastic about the 'added value' you can bring to using an existing data set.

Third, the privilege of working with a range of stakeholders, who may have very different perspectives, is that, as researchers, we have a ready source of comparative epistemological frameworks, theoretical insights and alternative interpretations to add analytical depth. The process of thinking through why there are different perspectives, or how to explain your interpretations to those from other backgrounds, is an essential element of actually doing analysis. Applied work, although it can involve time-consuming and at times frustrating debates around methods, findings and their implications, also provides a very real source of inspiration and insight that are not available to those who are working in isolation, or purely within the academy. The challenge is to ensure there is enough time and support for these debates to be productive and mutually beneficial.

Conclusion

Much qualitative research is done in the context of larger programmes, or alongside projects with goals such as evaluation, rather than as stand-alone 'pure' research. Tensions can arise from the different orientations of applied projects and qualitative research, particularly around the timescales, the nature of findings, and the methodological contribution. Doing qualitative research in practice therefore requires developing skills in collaboration, and communicating across boundaries. At a minimum, we have to collaborate with research participants from a range of professional and disciplinary backgrounds, and much health research is done in the context of various multidisciplinary and international collaborations. When qualitative researchers are seen as bringing merely a set of methods (a tool box of techniques that can be applied to a particular research question), this appears relatively unproblematic: the qualitative component of a project 'adds value' by addressing some issue such as users' views, an exploration of process, or observational description as 'colour' for a report. When qualitative methodology is integrated into a larger project in a more meaningful way, in that researchers bring the theoretical insights and methodological understandings of their disciplines to the research questions, there is a need for more detailed consideration of what each partner expects from the collaboration, and what each expects from the others.

KEY POINTS

- Qualitative methods for data collection are increasingly used in applied health research, but there are often challenges in using qualitative approaches.
- Fruitful collaborative relationships need a considerable investment of time and commitment to establish expectations at the outset over such issues as:
  - the relationships between the different methods used;
  - expected outputs;
  - how the findings will be disseminated;
  - what 'rights' each partner has to the data.

- Epistemological differences between qualitative research approaches and other, more positivist, approaches may pose particular challenges.
- National, disciplinary and professional differences are rarely neutral, and qualitative researchers may have to account for 'differences' more often than those from other backgrounds.

EXERCISE

The European Union is funding a scheme to improve housing and cut the number of excess winter deaths by offering energy efficiency interventions (such as more efficient and affordable heating, improvements in windows) in three partner countries. The interventions are to be evaluated by teams of researchers in each country.

List the disciplines that might need to be involved in a project of this kind and then describe some of the potential benefits and pitfalls that might be encountered. What differences in research perspective might you find and what impact might these have?

One expectation from the evaluation is that findings from the three countries will be compared. What difficulties are you likely to face in developing a protocol suitable for use in all three different countries?

FURTHER READING

Janes, C.R., Stall, R. and Gifford, S. (1986) *Anthropology and epi-demiology: interdisciplinary approaches to the study of health and disease*. Dordrecht: Reidel. There are a number of books on applied medical anthropology that explore the interface between anthropology and public health. This has chapters on the history of collaboration and a number of interesting case studies.

Seale, C., Gobo, G., Gubrium, J. and Silverman, D. (eds) (2004) *Qualitative Research Practice*. London: Sage. A collection of chapters on doing qualitative research with an emphasis on the 'craft' of doing research, and from the perspectives of those engaged in research practice. The text has useful practical advice on a range of methods and methodological approaches, and insights across the range of research activities through to publishing in journals.

10 Writing up Qualitative Work

CHAPTER SUMMARY

Writing is part of the process of doing qualitative research. It is not merely the report of analysis undertaken, but an essential element of that analysis. Qualitative health researchers need to develop their skills in writing for different audiences in order to disseminate their findings not only widely, but also appropriately. This chapter discusses three types of writing typically needed in a qualitative project: articles for health or biomedical journals, writing for social science colleagues, and reports for non-specialist audiences.

Introduction

Writing up a qualitative study can be a very different experience from that of writing up a quantitative one. In part this is because the writing, for most researchers, is part of the analysis. The process of writing (deciding what to include, what order to put it in, how to construct each sentence and paragraph) makes us think in new ways about the data, the connections within the data, and between the data and the broader literature. The very process of writing is part of triggering the 'sociological (or historical, or anthropological) imagination' and identifying the cross-cutting connections that embed your work within the discipline or substantive field of knowledge to which you are contributing. This is why it is good practice to begin writing as soon as possible, rather than as a separate task at the end of the project. This could include writing 'memos' (see Chapter 8) as part of the analysis, writing a reflective diary of the fieldwork process, or descriptive accounts of emerging analysis as the study progresses. Certainly with a substantial piece of writing (such as a PhD thesis) the writing cannot be left to the end; it is an essential *part* of the process of research, rather than a subsequent 'objective' account of that process.

The writing process

Few people find writing easy, and many of us struggle with both getting started and completing the task. Experiences of 'displacement' activities, such as cleaning the house, or filing papers, or making endless cups of coffee to 'get started', are common. We tend to think of these as ways of delaying the real work of writing, but one reassuring perspective incorporates these activities as an essential element *of* writing, rather than a prelude to it. In an interview, Roland Barthes (1985) argued that these practical, or what he called 'ceremonial', aspects of the physical act of writing should not be seen as trivial, and that we should pay attention to the preparatory activities and the materials needed to write. These might include particular settings (do you need to be at a clear desk, or surrounded by files and papers?), routines (do you find it easier to write in long uninterrupted stretches, or in short bursts?) and the tools needed (do you type straight to a PC, or prefer to draft out papers by pen in a notebook first?). On materials, for instance, Barthes discusses the importance of pens to him:

> I would say, for example, that I have an almost obsessive relation to writing instruments. I often switch from one pen to another just for the pleasure of it. I try out new ones ... I cannot keep myself from buying them. ... In short, I've tried everything ... except Bics, with which I feel absolutely no affinity. I would even say, a bit nastily, that there is a 'Bic style', which is really just for churning out copy. ... In the end, I always return to fine fountain pens. (Barthes 1985: 178)

Thus, seeming irrelevancies can be taken seriously as part of the task of writing itself, which includes activities such as thinking, planning, and giving yourself opportunities to make imaginative connections within your data. Barthes's descriptions of his writing routines in this interview also suggest some tactics for the difficult point most writers face at times, when there seems no way to begin, or to phrase a particular section. Switching materials may help, in that writing in a notebook if used to typing straight to a screen, or perhaps moving to a new location, may trigger new ideas or ways of thinking about your text.

At a more practical level, the techniques that 'work' to facilitate writing will be personal to you, but there are a number of suggestions that may be useful for getting started and completing the task:

- Draft a detailed structure first, with headings for all the sections you want to include.
- Don't begin at the beginning – it is easiest to write the introduction when you know what is in the body of the text. Start with the section you find easiest or most interesting.
- Think about a specific reader as you write, and about what you are trying to communicate to him or her.
- Try writing your ideas in an everyday, conversational language if you feel defeated by trying to write the 'formal' accounts straight away.
- Introduce regular deadlines. Break large writing tasks into smaller ones, and make sure you have deadlines for each one, by promising drafts or sections to supervisors or co-workers at regular points.

Writing for different audiences

There are a number of potential audiences for any study, particularly in the field of health research, which will require tailored writing styles and formats. Any or all of the following written outputs might be needed from one study:

- one-page summaries of the key findings for the research participants
- a short paper on the key findings for a practitioners' journal
- progress reports and final study report for the sponsors
- an executive summary for policy makers
- articles for biomedical peer-reviewed journals
- longer academic articles for social science peer-reviewed journals
- book chapters or a monograph
- a dissertation or thesis.

Both the content and the style of these papers and reports will be very different, and researchers need a wide range of communication skills to address different audiences in effective ways. Increasingly, researchers are being asked to ensure that potential users of research are informed about outcomes. Users might include practitioners, policy makers at various levels and voluntary sector groups with an interest in the topic. Participative projects will of course build in considerable attention to communication with research participants throughout the research process, but studies of most kinds will require at least the main results to be disseminated to participants or stakeholders in an appropriate way. Of course, writing for these diverse audiences is not just a matter of writing differently. In some cases we have to *think* differently to write different outputs, putting ourselves in the position of an interviewee, or a practitioner, to think through what the implications of our findings might be. Shifting gear between the different registers needed for these diverse audiences can be difficult, and you may need a gap between writing in different ways.

To illustrate some of these different ways of communicating, we look here at three types of writing you might typically need to do within a qualitative health project: writing for health journals, writing for social science colleagues, and writing for non-specialist audiences.

Writing for health journals

Many qualitative studies in the health field aim to communicate findings not just to other qualitative researchers, but to colleagues from other disciplines or to practitioners. Less lofty aims, such as meeting the institution's needs for good-quality peer-reviewed publications in mainstream journals, are also an incentive for publishing in biomedical and health journals as well as social science ones. In some ways, qualitative findings may be easier to convey to audiences of professionals than complex statistical data, simply because there is an immediacy about accounts of everyday health practices and beliefs that most practitioners can relate to, in terms of their own experiences. Writing for biomedical journals (like any other kind of writing) requires a sensitivity to the audience: what is interesting for practitioners or researchers in other disciplines in your findings and why should they want to read this paper?

The paper needs to be written with the precise readership of the journal in mind, and with a clear sense of what is being communicated to them. This will shape the content of the paper, in that you will focus on the implications for practice and future research in the area, and perhaps some recommendations for those working in the field. Writing up qualitative work for biomedical journals also entails some attention to format and style. Most biomedical journals (look, for instance, at the *British Medical Journal*, or the *Lancet*) will expect submitted papers to conform to a standard format designed primarily for quantitative reports, with the following types of headings:

- *Abstract*. Summary of around 150 words, giving the purpose of the study, the setting, your methods, main findings and conclusions.
- *Introduction*. A brief overview of the aim of study and how this follows from 'what is already known'.
- *Methods*. Methods of data collection and analysis, how the sample was selected, a description of the sample, any ethical issues.
- *Results*. The findings of the study, in text or tables.
- *Discussion*. The limitations and implications of the findings in light of other work, and any recommendations that follow on from these.

Each journal has its own guidelines for authors, often reprinted inside the back cover of each issue of the journal, or available from the journal's or publisher's web page. These will cover issues like the maximum length of an article, how to cite references and whether a structured abstract is needed. Many biomedical journals have adopted the 'Uniform requirements for manuscripts submitted to biomedical journals' (International Committee of Medical Journal Editors 1991), which determine how manuscripts should be prepared (that is, in double-spaced type, using one side of the page, with each section on a new page). These general requirements are also known as the *Vancouver style*, and include requirements for citations and references. In the Vancouver style, references should be cited by inserting an Arabic superscript number in the text when the reference is first used, then listing the full references in number order at the end of the paper.

In addition to these general requirements, most journals have a particular 'house style' that will be more or less constrictive. This influences matters of style such as whether research reports can be written in the first person, whether extensive quotes can be used, whether a detailed methods section is needed, and the preferred vocabulary. This can be gauged by reading the qualitative articles published in the journal. There may also be 'checklists' of criteria for qualitative articles submitted to the journal, which are discussed in Chapter 11. It is obviously sensible to write with these in mind where possible, as these may well be used by reviewers who will decide whether to recommend your submitted article to the editor for publication.

Of course, many qualitative studies will not fit into this format. It would not be profitable, for instance, to try to force a rich, nuanced description of a healing system from an ethnographic study into a structured format unless there were 'stand-alone' findings that could be separated out and clear messages for the journal readership. Indeed, some claim that the conventional formats developed for reporting the results of quantitative studies are generally too constraining for the adequate reporting of qualitative studies: Miles and Huberman (1994), for instance, argue that structured headings are in general inappropriate because:

> Normally we'd have other expectations for a qualitative report. For example, we might expect a close description of the history, the context, the major actors. ... We might look for a more 'circular' linkage between research questions, methods, data collection and interim analysis, as each new analysis opened up new leads. (Miles and Huberman 1994: 298)

However, in the health field many qualitative studies are designed to produce 'findings' that can be reported under standard headings. The extract from an abstract in Box 10.1 illustrates the kind of qualitative study that works well for a biomedical journal, in that the authors are able to report their findings under standard headings. This is from a paper by Chris Griffiths and colleagues (Griffiths et al. 2001) published in the *British Medical Journal*.

This study, from a multidisciplinary team (of a sociologist, anthropologist, and primary and secondary care professionals), was clearly designed to

---

Box 10.1 **Sample abstract from a qualitative study**

Influences on hospital admission for asthma in south Asian and white adults: qualitative interview study

Objective: To explore the reasons for an increased risk of hospital admission among south Asian patients with asthma.

Design: Qualitative interview study using modified critical incident technique and framework analysis. [...]

Main outcome measures: Patients' and health professionals' views on influences on admission, events leading to admission, general practices' organization and asthma strategies, doctor-patient relationship, and cultural attitudes to asthma.

Results: South Asian and white patients admitted to hospital coped differently with asthma. [...] Patients describing difficulty accessing primary care during asthma exacerbation were registered with practices with weak strategies for asthma care and were often south Asian. [...]

Conclusions: The different ways of coping with asthma exacerbations and accessing primary care may partly explain the increased risk of hospital admission in south Asian patients. [...]

---

address a problem that is recognizable in clinical practice (the observed increased risk of admission for asthma for some groups in the UK population) and produce findings relevant for practitioners and health promoters working in the area. The data, gathered from interviews, are relatively easy to summarize for readers, and the methodological techniques used (such as framework analysis) can be referred to without too much discussion. However, even for studies like this, where it is possible to divide text up neatly into aims, background, findings and conclusions, the nature of qualitative inquiry does present some particular challenges with this kind of writing. One is the use of quoted material. Whereas a qualitative report may need considerable context and detail to provide credibility and a 'flavour' of the rich, detailed analysis done, biomedical journals may expect brevity and will therefore see such material as extraneous. In this example, Griffiths and colleagues have included some brief examples from interviews in the text, and a longer selection in a separate box. Biomedical journals may also require the 'quantification' of results, for instance counts of how many respondents had particular attitudes, and rather more transparency about the actual procedures used to analyse the data than is typical in social science journals.

More difficult than these issues of style is the problem of representing the theoretical grounding of the data, and its broader meanings. The space constraints and the 'practical implications' orientation of a biomedical journal mean that it is very difficult to do anything other than hint at what the findings imply for a more conceptual understanding. For this, you will need a more appropriate qualitative format for representing the findings of your study, such as a monograph or a paper for one of the social science journals.

Writing for social science colleagues

There is a huge range of general journals within each of the social science disciplines that publish qualitative studies on health, including those dedicated to the 'medical' sub-disciplines (such as *Medical Anthropology, Medical Anthropology Quarterly, Social Theory and Health* and *Sociology of Health and Illness*) and also a number of interdisciplinary journals, such as *Social Science and Medicine* and *Qualitative Health Research*. The various social science disciplines have their own traditions of writing, and each journal has its own favoured styles and approaches. Some publish articles in a more self-consciously 'scientific' style, similar to that in health sciences, in which papers are organized with separate sections on background, literature, methods, findings and discussion and the tone of papers tends to be more 'objective' and neutral, although articles tend to be longer than in the biomedical journals, and include rather more theoretical material. In these, you might be expected to use Vancouver style references. More typically, a social science journal article will have a more narrative style, and will include far more discussion of how the study reported contributes to the discipline. This will require longer background and discussion sections, and the 'findings' section might draw on other literature. The authors need to locate their findings within the theoretical and perhaps methodological debates in the field, and demonstrate not just new empirical data, but how these data extend our conceptual understanding of a problem. Given the importance of situating material within the literature of the discipline, citations to other published work are important, and social science journals usually use what is known as the *Harvard* style for referencing (as found in this book) in which the author and date of publication are cited in the text, with the full list arranged alphabetically by author at the end of the article.

Some journals explicitly encourage more innovative narrative styles, or expect the material to be organized in an appropriate way for the message of the paper. This could be as a first-person narrative, say, or as a dialogue. The degree to which writing is expected to be reflexive is one key difference, with some qualitative journals encouraging personal, subjective styles in which the author's experiences of doing the research are an essential element of the text. Consider, for instance, the opening sentences of one article from the journal *Qualitative Inquiry*, which does encourage a wider range of styles (including, for instance, poems on occasion) than many journals:

> Steel doors slam behind me, announcing my progress through the security checks of the detention facility, locally called the 'jail for children', where I am conducting my dissertation research. ... Combining narrative and ethnographic methods, I hope to describe the relationship between juvenile delinquents and the public institutions charged with the social control of teenagers. ...

> But there's a problem: In 2 months of observing ... I haven't met anyone willing to sign my human subjects' release forms ... and agree to the interviews I've planned. Then I meet Clayboy. (VanderStaay 2003: 974)

This, taken from Steven VanderStaay's paper on his research with one teenage drug user in the United States, illustrates the differences between the conventions of biomedical writing and some social science texts. Note that this introduction is in the first person: VanderStaay places himself in the research story from the beginning. He also starts his paper by referring to problems: that two months into his fieldwork, he had failed to find anyone willing to sign the necessary consent forms. This is in stark contrast to the 'post hoc' write-up expected in more scientific styles, in which such problems might be mentioned in the discussion, but are not seen as relevant to the report itself.

The development of a specifically 'scientific' style (relatively plain, neutral, unadorned) separate from a 'literary' style (which uses metaphor and evocative language) is an outcome of post-Enlightenment ideas about science in the West: that it is essentially empirical, in that 'facts speak for themselves', and require transparent language rather than rhetoric to speak for them. Of course, 'scientific' language has its own stylistic persuasiveness. This is achieved through the use of phrases such as 'the findings demonstrate' or 'the study reveals' (which suggest that the facts unearthed 'speak for themselves' without the intervention of the researcher), and the rhetorical use of titles that pose questions to be answered, implying that these will be dealt with authoritatively by the author (Kitzinger 1987; Thorogood 1997). The use of tables of numbers and statistical tests and complex technical language is also a way of framing an article as 'scientific' and credible.

So, all writers use 'literary' strategies to increase the credibility of the written report, but in the social sciences it is more common to be explicit about this, and to acknowledge the 'craft' of writing. Kathy Charmaz (1999), for instance, talks about borrowing the strategies of fiction writers to improve writing through providing a context for the story, pulling the reader in, recreating the mood and adding surprise. Note how VanderStaay, in the extract quoted above, skillfully uses the conventions of storytelling (brief description of a dramatic setting and the quest, setbacks on the way, an unexpected lucky break: 'Then I meet Clayboy') to interest the reader, and also sets up some expectations. We understand that, as a researcher trying to complete his dissertation, VanderStaay is perhaps desperate at this point for anyone who will agree, and we understand that his meeting with Clayboy is a pivotal moment, in both his story and that of the research. Rather than a neutral, 'scientific' account of aims and methods, the author has introduced a story in which the 'findings' are clearly going to be closely integrated in and contextualized by the researcher's own role in producing them.

Much qualitative writing for health adopts a scientific style relatively uncritically, in part to establish credibility for audiences familiar with that format. Indeed, there are few examples like that from VanderStaay in the more health-orientated social science journals. In ethnography, in particular, though, there has been considerable debate about writing, and the forms that are appropriate for the textual representation of both the process of researching and descriptions of cultures as the outputs of that research. In part, this follows from a tradition in which personal narratives have had a legitimate place in the writing up of fieldwork, including stories about arriving at the fieldwork site and the challenges faced in learning the language, arranging access and the practicalities of living in the field. Two traditions in anthropology sit in tension: those that stress its 'scientific' status, separate from mere travellers' tales or journalistic anecdotes, and those that recognize subjective experiences as part of establishing the 'authenticity' of the ethnography. The ways in which particular kinds of narrative produce particular possible readings are the subject of debate within the discipline. James Clifford summarizes the various different ways in which ethnographers will choose to 'translate experience into text':

> One can 'write up' the results of an individual experience of research. This may generate a realistic account of the unwritten experience of another group or person. One can present this textualization as the outcome of observation, of interpretation, of dialogue. One can construct an ethnography composed of dialogues. One can feature multiple voices, or a single voice. One can portray the other as a stable, essential whole or one can show it to be the product of a narrative of discovery, in specific historical circumstances. (Clifford 1986a: 115)

That these are choices to be debated indicates the focus in ethnography on writing itself as part of the process of representation, rather than merely a tool through which 'findings' are reported for other audiences, but of course Clifford's choices – in theory – will apply to all kinds of writing, not just ethnography. The journal article, or research report, is not a neutral window to the data produced and gathered, but rather a specific narrative that has political effects of its own.

Writing for and disseminating to non-specialist audiences

You may have to feed back results to a number of stakeholders in the research process, such as research participants (interviewees, gatekeepers), potential users of your findings (policy makers, practitioners) and perhaps wider audiences with the help of the mass media. The incentives for doing this are various, including attempts to influence practice, sharing results with those who helped produce them, and perhaps political purposes, such as generating publicity for your project or department. A common criticism of researchers is that they are poor at communicating their findings in appropriate ways to non-specialist audiences. This is to some extent a matter of style: producing long reports full of technical terms is clearly not an adequate way of informing those who need to use the findings, and preparing summaries of findings for such audiences as research participants means considering some practical aspects of your writing such as:

- *Writing clear, accessible prose.* One way of checking this is to calculate the 'Fog Index' of your writing, as follows:
  - Calculate the average number of words per sentence.
  - Add the percentage of words of three or more syllables to this.
  - Multiply by 0.4.

  As a rule of thumb, if the result is a Fog Index of more than 12, general readers may find the text difficult. Some word processors have functions that check the readability of text for you. (The sentence that precedes these bullet points scores 24!)
- *Avoid jargon.* We use specialized language and abbreviations as a short-hand to communicate with colleagues, but forget that many of these terms mean nothing (or something rather different!) to non-specialists.
- *Care with vocabulary.* Following on from that, you must be sensitive to ways in which many research users will utilize particular vocabularies. The use of non-discriminatory language is essential in all communication, but you may need to take particular care over language with some groups of users. Most people living with particular illnesses will not want to be described as 'sufferers', for instance, and practitioners will expect their 'technical' vocabularies to be used accurately. Any research on politically sensitive topics, where language may be a site of contestation, will need particular care – see, for instance, Case Study 9.2 on the difficulties of terminology in the Middle East.
- *Appropriate translations.* Some audiences will need specialized translations, for instance into other languages or audio-tape. Below are some suggestions for non-textual forms of feedback, which may be more appropriate for some audiences.

The principles of writing for non-specialist audiences are, though, the same as writing for academic colleagues: you need to think about the reader, what they are likely to want to know, and how to communicate this to them. Research participants and gatekeepers may be interested in issues such as: how typical they were compared with other participants, what is going to happen to the results of the study, whether they will lead to any improvements in practice. The general public (if this is a project likely to attract wider attention) will be primarily interested in the novel or unusual findings, and press releases designed for the mass media will need to focus on what is new or unexpected.

Alternatives to written reports

So far, this chapter has focused on 'writing up' as the most common way in which the findings of qualitative studies are disseminated. It is worth remembering, though, that written output such as reports, journal articles and books may not be the most appropriate ways to represent your research, because either the 'message' or the 'audience' may be best served by other formats. When working in multidisciplinary settings, textual accounts of the research findings may be particularly difficult for others to access. Here, more visual representations of the findings may be called for, either within traditional prose text or by replacing it on, for instance, posters. Results can be tabulated, pictorial illustrations included, and diagrams can be used to represent the connections between findings. Oral presentations of qualitative research are needed for conferences and seminars, and are also a useful way of feeding back results to users such as community groups.

Websites can provide a flexible format for reporting and disseminating qualitative findings. It is now relatively easy to create links on web pages to written outputs from projects, but Internet sites can also allow a more creative use of qualitative data. One good example is the DIPEx (Database of Individual Patients' Experience) project (www.dipex.org), which is a multimedia website and CD-ROM aimed at patients, carers, health professionals and researchers (Herxheimer et al. 2000). This uses data from a series of qualitative interview studies with patients with serious illnesses to provide information about how people coped with symptoms, found support and decided between treatment options. The main findings from each component qualitative study are summarized under key headings for each disease, and extracts from interviews are available for users to read, listen to or watch on video clips. A searchable website, with links to further information and details on support services, provides an accessible way of making the findings from these studies available to users who might want to look for examples of people who have had similar experiences.

Web-based publishing also offers possibilities for utilizing non-literary forms of communication within academic papers. Hyperlinks, which allow a user of web-based materials to 'click' on a button or highlighted text and move to other points, provide options to include a wealth of other materials alongside the text of the report, such as interview transcripts and links to comments from other authors or to non-textual material. The journal *Sociological Research Online*, for instance, has included articles that have hyperlinks to photographs (Thoutenhoofd 1998) and video clips (Lomax and Casey 1998) as part of the paper. Amanda Coffey and colleagues (1996) discuss the particular advantages that hypertext may have for writing qualitative research, given the possibilities it provides for non-linear representations of research outputs, and potentially a more interactive relationship with readers:

> Many people working with qualitative data, whether they use fieldnotes, interviews, oral history or documentary sources, feel frustrated by the necessity of imposing a single linear order on those materials. It is, after all, part of the rationale of ethnographic and similar approaches that the [researcher] recognizes the complexity of social inter-relatedness. (Coffey et al. 1996: 8.5)

Some practical issues to consider when writing up

Any piece of writing, then, needs to take into account the audience, in terms of what they are likely to want to know and how best to communicate this. We now turn to some general issues that you might face when writing up qualitative work in the health field.

Authorship

So far, we have assumed that you are the sole author of a qualitative report. This will be true of a research degree thesis, and is still typical in many qualitative social science research projects, but increasingly rare in other health research contexts, where you may be writing with others, or at least with their input. Cultures of authorship differ across disciplines, departments and even individual research teams, with each having their own expectations over such issues as whether team or individual authorship is the norm, or whether supervisors routinely expect to be listed as an author on their students' work. Conflicts over authorship (who is entitled to be named as an author, which order should the names go in?) can be extremely destructive to research teams, and it is good practice to establish responsibilities for writing up material at the beginning of a project. Some of the issues to consider at early team meetings include:

- What outputs are expected?
- Who will take the lead on drafting each?
- Who will be a contributing author, and who will have rights to edit, or approve, submitted papers?
- Who will have access to the data after the project is completed?

There are a number of guidelines for establishing rights and responsibilities with regard to authorship. The Vancouver guidelines, discussed above as establishing general requirements for biomedical journals, suggest that the rule of thumb is that each author should be able to defend the paper publicly, but this principle is difficult to put into practice, particularly when reporting studies that have contributors from a number of specialist disciplines. One approach suggests a system more like 'film credits' (Smith 1997), in which the specific contribution of each author is listed (such as research design, drafting the final paper, statistical analysis), and a guarantor named, who can take overall responsibility for a paper. Erol Digusto (1994) has a more complex solution that might be useful for those in larger teams. He suggests a 'points' system, in which all members of a research team award a fixed number of points among the team under headings for each kind of contribution. These are then used to award authorship and position on the authorship list for the list of papers likely to come out of the project in a fair and transparent manner. In practice, at least at the current time, most research teams still make decisions about authorship in an ad hoc manner, and researchers need to develop skills in both explicit negotiations around authorship and writing with colleagues.

Selecting examples and quotes

The amount of quoted material and context you can include will depend on the length of the article and the style of the journal, but in principle you need to include enough for the reader to judge the credibility of your interpretations. However much space you have, though, you will inevitably have to select particular quotes, and perhaps extracts from them, from the entire data set. Choosing particularly evocative or coherent quotes to illustrate findings is fine so long as the content is representative, and the text should indicate whether the extract is typical, or deviant, or perhaps unrepresentatively eloquent. Quotes should be tagged in the text with appropriate identifiers (such as age, gender, or whatever categories are important to the research), or an interview code number if this would breach confidentiality (see below). This both provides context for the reader, and demonstrates that you have not just picked illustrative examples from a small number of interviews.

Even in longer pieces of writing, be wary of 'over-quoting' and expecting your data to do the work that you, as author, should be doing to interpret, explain and make an argument. The quotes are there as *evidence* for your argument. Long articles with many quotes and little text in between look under-analysed, and the reader will not necessarily make the connections between them that you (having done the analysis and the thinking!) will.

Reproducing quotes

In general, quotes in qualitative papers are reproduced verbatim from the interview transcript or fieldwork notes, with the grammar and vocabulary of the original. This can pose a dilemma of balancing readability with veracity, with decisions about how to render, for instance, slang expressions or regional accents. Clearly, some editing always goes on, as a quote reproduced phonetically, with all the pauses and non-verbal noises transcribed, would be almost unreadable, and certainly not give a 'flavour' of the spoken version. Unless reporting the results of a conversation analysis type study (see Chapter 6), most pauses and intonations are not shown, and the spelling (in English-language journals) is standard English, unless the words used by the respondent are dialect or abbreviated. Transcription conventions (see Box 4.3) are used to represent missing text or explanatory words provided by the author.

Quoting material in a different language from the original creates even more acute dilemmas, in deciding whether to reproduce word-for-word translations or attempt to preserve the cultural meanings and nuances of the original. The decision of course depends on what work the quoted material is intended to do within the text. If extracts are there simply to give voice to particular participants, the choice may be to reproduce a 'cultural' translation, which maintains the meaning intended (as far as possible) for a reader using another language. A more ethnographic analysis may require considerable explanatory material in addition to the quote, to alert the reader to the relevant context. This might include issues such as how and when similar metaphors are used in this cultural setting, whether this is a relatively formal mode of speaking, whether the particular phrases used are common idioms used rhetorically, or are particular to this respondent.

Maintaining confidentiality for participants

If you have assured participants of confidentiality in final reports, you need to pay particular attention to whether the details of the case studies or interviewees you have given could be used to identify them. Code numbers, or perhaps pseudonyms, can be used to tag quotes or extracts from fieldnotes. Pseudonyms for people and places have the advantage of suggesting context, if chosen to reflect the connotations of the original.

Some study designs will pose particular problems in terms of confidentiality. Case studies, particularly of atypical or innovative services or settings, may be difficult to disguise, and those in the field are likely to know such sites, and possibly even the individuals involved. It is particularly important in these cases to ensure that participants have read draft reports and are happy about publication before disseminating more widely.

Making limitations and implications clear

Qualitative research may be an in-depth exploration of one particular setting, or an interview study of a relatively small sample of participants. As we discussed in Chapter 8, the generalizability of these findings is likely to arise from the conceptual transferability of the concepts generated, rather than the statistical representativeness of the sample. Readers will expect some comment on both the limitations of how far they can transfer your findings, and what implications the findings will have for their own practice, research or theories about the world. Routine or ritualistic accounts of the 'limitations' of qualitative work (such as 'this study was based on a small sample') are unhelpful, but it is worth noting the potential threats to generalizability in the study. To take an example from the paper quoted in Box 10.1, note how Griffiths and colleagues (Griffiths et al. 2001) flag up both the potential theoretical limitations to their study and the evidence that might mitigate these:

> We are aware of the dangers of stereotyping behaviour in ethnic groups, as well as problems in aggregating groups into classifications which might obscure cultural differences. None the less, distinctions emerged in accounts of south Asians and white patients that are consistent with work ... and which could explain differences in admission. (Griffiths et al. 2001: 965)

Other limitations worth discussing are methodological limitations, such as explicit reminders for the reader that the study used interview data, and thus concerns *accounts* of phenomena, rather than any direct evidence of those phenomena, or reminders about how the specific context of the research may have shaped the particular findings.

As well as noting the limitations, the conclusion section should also draw out the implications for the intended readership. Implications for practice, or for further research, may be 'obvious' to the researchers, who are immersed in the topic and have detailed knowledge, but these usually need to be explicitly marked for the reader.

Telling a story

Finally, a good qualitative paper tells a story. It uses your analytical ideas, related to theory, to take the reader through what you have discovered in your data. In essence, you are not just summarizing your respondents' views, but are presenting your analysis of them. Even for the 'drier', more scientific styles of biomedical journals, it is important for the article to lead the reader through the story you want to tell, rather than leaving them to divine the most salient points, or the new ideas contributed, or the connections between the concepts discussed. The background section should make a good case for why your report is interesting, and how the study you have done meets a need, and why the reader should care about your findings and interpretation. The findings should flow in the most coherent way possible, rather than be merely a list of 'themes' or points you want to make. A list of points suggests that the analysis is incomplete, and more work needs doing to make a tight argument about 'what is going on'. The discussion section should draw out the findings, in the light of what was already known, and frame the new discoveries and their implications for the reader. However well done the research was, it will not contribute to theory or practice if you cannot communicate the ideas to others in a way that engages them.

Conclusion

Many researchers find writing a challenge, at least for some kinds of output. For qualitative researchers, the process of writing is part of the work of analysis, rather than merely a report of it, and it is work. For publication, this can be particularly frustrating work, with most journals having high rejection rates and very few papers accepted on first submission (Loseke and Cahill 2004). Authors will typically revise manuscripts many, many times before submission. An essential skill for all writers is that of learning from feedback, and sharing drafts with colleagues who can be trusted to give good critical feedback is vital. Ask them to comment on: where your argument needed tightening; where you have made assertions with no evidence; where it is not clear why you have introduced a point, or followed it with another. Remember that, with written outputs, you as author are not present with the reader to take them through your argument: it has to stand alone as a written text, with enough 'signposting' throughout the story to tell them why they are being presented with this point, or this argument, at this moment, and why they should care.

Disseminating the findings of qualitative health research increasingly relies on an ability to produce a range of different written texts, and sometimes to think more imaginatively about other formats for reporting. Qualitative health researchers working in multi-disciplinary settings may face a 'double burden' of having to contribute to their discipline (for instance, in writing for mainstream social science journals, or producing monographs) as well as articles for biomedical journals. This is an opportunity, though, as well as a burden. In a practical sense, the outputs of qualitative health research are perhaps more likely to reach those in a position to utilize them than in other qualitative areas of research. In terms of theoretical development, being forced to think through the meaning of research findings from a number of perspectives is a real advantage in ensuring that qualitative data are fully analysed and exploited.

KEY POINTS

- Writing is an essential part of the process of qualitative analysis, and should begin early in the study.
- Qualitative researchers need to develop skills in addressing a range of specific audiences.
- This involves attention to both style and content.

EXERCISE

Take the observations you did for Exercise 2 in Chapter 6. Write up a short account of these in two different styles. Try writing one in the style of a biomedical journal, and one in a more sociological style. Consider the differences between these two accounts in terms of: vocabulary, structure, whether you wrote in the first person, whether you were focusing on different aspects of your observations.

FURTHER READING

Charmaz, K. (2006) *Constructing grounded theory: a practical guide through qualitative analysis*. London: Sage. This is a general text taking the reader through the steps of Charmaz's approach to grounded theory, but Charmaz takes the craft of writing seriously, and there is much insightful advice throughout this book for those using any style of qualitative research wanting to improve their written outputs.

Hall, G.M. (2003) *How to write a paper* (3rd edn). London: BMJ Books. Taken from short articles in the *British Medical Journal*. Although it does not deal specifically with the demands of writing up qualitative work, this is an excellent guide to the general issues of writing for biomedical journals, with contributions from several journal editors on how to write clearly and maximize your chances of being published.

Woods, P. (1999) *Successful writing for qualitative researchers*. London: Routledge. This is a practical text on issues of style and the problems typically faced in writing up qualitative research for social science journals. Includes chapters on both 'standard' and alternative journal formats, with examples largely taken from the sociology of education.

11 Reading and Appraising Qualitative Outputs

CHAPTER SUMMARY

Doing research entails reading the research outputs of others, both to locate our own findings within existing bodies of knowledge, and to develop methodological skills through exposure to as wide a range of material as possible. Reading is a critical activity, in that researchers have to evaluate qualitative work in the context of their own research. In some areas of health research, the formalization of critical appraisal has been advocated, although the application of 'quality checklists' to qualitative research remains contentious.

Introduction

In the previous chapter, we noted that if you are writing for colleagues in the social sciences, demonstrating how your study contributes to the wider discipline or topic is essential. Chapter 8 also touched on the importance of reading for developing the 'social science imagination' that is essential for insightful analysis. This clearly entails a broad reading background: to do good qualitative work requires a familiarity with both the traditional canon of your own discipline, and the more recent relevant work in your topic area.

Reading the research outputs of others is, however, not just done to produce the 'Literature Review' chapter of a thesis, or the background section of a research report. It is an essential element of learning and developing method-ological skills. We read journal articles, books and research reports not just to add to our store of empirical knowledge, but to see how others have addressed methodological challenges, or to spark off connections between our own areas of research and those of others. Reading is not a passive task. To read for research involves critical appraisal, in that the aim is to evaluate what you read in terms of the research you have undertaken, or propose to do. This chapter goes on to discuss whether this kind of appraisal can (or should) be formalized for qualitative research, but first we turn to the more general issues of reading in the context of qualitative research.

We bring to reading our own experiences and frameworks of understand-ing, and re-reading qualitative work often brings different understandings at different points in a research career. There is no single 'true' reading of any text, but a multiple number of possible readings. These change, for instance, over time with the shifting political and social contexts framing particular readings of texts. James Clifford, after discussing the ways in which classic ethnographies now appear (through decades of feminist scholarship) to be 'biased' in terms of their focus on the cultural domains of men, notes:

> In recognising such biases, however, it is well to recall that our own 'full' versions will themselves inevitably appear partial: and if many cultural portrayals now seem more limited than they once did, this is an index of the contingency and historical movement of all readings. No one reads from a neutral or final position. (Clifford 1986b: 18)

He goes on to note that this implies that the notion of identifying 'gaps' in the literature as a rationale for research is a rather limited one. Such gaps will be filled, but in doing so others are revealed, given that there is no possible com-plete truth that can be read. The 'canon' of literature in whatever field we are researching is not an unchanging corpus of facts to which new findings are accrued, but a shifting field of possible readings. The implications of this for reading for any specific project are twofold. First, it is important not to rely purely on mechanical searches of databases of literature. The use of elec-tronic databases of abstracts (such as PubMed or Medline) is becoming increasingly popular in health research. They do have a very useful function, in generating a number (often a dauntingly large pile!) of useful leads, but this cannot be taken to be the sum total of 'the literature' worth reviewing. Such a comprehensive undertaking is impossible. In doing qualitative work, it is worth reading both widely and imaginatively – including 'classic' works as well as the latest findings in the field, and research reports from outside the narrow field of interest. Readings likely to be of interest to health researchers will come from a number of sources, including books and social science jour-nals (which may not be abstracted on electronic databases), from social sci-ences research in topics other than health, and also from 'non-research' sources, such as fiction and journalism.

A second implication is that the outcomes of reading are not just a store of new 'facts' to add to our understanding of the topic, but are rather more flexible and contingent. One article might suggest new concepts we can adapt, a monograph might provide a methodological insight, and a novel may spark off a new way of thinking about our data. Re-reading any of these sources will generate different insights at different points in a research career. There is an increasing tendency to look only for the most recent research articles, and to assume that anything published more than ten years ago will have little relevance. While this may be true if working in fast-moving scientific fields, it is worth remembering that human behaviour changes rather slowly. There is often much of value in the 'classic' social science articles and books, and it is usually worth following up original sources where possible, rather than relying on textbook summaries or reviews, as your reading will be framed by the particular problems and concepts that concern you in the context of your own research.

Reading qualitative research, and reading for qualitative research, is as incremental as all other stages of the research process. Reading cannot be restricted to the start of a project, with perhaps a brief check to update the literature review before submitting a paper or handing in a dissertation. Like analysis and writing, it has to be integrated through the whole research process. Early data analysis will generate new ideas and concepts to follow up in the literature, and wide reading throughout the stages of fieldwork and analysis will help develop analytical ideas about the data.

Reading critically

In qualitative research, the result of reading the literature should, then, be rather more than merely summarizing the key points of previous researchers and then listing them, or identifying the empirical 'gaps' in what has been written. Indeed, Harry Wolcott (2002) argues that a traditional literature review may be inappropriate for qualitative research, given that it is merely a device to prove how 'learned' the writer is, and he suggests that we should instead just use literature as and when it is needed within our arguments. However, many research outputs (whether PhD theses or journal articles) will demand something that looks like a literature review. Whether written up as a traditional 'stand-alone' chapter or section, or integrated throughout a piece of writing, there are some specific tasks that the qualitative review should do. For a research degree thesis, one task of the review is still to demonstrate the writer's ability to critically appraise the literature. For all research, though, the key one is to locate your own particular study and its findings in terms of the broader scholarship in your discipline (or disciplines), and you therefore need to *use* the literature to answer a number of questions, such as:

- What theoretical approach(es) does this research question arise from?
- What debates are current within this field, and how does this study contribute to them?

- What areas of consensus are there? That is, what is the received wisdom in the field, what everyone believes to be true?
- What shortcomings in previous scholarship are recognized?

Reading, and writing up your review of the literature, should be a critical exercise that helps a reader of your research to see exactly why your study was important (theoretically or practically) and how it builds on previous scholarship, by contributing to debates, undermining 'what is known', or extending understanding. Reviewing the relevant literature for any particular research project requires, then, a 'respectfully critical' approach, which balances an awareness of previous contributions with an appraisal of them. 'Respect' can be particularly difficult in fields like health, where the literature you come across comes from such a wide range of disciplines and theoretical perspectives, some of which may be unfamiliar. Chris Hart, in his (1998) book on carrying out literature reviews in the social sciences, discusses the challenges of coming to this respectful approach when faced with what seem unnecessarily 'difficult' texts:

> ... competence in reading research is not easily acquired. ... It takes time and a willingness to face challenges, acquire new understandings and have sufficient openness of mind to appreciate that there are other views of the world. ... This means not categorizing the text using prejudicial perceptions of the study discipline, but instead placing the research in the context of norms of the discipline. (Hart 1998: 11)

Critical appraisal involves, then, understanding research outputs in their own terms, and persevering with what can seem at first sight to be jargon-filled or overly complex accounts from unfamiliar fields. In addition to being 'respectful', though, reading for research needs to be evaluative, in identifying both the contributions and the shortcomings of what has gone before. Evaluation entails appraising qualitative research in its own terms (was the methodological approach appropriate for the question? Is the analysis credible?) and also in terms of broader questions about its contribution to knowledge.

Appraising empirical work: are criteria possible?

We all evaluate or appraise work when we read it, in deciding whether it is well written, useful, credible or flawed. This appraisal is done for particular purposes. Journal reviewers are judging whether the manuscript is appropriate for the journal readership, meets certain (sometimes formal) criteria of 'sound' research and is written in an acceptable style. PhD students will judge whether particular articles are relevant for their topic or important to the field they are studying. One question that has divided qualitative researchers is whether we should try to formalize these implicit criteria that are used to make these kinds of appraisals. A key problem, of course, is that the different epistemological approaches, theoretical starting points and methodological choices made by qualitative researchers would imply rather different criteria, if we were being 'respectful' and judging qualitative outputs in their own terms. Is it possible to come to any consensus about what constitutes 'quality' in written accounts of qualitative research?

The increasing interest in using the findings from qualitative research in health has generated substantial interest in trying to do just this. The incentives for attempting what seems to be an impossible task come from a number of directions:

- *The growing interest in 'evidence-based health care'*. In the field of health, there has been a powerful movement for using research evidence to inform both policy and clinical decision making (Sackett et al. 1996; Gray 1997). If qualitative findings are to be included in an 'evidence base' (Green and Britten 1998), it has been argued that we need some way of appraising the quality of evidence from these studies in order to synthesize empirical findings (Mays et al. 2001).
- *The increasing acceptability of qualitative work to biomedical journal editors.* Given the lack of training in social sciences methodology of many journal editors and reviewers, there has been a demand for criteria to help them make decisions about the quality of articles submitted for publication.
- *Interest in multidisciplinary studies in health care.* When working across disciplines, it can be helpful for those from non-social science traditions to have guidelines for reading unfamiliar types of literature, to suggest how they might evaluate the validity and usefulness of contributions that use unfamiliar methodologies. The Critical Appraisal Skills Programme (CASP), for instance, introduces its assessment tool for qualitative research saying that it has 'been developed for those unfamiliar with qualitative research' (CASP 2001).

Over the last decade, a number of 'checklists' for appraising qualitative empirical articles have been generated, in part to meet the needs identified above (see, for instance, Boulton et al. 1996; Popay et al. 1998; Mays and Pope 1999; Blaxter 2000; CASP 2001). Dixon-Woods and colleagues, in their review of the problems of such checklists, identified over 100 proposals for quality criteria, with 'some adopting non-reconcilable positions on a number of issues' (Dixon-Woods et al. 2004: 224). The growing interest in systematic reviews of qualitative research (discussed in Chapter 7) has been one incentive for producing such checklists, given the need to assess the quality of contributing studies. The use of 'checklists' to appraise qualitative work does raise a number of questions:

- Given the range of designs and approaches in qualitative research, is it desirable to try to reach a consensus on what the `criteria of quality' should be?
- If it is desirable, is it possible to 'operationalize' the procedures readers use when judging quality? That is, is it possible to reify the elements of quality in such a way that they can be clearly described as 'quality criteria' for readers

to evaluate the research, rather than merely what has been included in the report? This is essentially a question about the *validity* of checklists.

- If it is desirable and possible, how far would different readers agree on whether criteria had been met or not? That is, is it possible to develop *reliable* checklists, which could be used to reach a consensus on the quality of an empirical report of qualitative work?

In general terms, it is probably impossible to develop a consensus view on what the criteria of good quality should be for all empirical qualitative work. The different epistemological starting points, methodological approaches and disciplinary traditions would all imply rather different evaluations of what 'good research' would look like. However, most checklists are not aiming to identify criteria for 'quality' per se, but rather criteria for *appropriateness* for particular uses. These uses might include publication in a particular journal, or perhaps inclusion in a systematic review of the qualitative evidence on a particular topic. For use in a systematic review, the questions around the reliability of guidelines could be addressed through using more than one reviewer, so that the degree of consensus on how far each paper considered met the criteria could be measured.

Appraisal criteria

The various checklists that have been developed cover a number of common issues, although obviously there are differences reflecting the different functions they were designed to perform. Mildred Blaxter (2000), on behalf of the UK Medical Sociology Group, developed the list that is summarized in Box 11.1, for circulation to medical journal editors to assist them in appraising qualitative work. They were not designed to be comprehensive or exhaustive, and not all researchers would agree on these as markers of quality, but they do cover the main topics that readers using literature to inform a review for evidence, or judging the appropriateness of findings for a general health care audience, might need to consider.

Many of the criteria summarized in Box 11.1 were discussed in Chapter 8 as elements of rigorous analysis. They are, at this level, not particularly contentious – especially if it is remembered that they are aiming not to legislate for what qualitative work *should* look like, but merely to highlight questions that readers of particular sorts (such as editors of biomedical journals, or reviewers carrying out a literature review for policy making) might want to consider in judging whether the research has been conducted and reported appropriately. However, the use of such 'checklists' has prompted debate about what is 'lost' from the qualitative tradition in attempting to formalize good practice guidelines in this way.

A first criticism is that they do not reflect current practice. Mary Boulton and colleagues (Boulton et al. 1996) searched for all the qualitative reports in five years of publishing from seven medical journals, and found 70 examples that had used qualitative methods of data collection and analysis. Of these, they

Box 11.1	Some criteria for the evaluation of qualitative research papers
Criteria	**Examples**
Research design: Are the methods appropriate for the research question?	Does the research seek to understand processes or structures, or illuminate subjective experiences or meanings?
Theory: Is the connection to an existing body of knowledge or theory clear?	Is there adequate reference to the literature? Does the work cohere with, or critically address, existing theory?
Transparency of procedures: Are there clear accounts of the sampling strategy, data collection and analysis?	Is the selection of cases or participants theoretically justified?
Has the relationship between fieldworkers' research and participants been considered?	How did research participants perceive the research? Were careful records kept?
Was data collection and record-keeping systematic?	Were full records or transcripts used, if appropriate?
Analysis: Is reference made to acceptable procedures for analysis?	Is it clear how analysis was done? Has reliability been considered?
How systematic was the analysis? Is there adequate discussion of how themes, concepts or categories were derived from the data?	What steps were taken to guard against selectivity in the use of data?
Is there adequate discussion of the evidence for and against the researcher's arguments?	Are negative data given? Has there been a search for 'deviant cases'?
Presentation: Is the research clearly contextualized?	Is there relevant information about the settings and participants?
Are the data presented systematically?	Are the cases or variables integrated into their social context, rather than abstracted and decontextualized?

(Continued)

Is there a clear distinction between data and interpretation?	Are quotations, fieldnotes, etc., identified such that the reader can judge the range of evidence being used?
Is the author's own position clearly stated?	Do the conclusions follow from the data? Has the impact of this on the research been explored?
Value: Are the results credible and appropriate?	Do they address the research question? Are they plausible and coherent? Are they important, either theoretically or practically?
Ethics: Have ethical issues been adequately considered?	Has the issue of confidentiality been considered? Have the consequences of the work been considered?

found that the majority appropriately used qualitative methods for the research question, but fewer would meet other quality criteria. Using a similar list to that summarized in Box 11.1, Boulton and colleagues found that about half of the papers met most of the criteria, but that there were typically shortcomings over such criteria as: providing sufficient original material to satisfy the reader about the relationship between data and interpretation, steps to improve validity of the analysis, steps to improve reliability, and the processes of data analysis.

A second possible criticism of the application of checklists is that the more interpretative elements of analysis, which, arguably, result in interesting and more conceptually satisfying findings, are rather difficult to describe. Boulton and colleagues note that even the more mundane processes of analysis (how coding schemes were developed and applied, for instance) can be very difficult to describe, but they argue that this is an essential element of providing credible evidence.

Third, as we noted in Chapter 8, few of the 'classic' qualitative studies that have had an impact on the field of health and illness, and reported in monographs or social science journals, would meet the kinds of criteria suggested above. Boulton and colleagues consider the concern that quality criteria would 'inhibit more purely creative and imaginative uses of qualitative methods ... and rule governed research would less frequently produce the startling narrative found in the works of, say, Goffman or Becker' (Boulton et al. 1996: 178). However, they find this an unconvincing argument, at least when applied to the kinds of qualitative research reported in health journals. As they note, little of the work they reviewed 'aspired to such creative use of the qualitative method', and on balance they argue that there are advantages in moving towards consensus and transparency around how we judge the quality of qualitative reports.

Finally, a practical shortcoming of criteria checklists is that adequate space for addressing all the issues covered in guidelines (locating the study in a body of theory, context, details of the analysis, reflexivity) is rarely available in a medical journal, which might allow 2,000 words. One response some journals have to this problem is to provide longer web-based versions, in which further details of, say, analysis procedures can be discussed.

A more fundamental problem with guidelines is perhaps the range of qualitative methodological approaches that generates useful findings for health, and the danger that producing checklists for journals to use will restrict the range of research undertaken, as being able to publish findings is one factor in deciding how and what to research. There are resulting problems with researchers 'writing to the guidelines' in rather unreflective and routine ways. It is not uncommon, for instance, to come across such claims in medical journal qualitative papers as 'Reliability was maximized by using two people to code the data' or 'Grounded theory was used to analyse the data'. Such sentences tell the reader very little (how did the two coders develop their conceptual coding scheme from their discussions? In what ways did a grounded theory approach inform the design and analysis of the study?), and there is a sense that they have been inserted to 'tick the box on a checklist' and maximize the chances of publication, rather than adopted to maximize the validity of the analysis.

It could also be noted that the guidelines might work relatively well for small-scale interview studies that have been analysed using thematic content analysis, which do form the bulk of qualitative contributions to medical journals (Boulton et al. 1996), but are perhaps considerably less useful for other study designs (such as ethnographic studies, complex action research projects), or other analytical approaches (such as conversation analysis, the findings from a 'saturated' grounded theory study). Dixon-Woods et al. (2004) suggest a useful compromise of a series of prompts for appraising qualitative research which are generic, but which could be followed up with more specific prompts for different methodologies. However, this does not perhaps deal with the more fundamental objections to the undue focus on empirical findings rather than theoretical insight. Ethnographers, in particular, have debated the issue of criteria for qualitative writing, and in general have been less accepting of the 'checklist' approach than qualitative health service researchers.

Criteria in ethnography

Reviewing the various positions in the debate on 'criteria' for appraisal in ethnography, Martyn Hammersley (1992b: 57–68) outlines three possible positions, which could be summarized as:

1   Given that qualitative research does not start from a positivist position, there can be no privileged position from which to assess the 'truth' or

trustworthiness of a particular account. Therefore, the idea of quality criteria is a logical impossibility.

2   Ethnography, in claiming to produce 'scientific' findings, should be judged in terms of the same criteria that any research is judged by.

3   Ethnography, as an alternative paradigm, and as drawing on non-positivistic epistemological underpinnings, requires a particular set of criteria for judging quality.

Rejecting the first two, on the grounds that the relativism of (1) would undercut the basis of rational discussion and that the kinds of models implied by (2) are those of quantitative research, with concepts that are inadequate for judging qualitative, non-experimental studies, he develops some suggestions under (3). His argument for the need for criteria is that he believes that the aim of ethnographic research should be to 'provide information that is both true and relevant to some legitimate public concern' (Hammersley 1992b: 68), and that criteria should therefore relate to both validity and relevance. On the first, validity (the 'truth' of the account), he argues that ethnographic writing should be judged in terms of plausibility and credibility. The reader essentially asks: are the findings plausible, and is there sufficient evidence provided to render the claims made credible? Clearly, the less plausible findings are (in that they are, say, out of line with our expectations or the accepted consensus), the more evidence a reader will need to be convinced of their credibility. Here, Hammersley demonstrates the need for sensitivity to the needs of different audiences: to make findings credible for, say, general practitioners compared with a patients' organization, we would probably need to include different levels of detail on the various sorts of evidence from the study. His second criterion is 'relevance', in terms of the importance of the topic and how it contributes to the literature. These criteria have considerable appeal to areas such as health care ethnography, where (multidisciplinary) audiences are generally demanding of both credibility and relevance.

Hammersley stays at the level of the 'evidence' in discussing criteria for assessing the quality of ethnographic work in terms of what it contributes. Others have attempted to integrate the aesthetic criteria that in practice are a large element of our reaction to a particular piece of work. In judging whether a piece of research is credible or not, we are as likely to be persuaded by writing style and rhetorical skill as any more 'objective' notions of the strength of evidence. Laurel Richardson (2000), in a bid to combine both 'scientific' and 'literary' criteria for judging qualitative work, outlines five criteria that she uses when reviewing papers and monographs:

• substantive contribution to our understanding of social life
• aesthetic merit
• reflexivity, including an account of how the text came to be written, whether there is enough about the author to judge their point of view and ethical issues

- impact – does it have an emotional and intellectual impact on the reader?
- expression of a reality – is it credible?

This is an attempt to see the aims of writing up as broader than merely adding (valid) empirical evidence to what is known about a topic. Other ethnographic writers go further, with arguments under Hammersley's first position: that it is impossible to come up with 'objective' criteria for appraising qualitative research. Arthur Bochner (2000), for instance, argues that the obsession with criteria is evidence of 'our insecurities about our scientific stature', and an unwillingness to admit that the phenomena that qualitative researchers study are 'messy, complicated, uncertain and soft'. Criteria focus the researcher towards rigour rather than imagination, and questions of 'truth' rather than possibility. Bochner is not advocating an 'anything goes' approach, but rather a concern with the narratives that, for him, are the core of research, and the unique contribution of ethnography. Thus, in appraising writing, he reports six elements of narratives that are important for him. These link experiences and meanings, and bring in the imaginative and poetic aspects of the writing. These are summarized in Box 11.2.

Box 11.2   Bochner's criteria for judging 'poetic social science'

- Detail, of the commonplace, of feelings as well as facts.
- Narratives that are structurally complex and take account of time as it is experienced.
- A sense of the author, their subjectivity and 'emotional credibility'.
- Stories that tell about believable journeys through the life course.
- Ethical self-consciousness: respect for others in the field, and for the moral dimensions of the story.
- A story that moves the reader at an emotional as well as a rational level.

Source: Adapted from Bochner (2000).

Reading qualitative research for health, we are often drawn to the criteria of rigour summarized in Box 11.1, for these are framed in ways that are familiar to colleagues from other disciplines, and orientated towards producing 'evidence' that is 'useful' (because it is credible) for practice. However, Bochner's alternative suggestions are a reminder that what qualitative research often aims to provide is not evidence, but insight, and not credibility, but possibility. Reading widely, and appraising in ways appropriate to both our disparate research needs and the aims of the writer, is the best way of ensuring that our own research can contribute in terms of both evidence and insight.

Conclusion

The debate about criteria for evaluating qualitative research centres on a division about what research is for: whether to add to an evidence base, in which case we need criteria in order to judge the validity and usefulness of that evidence, or whether to provide a more unique, qualitative contribution to our understanding of health, which involves an insightful understanding of concepts of health and illness in terms of people's lived experience. The former perspective is perhaps typical of qualitative health services research, whereas the latter is debated most heatedly in ethnography. Most researchers will shift between the two perspectives, and of course will utilize the arguments of each rhetorically at times, in order to persuade particular audiences of the value of their methods.

In conclusion, there is a now a huge qualitative health research literature, and an even wider range of potentially useful readings for qualitative health researchers. In this chapter we have suggested that doing 'good' qualitative research in health involves a familiarity with this literature, and a respectful appraisal of it in terms of how past scholarship has contributed to the questions we ask and how we consider answering them. A broad reading experience is an essential precondition for contributing your own insights to the field of qualitative research in health.

KEY POINTS

- Doing good qualitative work requires broad reading.
- Reading for research should be both respectful and critical.
- There is considerable debate as to whether criteria for assessing the quality of qualitative work are possible or desirable.

EXERCISE

Choose two qualitative articles you have enjoyed, one from a social science journal and one from a biomedical journal. Assess them both in terms first of the criteria summarized in Box 11.1 and then in Box 11.2. Did the 'scores' reflect your own views of the usefulness, quality or contribution of the articles? If possible, compare your evaluations with those of a colleague. How reliable are such guidelines?

FURTHER READING

Clifford, J. and Marcus, G. (1986) *Writing culture: the poetics and politics of ethnography*. Berkeley: University of California Press. A collection of essays on the topic of representation in ethnography, which explore, from a number of perspectives, the status of texts and authors. Interesting reading for those looking to challenge the ways in which they read qualitative products, and to examine at texts in their literary, political and ethical contexts.

Hart, C. (1998) *Doing a literature review: releasing the social science research imagination*. London: Sage. Aimed at postgraduate students needing to do a literature review for a dissertation or thesis, this is also an excellent text for other researchers on what the aims of reading should be and how we can communicate material gathered from reviews.

Glossary

Action research A study in which the aim is to change practice, rather than (or as well as) to describe, analyse or evaluate practice.

Case study In-depth study undertaken of one particular 'case', which could be a site, individual or policy.

CAQDAS Computer Assisted Qualitative Data Analysis Software. A number of packages have now been developed to aid in the management and analysis of qualitative data.

Coding Process of assigning labels ('codes') to extracts of data. In framework analysis this process is called 'indexing'.

Coding scheme An emerging list, or more detailed framework, of the names and descriptions of codes that will be used to code and analyse the data.

Constant comparative method The use of comparisons at every stage of analysis; central to the methodological approach of grounded theory.

Constructionist approach An epistemological approach which assumes that there are no stable, pre-existing phenomena (such as disease categories, or biological genders, for instance) but seeks instead to address questions of how those phenomena are created through social processes.

Conversation analysis Detailed analysis of the form and content of talk to address questions of how meaning is actively created by social actors.

Covert observation Observation in research conducted without the knowledge of those observed. This raises a number of ethical issues that need to be considered.

Critical incidents Those incidents that have a significant positive or negative effect. Asking about 'critical incidents' is a useful way of generating data about those factors that contribute most to, for instance, satisfaction or dissatisfaction with services.

Deviant cases Examples from a data set that do not fit emerging hypotheses. In grounded theory approaches, these are deliberately sought out to challenge developing theory about the data.

Discourse analysis   This phrase is used in a number of ways; sometimes to describe techniques to analyse micro level discourses (e.g., everyday talk), but also to describe the analysis of macro-level discourse, such as 'biomedicine'.

Emic   In anthropology, emic codes are those utilized by the participants themselves to describe the world. An emic understanding is one from the perspective of those you are studying.

Epistemology   A branch of philosophy concerned with *knowing*; including what the nature of knowledge is, how we come to know what we know, and how we demonstrate the legitimacy of that knowledge.

Ethnomethodology   An approach to research developed by the sociologist Harold Garfinkel which is directed at questions of how social order is produced through analysing how people make sense of the world.

Etic   In anthropology, etic codes are the analytical codes the researcher develops to explain what is going on.

Framework analysis   A structured approach to qualitative analysis developed by the National Centre for Social Research that is particularly useful for applied policy studies.

Gatekeepers   In fieldwork, those people who can facilitate or give permission for you to enter the field or approach participants.

Generalizability   The extent to which the findings of a study can be extended to other settings, populations or topics.

Grounded theory   An approach to qualitative research based on 'discovering' theory from data, with an associated set of explicit techniques for analysing data, developed by Anselm Strauss, Barney Glaser and their colleagues and students.

In-depth interviews   Qualitative research interviews with an aim of allowing the respondent to speak at length, in detail, in ways in which they are most comfortable, on a given topic. They may have a topic guide, but not a strict, pre-determined schedule of questions.

Informed consent   The principle that participants in a study should be informed about the risks, benefits and purposes of their participation before deciding whether or not to take part, and that this participation should be freely chosen.

Meta-ethnography   A technique for integrating the findings from a set of qualitative research on related topics by subjecting the findings to secondary analysis in order to derive new insights.

Methodology   The study of methods, including the philosophical principles that inform different approaches as well as the technical issues of how to generate and analyse data. To describe the 'methodology' rather than the 'methods' of a study implies an account of the principles by which particular approaches were taken, rather than just a recipe of the techniques used.

Narrative analysis   Approaches to analysis that assume that accounts can be treated as 'narratives', with particular structures and styles.

Participant observation   Study involving the researcher observing social life from the perspective of a 'participant' within the field. This describes the methodological approach of most traditional anthropology, in which the anthropologist lived or worked in the setting they were researching over long periods of time.

Phenomenology   The study of phenomena, as they are experienced through consciousness, and a methodological approach that addresses the 'essences' of phenomena.

Positivism   Epistemological approach to research which assumes a stable reality that can be known and understood through empirical methods. More typical in quantitative than qualitative methodologies.

Pseudo-patient studies   Also called 'simulated client studies', these involve researchers acting as patients in order to study what goes on in health care encounters.

Purposive sample   A sample in which participants are selected 'purposefully' in order to include a pre-determined range.

RCT (Randomized controlled trial)   Experimental research design in which one group of cases (which could be patients, or villages, or any other unit) receive an intervention (such as a medicine, or a social programme) and another group (the 'controls') do not. Membership of each group is randomly assigned. In a placebo controlled RCT, the control group receive an alternative assumed to have no therapeutic effect.

Reflexivity   The process of reflecting on both your own effect on the data generated as a participant in the field, and on the social and cultural processes of the research itself (how and why it is possible to ask this question, now, for instance).

Relativism   A belief that there can be different perspectives on reality or truth, or in *constructionist* accounts, that there can be different realities, and that there are no logical grounds for privileging one particular account of reality (such as a biomedical one) above others.

Reliability   In quantitative methods, this refers to the stability of measures. In qualitative work it refers to issues such as accuracy of reporting, consistency of coding, and thoroughness of analysis.

Respondent validation   Also called member checking, an exercise of taking findings back to participants in the study for feedback on the interpretation of the data. May be useful as a source of further data, but there are limits to how far this will contribute to validation.

Saturation   In grounded theory approaches this is the point where new data are not adding to emerging theory.

Semi-structured interviews   Interviews which have a predetermined *topic guide*, but the interviewer has flexibility over how to and in what order, to ask the questions.

Systematic review   Review of the literature which has an explicit strategy for searching for and including studies, and seeks to answer a specific research question.

Theoretical sample   In grounded theory, a sample selected iteratively, initially on the basis of existing theory about who will be informative, and then on the basis of ongoing analysis. Sampling continues to the point of *saturation.*

Topic guide   List of questions or topics to cover during an interview or group discussion.

Transferability   This concept is often preferred to *generalizability* in qualitative research as it refers to the extension of *conceptual* rather than *empirical* findings to other settings.

Triangulation   A process of using multiple methods or data sets to increase the *validity* of findings, on the assumption that findings are more credible if they are consistent with others.

Validity   This refers to the 'truth' of findings, and in qualitative research involves attention to the quality of analysis and techniques to aid the credibility of interpretation.

References

Adams, S., Pill, R. and Jones, A. (1997) 'Medication, chronic illness and identity: the perspective of people with asthma', *Social Science and Medicine*, 45: 189–201.

Adamson, C. (1997) 'Existential and clinical uncertainty in the medical encounter: an idiographic account of an illness trajectory defined by inflammatory bowel disease and avascular necrosis', *Sociology of Health and Illness*, 19: 133–59.

Agar, M.H. (1980) *The professional stranger: an informal introduction to ethnography.* San Diego, CA: Academic Press.

Andrews, L., Stocking, C., Krizek, T., et al. (1997) 'An alternative strategy for studying adverse events in medical care', *Lancet*, 349: 309–13.

Andrews, M., Squire, C. and Tamboukou, M. (2008) (eds) *Doing narrative research.* London: Sage.

Annandale, E. (1998) *The sociology of health and medicine.* London: Polity.

Annett, H. and Rifkin, S. (1995) *Guidelines for rapid participatory appraisals to assess community health needs.* Geneva: World Health Organization.

Armstrong, D. (1986) 'The invention of infant mortality', *Sociology of Health and Illness*, 8: 211–32.

ASA (Association of Social Anthropologists) (1987) *Ethical guidelines for good practice.* London: Association of Social Anthropologists.

Atkins, S., Lewin, S., Smith, H. et al. (2008) 'Conducting a meta-ethnography of qualitative literature: lessons learnt', *BMC Medical Research Methodology*, 8: 21.

Atkinson, P. (1995) *Medical talk and medical work: the liturgy of the clinic.* London: Sage.

Backhouse, G. (2002) 'How preserving confidentiality in qualitative health research can be compatible with preserving data for future use', *Medical Sociology News*, 28(2): 32–5.

Baker, R. and Hinton, R. (1999) 'Do focus groups facilitate meaningful participation in social research?', in R. Barbour and J. Kitzinger (eds), *Developing focus group research: politics, theory and practice.* London: Sage, pp. 79–98.

Barnard, M. (2005) 'Discomforting research: colliding moralities and looking for "truth" in a study of parental drug problems', *Sociology of Health and Illness*, 27(1):1–19.

Barrett, G. and Wellings, K. (2002) 'What is a "planned" pregnancy? Empirical data from a British study', *Social Science and Medicine* 55: 545–57, and Barrett, G., Personal communication.

Barthes, R. (1985) 'An almost obsessive relation to writing instruments', in *The Grain of the Voice*: Interview 1962–1980 (translator L. Coverdale). New York: Hill & Wang, pp. 177–82.

Basch, C.E. (1987) 'Focus group interview: an underutilized research technique for improving theory and practice in health education', *Health Education Quarterly*, 14: 411–48.

Baum, F. (1995) 'Researching public health: behind the qualitative-quantitative methodological debate', *Social Science and Medicine*, 40: 459–68.

Bazeley, P. (2007) *Qualitative data analysis with NVivo.* London: Sage.

Beauchamp, T.L. and Childress, J.F. (1983) *Principles of biomedical ethics* (2nd edn). Oxford: Oxford University Press.

Becker, H. (1967) 'Whose side are we on?', *Social Problems*, 14: 239–47.

Becker, H. and Geer, B. (1957) 'Participant observation and interviewing: a comparison', *Human Organization*, 16: 28–32.

Becker, M.H. (1974) 'The health belief model and personal health behaviour', *Health Education Monographs*, 2: 324–508.

Beckerleg, S., Lewando-Hundt, G.A., Borkan, J.M., Abu Saad, K.J. and Belmaker, I. (1997) 'Eliciting local voices using natural group interviews', *Anthropology and Medicine*, 4: 273–88.

Bendelow, G. (1993) 'Using visual imagery to analyse gender differences in perception of pain', in C. Renzetti and R. Lee (eds), *Researching sensitive subjects*. London: Sage, pp. 212–29.

Berger, P.L. and Luckman, T. (1967) *The social construction of reality*. Harmondsworth: Penguin.

Black, N. (1994) 'Why we need qualitative research', *Journal of Epidemiology and Community Health*, 48: 425–6.

Blaxter, M. (2000) 'Criteria for qualitative research', *Medical Sociology News*, 26: 34–7.

Bloor, M., Fincham, B. and Sampson, H. (2007) *Qualiti (NCRM) Commissioned Inquiry into the risk to well-being of researchers in qualitative research*. Cardiff: Cardiff University.

Bloor, M., Frankland, J., Thomas, M. and Robson, K. (2001) *Focus groups in social research*. London: Sage.

Bochner, A.P. (2000) 'Criteria against ourselves', *Qualitative Inquiry*, 6: 266–72.

Bond, S. and Bond, J. (1982) 'A Delphi study of clinical nursing research priorities', *Journal of Advanced Nursing*, 7: 565–75.

Boulton, M., Fitzpatrick, R. and Swinburne, C. (1996) 'Qualitative research in health care. II. A structured review and evaluation of studies', *Journal of Evaluation in Clinical Practice*, 2: 171–9.

Bowden, A., Fox-Rushby, J.A., Nyandieka, L. and Wanjau, J. (2002) 'Methods for pre-testing and piloting survey questions: illustrations from the KENQOL survey of health-related quality of life', *Health Policy and Planning*, 17: 322–30.

Bowker, G.C. and Star, S.L. (1999) *Sorting things out: classification and its consequences*. Cambridge, MA: MIT Press.

Bowler, I. (1995) 'Further notes on record taking and making in maternity care: the case of south Asian descent women', *Sociological Review*, 43: 36–51.

Brikci, N. and Green, J. (2007) *A guide to using qualitative methods*. London: MSF UK.

Britten, N., Campbell, R., Pope, C., Donovan, J., Morgan, M. and Pill, R. (2002) 'Using meta-ethnography to synthesise qualitative research: a worked example', *Journal of Health Services Research and Policy*, 7: 209–15.

Bryman, A. (1988) *Quantity and quality in social research*. London: Routledge.

BSA (British Sociological Association) (1992) 'BSA statement of ethical practice', *Sociology*, 26: 703–7.

Bulmer, M. (1982) 'The research ethics of pseudo-patient studies: a new look at the merits of covert ethnographic methods', *Sociological Review*, 30: 627–46.

Bulmer, M. (1984) *Sociological research methods: an introduction* (2nd edn). Basingstoke: Macmillan.

Burghart, R. (1993) 'His Lordship at the Cobblers' well', in M. Hobart (ed.), *An anthropological critique of development*. London: Routledge, pp. 77–99.

Bury, M. (1982) 'Chronic illness as biographic disruption', *Sociology of Health and Illness* 4: 167–82.

Bury, M. (1986) 'Social constructionism and the development of medical sociology', *Sociology of Health and Illness*, 8: 137–69.

Busby, H. (2000) 'Writing about health and sickness: an analysis of contemporary autobiographical writing from the British Mass-Observation Archive', *Sociological Research Online*, 5(2) (www.socresonline.org.uk/5/2/busby.html).

Butler, J. (1990) *Gender trouble: feminism and the subversion of identity*. New York: Routledge.

Carmel, S. (2003) *High technology medicine in practice: the organisation of work in Intensive Care*. PhD Thesis, University of London.

CASP (Critical Appraisal Skills Programme) (2001) 10 Questions to help you make sense of qualitative research. Public Health Resource Unit. www.phru.nhs.uk/Pages/PHD/CASP.htm (accessed 9 July 2008).

Cassell, J. (1980) 'Ethical principles for conducting fieldwork', *American Anthropologist*, 82: 28–41.

Chamberlayne, P., Bornat, J. and Wengraf, T. (eds) (2000) *The turn to biographical methods in social science* London: Routledge.

Chambers, R. (1994) 'Participatory rural appraisal (PRA): analysis of experience', *World Development*, 22(9): 1253–68.

Chard, J.A., Lilford, R.J. and Court, B.V. (1997) 'Qualitative medical sociology: what are its crowning achievements?', *Journal of the Royal Society of Medicine*, 90: 604–9.

Charmaz, K. (1999) 'Stories of suffering: subjective tales and research narratives', *Qualitative Health Research*, 9: 362–82.

Charmaz, K (2006) *Constructing grounded theory: a practical guide through qualitative analysis*. London: Sage.

Charon, R. (2006) *Narrative medicine: honoring the stories of illness*. New York: Oxford University Press.

CIOMS (1991) *Ethics and epidemiology: international guidelines (Proceedings of the XXVth CIOMS Conference, 1990, Geneva)*. Geneva: Council for International Organizations of Medical Science.

Clark, J. and Mishler, E. (1992), 'Attending to patients' stories: reframing the clinical task', *Sociology of Health and Illness*, 14: 344–72.

Clifford, J. (1986a) 'On ethnographic allegory', in J. Clifford and G. Marcus (eds), *Writing culture: the poetics and politics of ethnography*. Berkeley: University of California Press, pp. 98–121.

Clifford, J. (1986b) 'Introduction: partial truths', in J. Clifford and G. Marcus (eds), *Writing culture: the poetics and politics of ethnography*. Berkeley: University of California Press, pp. 1–26.

Coffey, A., Holbrook, B. and Atkinson, P. (1996) 'Qualitative data analysis: technologies and representations', *Sociological Research Online*, 1(1) (www.socresonline.org.uk/socresonline/1/1/4.html).

Cooke, B. and Kothari, U. (2001) *Participation: the new tyranny*. London: Zed Books.

Coreil, J. (1995) 'Group interview methods in community health research', *Medical Anthropology*, 16: 193–210.

Cornwell, J. (1984) *Hard earned lives: accounts of health and illness from East London*. London: Tavistock.

Cortazzi, M. and Jin, L. (1997) 'Communication for learning across cultures', in D. McNamara and R. Harris (eds), *Overseas students in higher education: issues in teaching and learning*. London: Routledge, pp. 76–90.

Corti, L. and Thompson, P. (2004) 'Secondary analysis of archived data' in Seale, C., Gobo, G., Gubrium, J.F. and Silverman, D. (eds), *Qualitative research practice* London: Sage, pp. 297–313.

Cosby, N., Kelly, J.M. and Shaefer, P. (1986) 'Citizens' panels: a new approach to citizen participation', *Public Administration Review*, 46: 170–8.

Craig, G., Corden, A. and Thornton, P. (2000) *Safety in social research* (Social Research Update 29). Guildford: University of Surrey.

Danziger, R. (1998) 'HIV testing for HIV prevention: a comparative analysis of policies in Britain, Hungary and Sweden', *AIDS Care*, 10: 563–70.

Davison, C., Davey Smith, G. and Frankel, S. (1991) 'Lay epidemiology and the prevention paradox: the implications of coronary candidacy for health education', *Sociology of Health and Illness*, 13: 1–19.

Denzin, N.K. (1971) 'The logic of naturalistic inquiry', *Social Forces*, 50: 166–82.

Denzin, N.K. (1989a) *Interpretative biography* (Qualitative Research Methods Series 17). Newbury Park, CA: Sage.

Denzin, N.K. (1989b) 'Strategies of multiple triangulation', in *The research act: a theoretical introduction* (3rd edn). Englewood Cliffs, NJ: Prentice-Hall, pp. 234–47.

Denzin, N.K. (1994) 'The art and politics of interpretation', in N.K. Denzin and Y.S. Lincoln (eds), *Handbook of qualitative research*. London: Sage, pp. 500–15.

Denzin, N.K. and Lincoln, Y.S. (1998) 'Introduction: entering the field of qualitative research', in N.K. Denzin and Y.S. Lincoln (eds), *Strategies of qualitative inquiry*. Thousand Oaks, CA: Sage, pp. 1–34.

Desvouges, W.H. and Smith, V.K. (1988) 'Focus groups and risk communication: the "science" of listening to data', *Risk Analysis*, 8: 479–84.

Dexter, L.A. (1970) *Elite and specialized interviewing*. Evanston, IL: Northwestern University Press.

DiGiacomo, S. (1999) 'Can there be a cultural epidemiology?', *Medical Anthropology Quarterly*, 13: 436–57.

Digusto, E. (1994) 'Equity in authorship: a strategy for assigning credit when publishing', *Social Science and Medicine*, 38: 55–8.

Dixon-Woods, M., Shaw, R.L., Agarwal, S. and Smith, J.A. (2004) 'The problem of appraising qualitative research', *Quality and Safety in Health Care* 13: 223–25.

DOH (Department of Health) (2001) *Governance arrangements for NHS Research Ethics Committees*. London: DOH.

Draper, A., Green, J. and Dowler, E. (2002) *Public perceptions of BSE and CJD risk in Europe. Final Report for Task 1: Inter-country results and comparisons*. Geneva: WHO.

Edwards, R. (1990) 'Connecting method and epistemology: a white woman interviewing black women', *Women's Studies International Forum*, 13: 477–90.

Ehrich, K. (2001) 'It could be you', *Medical Sociology News*, 27: 23–4.

Esbensen, T.B., Dykes, S.K. and Hallberg, I.R. (2004) 'The meaning of having to live with cancer in old age', *European Journal of Cancer Care*, 13: 399–408.

Esposito, N. (2001) 'From meaning to meaning: the influence of translation techniques on non-English focus group research', *Qualitative Health Research*, 11: 568–79.

Evans, M., Stoddart, H., Condon, L., Freeman, E., Grizzell, M. and Mullen, R. (2001) 'Parents' perspectives on the MMR immunisation: a focus group study', *British Journal of General Practice*, 51: 904–10.

Evans, M.J. and Hallet, C.E. (2007) 'Living with dying: a hermeneutic phenomenological study of the work of hospice nurses', *Journal of Clinical Nursing*, 16: 742–51.

Fahim, H. (ed.) (1982) *Indigenous anthropology in non-Western countries*. Durham, NC: Carolina Academic Press.

Fielding, N. (1994) 'Getting into computer-aided qualitative data analysis', *ESRC Data Archive Bulletin* (September).

Fielding, N. (1995) 'Choosing the right qualitative software package', *ESRC Data Archive Bulletin*, 58 (May).

Finch, J. (1984) '"It's great to have someone to talk to": ethics and politics of interviewing women', in C. Bell and H. Roberts (eds), *Social researching: politics, problems and practice*. London: Routledge, pp. 70–87.

Fineman, N. (1991) 'The social construction of noncompliance: a study of health care and social service providers in everyday practice', *Sociology of Health and Illness*, 13: 354–75.

Frank, A.W. (1997) *The wounded story-teller: body, illness and ethics*. Chicago: University of Chicago Press.

Fox, N., Ward, K., and O'Rourke, A. (2005) 'Pro-anorexia, weight loss drugs and the internet: an "anti-recovery" explanatory model of anorexia', *Sociology of Health and Illness* 27: 944–71.

Gabbay, J. (1982) 'Asthma attacked?', in P. Wright and A. Treacher (eds), *The problems of medical knowledge: examining the social construction of medicine*. Edinburgh: Edinburgh University Press, pp. 23–48.

Gallagher, M., Hares, T., Spencer, J., Bradshaw, C. and Webb, I. (1993) 'The Nominal Group Technique: a research tool for general practice?', *Family Practice*, 10: 76–81.

Garfinkel, H. (1967) *Studies in ethnomethodology*. Englewood Cliffs, NJ: Prentice-Hall.

Geneau, R., Massae, P., Courtright, P., Lewallen, S. (2008) 'Using qualitative methods to understand the determinants of patients' willingness to pay for cataract surgery: A study of Tanzania', *Social Science and Medicine* 66: 558–68.

Gibbs, G (2007) *Analysing qualitative data*. London: Sage.

Gillon, R. (ed.) (1994) *Principles of health care ethics*. Chichester: John Wiley.

Glaser, B. and Strauss, A. (1967) *The discovery of grounded theory: strategies for qualitative research*. Chicago: Aldine.

Godin, B. and Gingras, Y. (2000) 'Impact of collaborative work on academic science', *Science and Public Policy*, 27: 65–73.

Goffman, E. (1963) *Stigma: notes on the management of a spoiled identity*. Englewood Cliffs, NJ: Prentice-Hall.

Goffman, E. (1968) *Asylums: essays on the social situation of mental patients and other inmates*. New York: Doubleday.

Gold, R.L. (1958) 'Roles in sociological field observation', *Social Forces*, 36: 217–23.

Gorard, S. (2002) *Ethics and equity: pursuing the perspectives of non-participants* (Social Research Update 39). Guildford: University of Surrey.

Gordon, D. (1988) 'Tenacious assumptions in Western medicine', in M. Lock and D. Gordon (eds), *Biomedicine examined*. Dordrecht: Kluwer Academic Publishers, pp. 19–56.

Graham, H. (1987) 'Women's smoking and family health', *Social Science and Medicine*, 25: 47–56.

Gray, J.A.M. (1997) *Evidence based health care: how to make health policy and management decisions*. Edinburgh: Churchill Livingstone.

Green, J. (1993a) 'The views of single handed general practitioners: a qualitative study', *British Medical Journal*, 307: 607–10.

Green, J. (1993b) *The problems faced by single handed general practitioners: study report*. London: Department of General Practice, UMDS.

Green, J. (1997) *Risk and misfortune*. London: UCL Press.

Green, J. (1999) 'From accidents to risk: public health and preventable injury', *Health, Risk and Society*, 1: 25–39.

Green, J. and Britten, N. (1998) 'Qualitative research and evidence based medicine', *British Medical Journal*, 316: 1230–4.

Green, J. and Hart, L. (1999) 'The impact of context on data', in R. Barbour and J. Kitzinger (eds), *Developing focus group research: politics, theory and practice*. London: Sage, pp. 21–35.

Green, J., Free, C. and Newman, T. (2002a) *Bilingual children/monolingual parents*. Final Report for ESRC, award number R000223433.

Green, J., Siddall, H. and Murdoch, I. (2002b) 'Learning to live with glaucoma: a qualitative study of diagnosis and the impact of sight loss', *Social Science and Medicine*, 55: 257–67.

Green, J., Draper, A. and Dowler, E. (2003) 'Short cuts to safety: risk and "rules of thumb" in accounts of food choice', *Health, Risk and Society*, 5: 33–52.

Greenhalgh, T. and Hurwitz, B. (1998) *Narrative based medicine: dialogue and discourse in clinical practice*. London: BMJ Books.

Griffiths, C., Kaur, G., Gantley, M., Feder, G., Hillier, S., Goddard, J. and Packe, G. (2001) 'Influences on hospital admission for asthma in south Asian and white adults: qualitative interview study', *British Medical Journal*, 323: 962–6.

Grinyer, A. (2002) *The anonymity of research participants: assumptions, ethics and practicalities* (Social Research Update 36). Guildford: University of Surrey.

Hahn, C. (2008) *Doing qualitative research using your computer.* London: Sage.

Hakim, C. (1982) *Secondary analysis in social research.* London: Allen & Unwin.

Hammersley, M. (1992a) 'So, what are case studies?', in *What's wrong with ethnography?* London: Routledge, pp. 183–200.

Hammersley, M. (1992b) 'By what criteria should ethnographic work be judged?', in *What's wrong with ethnography?* London: Routledge, pp. 57–82.

Hammersley, M. and Atkinson, P. (1983) *Ethnography: principles in practice.* London: Routledge.

Haraway, D. (1991) *Simians, cyborgs, and women: the re-invention of nature.* New York: Routledge.

Hardey, M. (1999) 'Doctor in the house: the internet as a source of lay health knowledge and the challenge to expertise', *Sociology of Health and Illness*, 21: 820–35.

Harding, S. (1986) *The science question in feminism.* Milton Keynes: Open University Press.

Harrison, B. (1996) 'Every picture "tells a story": uses of the visual in sociological research', in E.S. Lyon and J. Busfield (eds), *Methodological imaginations.* London: Macmillan, pp. 75–94.

Hart, C. (1998) *Doing a literature review: releasing the social science research imagination.* London: Sage.

Hart, E. and Bond, M. (1995) *Action research for health and social care: a guide to practice.* Buckingham: Open University Press.

Harvey, L. (1990) *Critical social research.* London: Unwin Hyman.

HCPO (Hopi Cultural Preservation Office) (2001) *HCPO policy and research* (www.nau.edu/~hcpo-p/hcpo/index.html).

Helman, C.G. (1978) 'Feed a cold, starve a fever', *Culture, Medicine and Psychiatry*, 2: 107–37.

Helman, C.G. (1984) *Culture, health and illness.* Bristol: Wright.

Henderson, L., Kitzinger, J. and Green, J. (2000) 'Representing infant feeding: content analysis of British media portrayals of bottle feeding and breast feeding', *British Medical Journal*, 321: 1196–8.

Henderson, L.J. (1935) 'Physician and patient as a social system', *New England Journal of Medicine*, 212: 819–23.

Herxheimer, A., McPherson, A., Miller, R., Shepperd, S., Yaphe, J. and Ziebland, S. (2000) 'Database of patients' experiences (DIPEx): a multi-media approach to sharing experiences and information', *Lancet*, 355: 1540–3.

Hinton, T. (1994) 'Researching homelessness and access to health care', *Critical Public Health*, 5: 33–8.

Holden, P. (1991) 'Colonial sisters: nurses in Uganda', in P. Holden and J. Littlewood (eds), *Anthropology and nursing.* London: Routledge, pp. 67–83.

Holstein, J. and Gubrium, J. (1998) 'Phenomenology, ethnomethodology and interpretive practice' in Denzin, N.K. and Lincoln, Y.S. (eds), *Strategies of Qualitative Inquiry.* Thousand Oaks: Sage.

Homan, R. (1991) *The ethics of social research.* London: Longman.

Hughes, D. (1989) 'Paper and people: the work of the casualty reception clerk', *Sociology of Health and Illness*, 11: 382–408.

Husserl, E. (1970) *Logical investigation.* New York: Humanities Press.

Inhorn, M. (1995) 'Medical anthropology and epidemiology: divergences or convergences?', *Social Science and Medicine*, 40: 285–90.

International Committee of Medical Journal Editors (1991) 'Uniform requirements for manuscripts submitted to biomedical journals', *British Medical Journal*, 302: 338–41.

Irigaray, L. (1985) *The sex which is not one*, trans. Catherine Porter with Carolyn Burke. Ithaca, NY: Cornell University Press.

James, M. (1994) 'Historical research methods', in K. McConway (ed.), *Studying health and disease.* Buckingham: Open University Press.

Jeffrey, R. (1979) 'Normal rubbish: deviant patients in casualty departments', *Sociology of Health and Illness*, 1: 90–107.

Jewkes, R., Abrahams, N. and Mvo, Z. (1998) 'Why do nurses abuse patients? Reflections from South African nursing obstetric services', *Social Science and Medicine*, 47: 1781–95.

Jones, K. (2004) 'Mission drift in qualitative research, or moving toward systematic review of qualitative studies, moving back to a more systematic narrative review'. *The Qualitative Report*, 9(1): 95–112.

Katainen, A. (2006) 'Challenging the imperative of health? Smoking and justification of risk taking', *Critical Public Health*, 16: 295–305.

Kaufert, P. (1988) 'Menopause as process or event: the creation of definitions in bio-medicine', in M. Lock and D. Gordon (eds), *Biomedicine examined.* Dordrecht: Kluwer Academic Publishers, pp. 331–50.

Kelly, M.J. (2004) 'Qualitative evaluation research' in C. Seale, G. Gobo, J.F. Gubrium, and D. Silverman, (eds), *Qualitative Research Practice.* London: Sage.

Kendall, C., Foote, D. and Martorell, R. (1984) 'Ethnomedicine and oral rehydration therapy: a case study of ethnomedical investigation and program planning', *Social Science and Medicine*, 19: 253–60.

Khan, M.E. and Manderson, L. (1992) 'Focus groups in tropical diseases research', *Health Policy and Planning*, 7: 56–66.

Kitzinger, C. (1987) *The social construction of lesbianism.* London: Sage.

Kitzinger, J. (1990) 'Audience understandings of AIDS messages: a discussion of methods', *Sociology of Health and Illness*, 12: 319–35.

Kitzinger, J. (1994) 'The methodology of focus groups: the importance of interaction between the research participants', *Sociology of Health and Illness*, 16: 103–21.

Kleinman, A. (1973) 'Toward a comparative study of medical systems: an integrated approach to the study of the relationship of medicine and culture', *Science, Medicine and Man*, 1: 55–65.

Koch, T. and Kralik, D. (2006) *Participatory action research in health care.* Oxford: Blackwell Publishing.

Krueger, R. and Casey, M.A. (2000) *Focus groups: a practical guide for applied research* (3rd edn). Thousand Oaks, CA: Sage.

Labov, W. and Waletzky, J. (1967) 'Narrative analysis: oral versions of personal experience', *Journal of Narrative and Life History*, 7: 3–38.

Lacerda, E. (2008) *Water pollution and health: a case study of a participatory research journey with a marisqueira community in Northeast Brazil.* PhD Thesis, University of London.

Lambert, H. (1998) 'Methods and meanings in anthropological, epidemiological and clinical encounters: the case of sexually transmitted disease and human immunodeficiency virus control and prevention in India', *Tropical Medicine and International Health*, 3(12): 1002–10.

Lawler, J. (1991) *Behind the screens: nursing, somology and the problem of the body.* London: Churchill Livingstone.

Lawson, A. (1991) 'Whose side are we on now? Ethical issues in social research and medical practice', *Social Science and Medicine*, 32: 591–9.

Lenaghan, J. (1999) 'Involving the public in rationing decisions: the experience of citizens' juries', *Health Policy*, 49: 45–61.

Lévi-Strauss, C. (1966) *The savage mind.* Chicago: University of Chicago Press.

Lewando-Hundt, G. (2000) 'Multiple scripts and contested discourse in disseminating research findings', *Social Policy and Administration*, 34: 419–33.

Lewando-Hundt, G. (2001) '"Good" reasons for "bad" records: the social, political and cultural context of vital registration', in M. MacLachlan (ed.), *Cultivating health: cultural perspectives on promoting health.* Chichester: John Wiley, pp. 37–53.

Lewando-Hundt, G., Abed, Y., Skeik, M., Beckerleg, S. and El Alem, A. (1999) 'Addressing birth in Gaza: using qualitative methods to improve vital registration', *Social Science and Medicine*, 48: 833–43.

Lewin, K. (1946) 'Action research and minority problems' *Journal of Social Issues.* 2: 34–46.

Lewin, S., Daniels, K., Dick, J., Zwarenstein, M. and van der Walt, H. (2002) *A qualitative evaluation of the Kopana TB training intervention.* Internal Report, Health Systems Research Unit, Medical Research Council of South Africa.

Lewins, A. and Silver, C. (2007) *Using software in qualitative research: a step by step guide.* London: Sage.

Leydon, G. and Green, J. (2001) *The management of information in out-patient oncology consultations.* Final Report for ESRC, award number R000223142.

Leydon, G., Boulton, M., Moynihan, C., Jones, A., Mossman, J., Boudioni, M. and McPherson, K. (2000) 'Cancer patients' information needs and help seeking behaviour: an in-depth interview study', *British Medical Journal*, 320: 909–13.

Lofland, J. (1971) *Analyzing social settings.* Belmont, CA: Wadsworth Publishing Company.

Lomax, H. and Casey, N. (1998) 'Recording social life: reflexivity and video methodology', *Sociological Research Online* 3(2) (www.socresonline.org.uk/socresonline/3/2/1.html).

Loseke, D. and Cahill, S.E. (2004) 'Publishing qualitative manuscripts: lessons learned' in Seale, C., Gobo, G., Gubrium, J.F. and Silverman, D. (eds), *Qualitative research practice* London: Sage.

Lupton, D. (1994) *Medicine as culture: illness, disease and the body in Western society.* London: Sage.

Madden, J.M., Quick, J.D., Ross-Degnan, D. and Kafle, K.K. (1997) 'Undercover careseekers: simulated clients in the study of health provider behaviour in developing countries', *Social Science and Medicine*, 45: 1465–82.

Martin, G. P. (2008) '"Ordinary people only": knowledge, representativeness, and the publics of public participation in health care', *Sociology of Health and Illness*, 30: 35–54.

Mason, J. (1996) *Qualitative researching.* London: Sage.

Maynard, D. (1991) 'Interaction and asymmetry in clinical discourse', *American Journal of Sociology*, 97: 448–95.

Mays, N. and Pope, C. (1999) 'Quality in qualitative health research', in C. Pope and N. Mays (eds), *Qualitative research in health care* (2nd edn). London: BMJ Books, pp. 89–101.

Mays, N., Roberts, E. and Popay, J. (2001) 'Synthesising research evidence', in N. Fulop, P. Allen, A. Clarke and N. Black, (eds), *Studying the organisation and delivery of health services: research methods.* London: Routledge.

Meyer, J. (2000) 'Using qualitative methods in health related action research'. *British Medical Journal*, 320: 178–81.

Meyer, J.(1993) 'New paradigm research in practice: the trials and tribulations of action research', *Journal of Advanced Nursing*, 18: 106–72.

Meyer, J.(1997) 'Action research in health care practice: nature, present concerns and future possibilities', *Nursing Times Research*, 2: 175–84.

Milburn, K., Fraser, E., Secker, J. and Pavis, S. (1995) 'Combining methods in health promotion research: some considerations about appropriate use', *Health Education Journal*, 54: 347–56.

Miles, M.B. and Huberman, A.M. (1994) *Qualitative data analysis: an expanded sourcebook* (2nd edn). Thousand Oaks, CA: Sage.

Mills, E., Jahad, A.R., Ross, C. and Wilson, K. (2005) 'Systematic review of qualitative studies exploring parental beliefs and attitudes toward childhood vaccination identifies common barriers to vaccination'. *Journal of Clinical Epidemiology*, 58: 1081–8.

Monaghan, L.F. (2003) 'Danger on the doors: bodily risk in a demonised occupation', *Health, Risk and Society*, 5: 11–32.

Montgomery, C.M., Lees, S., Stadler, J., Morar, N.S., Ssali, A., Mwanza, B., Mntambo, M., Phillips, J., Watts, C. and Pool, R. (2008) 'The role of partnership dynamics in determining the acceptability of condoms and microbicides', *AIDS Care*, 20(6): 733–40.

Morrow, V. and Richards, M. (1996) 'The ethics of social research with children: an overview', *Children and Society*, 10: 90–105.

Morse, J. (2002) 'A comment on comments', *Qualitative Health Research*, 12: 3–4.

Munodawafa, D., Gwede, C. and Mubayira, C. (1995) 'Using focus groups to develop HIV education among adolescent females in Zimbabwe', *Health Promotion International*, 10: 85–92.

Murphy, M.K., Black, N., Lamping, D.L., McKee, C.M., Sanderson, C.F.B., Askham, J., and Marteau, T. (1998) 'Consensus development methods, and their use in clinical guideline development', *Health Technology Assessment*, 2(3): 1–88.

Murphy, E., Dingwall, R., Greatbatch, D. et al. (1998) 'Qualitative research methods in health technology assessment: a review of the literature', *Health Technology Assessment*, 2(16): 1–276.

Murphy, E. and Dingwall, R. (2003) *Qualitative methods and health policy research*. New York: Aldine de Gruyter.

NCB (Nuffield Council on Bioethics) (2003) *The ethics of research related to health care in developing countries*. London: Nuffield Foundation.

Nettleton, S. (1992) *Power, pain and dentistry*. Buckingham: Open University Press.

Noblit, G.W. and Hare, R.D. (1988) *Meta-ethnography: synthesizing qualitative studies*. Newbury Park, CA: Sage.

Ntau, C.G. (2002) 'Medical careers of Botswana doctors' (Report from the Phil Strong Prize), *Medical Sociology News*, 28(3): 9–12.

Oakley, A. (1981) 'Interviewing women: a contradiction in terms?', in H. Roberts (ed.), *Doing feminist research*. London: Routledge, pp. 30–61.

Oakley, A. (1990) 'Who's afraid of randomised controlled trials?', in H. Roberts (ed.), *Women's health counts*. London: Routledge, pp. 167–94.

Ogden, J.A. and Porter, J.D.H. (2000) 'The politics of partnership in tropical public health: researching tuberculosis control in India', *Social Policy and Administration*, 34: 377–91.

Oinas, E. (1998) 'Medicalisation by whom? Accounts of menstruation conveyed by young women and medical experts in medical advisory columns', *Sociology of Health and Illness*, 20: 52–70.

O'Laughlin, B. (1998) 'Interpreting institutional discourses', in Thomas, A., Chataway, J. and M. Wuyts (eds), *Finding out fast: investigative skills for policy and development*. London: Sage, pp. 107–26.

Opala, J. and Boillot, F. (1996) 'Leprosy among the Limba: illness and healing in the context of world view', *Social Science and Medicine*, 42: 3–19.

Paine, K., Hart, G., Jawo, M., Ceesay, S., Jallow, M., Merison, L., Walraven, G., McAdam, K. and Shaw, M. (2002) '"Before we were sleeping, now we are awake": preliminary evaluation of the Stepping Stones sexual health programme in The Gambia', *African Journal of AIDS Research*, 1: 41–52.

Palmer, D. (2000) 'Identifying delusional discourse: issues of rationality, reality and power', *Sociology of Health and Illness*, 22: 661–78.

Patterson, M. (2008) 'Narratives of events: Labovian narrative analysis and its limitations'. In M. Andrews, C. Squire and M. Tamboukou, (eds), *Doing narrative research*. London: Sage, pp. 22–40.

Patton, M.Q. (1990) *Qualitative evaluation and research methods* (2nd edn). Newbury Park, CA: Sage.

Pelto, P.J. and Pelto, G.H. (1992) 'Developing applied medical anthropology in third world countries: problems and action', *Social Science and Medicine*, 35: 1389–95.

Peräkylä, A. and Silverman, D. (1991) 'Reinterpreting speech exchange systems: communication formats in AIDS counselling', *Sociology*, 25: 627–51.

Petticrew, M. (2001) 'Systematic reviews from astronomy to zoology: myths and misconceptions', *British Medical Journal*, 322: 89–101.

Pinder, R. (2007) 'On movement and stillness', *Ethnography*, 8(1): 99–116.

Plummer, K. (1983) *Documents of life: an introduction to the problems and literature of a humanistic method*. London: Unwin Hyman.

Pool, R. (1994) *Dialogue and the interpretation of illness: conversations in a Cameroon village*. Oxford: Berg.

Popay, J., Rogers, A. and Williams, G. (1998) 'Rationale and standards for the systematic review of qualitative literature in health services research', *Qualitative Health Research*, 8: 341–51.

Pope, C. (1991) 'Trouble in store: some thoughts on the management of waiting lists', *Sociology of Health and Illness*, 13: 193–212.

Pope, C. (2002) 'Contingency in everyday surgical work', *Sociology of Health and Illness*, 24: 369–84.

Potter, J. and Wetherell, M. (1987) *Discourse and social psychology: beyond attitudes and behaviour*. London: Sage.

Pound, P., Britten, N., Morgan, M., Yardley, L., Pope, C., Daker-White, and Campbell, R. (2005) 'Resisting medicines: a synthesis of qualitative studies of medicine taking', *Social Science and Medicine*, 61: 133–55.

Prior, L., Chun, P.L. and Huat, S.B. (2000) 'Beliefs and accounts of illness: views from two Cantonese-speaking communities in England', *Sociology of Health and Illness*, 22: 815–39.

Prior, P. (1995) 'Surviving psychiatric institutionalisation: a case study', *Sociology of Health and Illness*, 17: 651–67.

Rapley, T.J. (2001) 'The art(fulness) of open-ended interviewing: some considerations on analysing interviews', *Qualitative Research*, 1: 303–23.

Reason, P. (1998) 'Three approaches to participative inquiry', in N.K. Denzin and Y.S. Lincoln (eds), *Strategies of qualitative inquiry*. London: Sage, pp. 261–91.

Richards, L. (1999) *Using NVivo in qualitative research*. London: Sage.

Richardson, L. (2000) 'Evaluating ethnography', *Qualitative Inquiry*, 6: 253–5.

Richman, J. (2000) 'Coming out of intensive care crazy: dreams of affliction', *Qualitative Health Research*, 10: 84–102.

Riessman, C.K. (2005) 'Exporting ethics: a narrative about narrative research in South India', *health: an interdisciplinary journal for the social study of health, illness and medicine*, 9(4): 473–90.

Riessman, C.K. (2008) *Narrative methods for the human sciences*. Thousand Oaks, CA: Sage.

Rifkin, S. (1996) 'Rapid rural appraisal: its use and value for health planners and managers', *Public Administration*, 74: 509–26.

Riley, T., Hawe, P. and Shiell, A. (2005) 'Contested ground: how should qualitative evidence inform the conduct of a community intervention trial?', *Journal of Health Services Research Policy*, 10(2): 103–10.

Ritchie, J. and Spencer, L. (1994) 'Qualitative data analysis for applied policy research', in A. Bryman and R.G. Burgess (eds), *Analyzing qualitative data*. London: Routledge, pp. 173–94.

Rogers, A. and Pilgrim, D. (1995) 'The risk of resistance: perspectives on the mass childhood immunisation programme', in J. Gabe (ed.), *Medicine, health and risk: sociological approaches*. Oxford: Blackwell, pp. 73–90.

Rosenhan, D.L. (1973) 'On being sane in insane places', *Science*, 179: 250–8.

Rowe, G. and Frewer, L.J. (2000) 'Public participation methods: a framework for evaluation', *Science, Technology and Human Value*, 25: 3–29.

Sackett, D.L., Rosenberg, W., Gray, J.A.M., Hayne, R.B. and Richardson, W.S. (1996) 'Evidence based medicine: what it is and what it isn't', *British Medical Journal*, 312: 71–2.

Sacks, H. (1989) 'Lecture four: an impromptu survey of the literature', *Human Studies*, 12: 253–9.

Scheper-Hughes, N. (1979) *Saints, scholars and schizophrenics: mental illness in Northern Ireland*. Berkeley: University of California Press.

Scheper-Hughes, N. (2000) 'Ire in Ireland', *Ethnography*, 1: 117–40.

Schneider, H. and Palmer, N. (2002) 'Getting to the truth? Researching user views of primary health care', *Health Policy and Planning*, 17: 32–41.

Schutz, A. (1964) *Studies in social theory*. The Hague: Martinus Nijhoft.

Schutz, A. (1970) *On phenomenology and social relations*. Chicago: University of Chicago Press.

Schwartzman, H. (1993) *Ethnography in organizations*. (Qualitative Research Methods Series 27). London: Sage.

Scott, P. (1999) 'Black people's health: ethnic status and research issues', in S. Hood, B. Mayall and S. Oliver (eds), *Critical issues in social research*. Buckingham: Open University Press, pp. 80–93.

Scrimshaw, S.C.M. and Hurtado, E. (1988) 'Anthropological involvement in the Central American diarrheal disease control project', *Social Science and Medicine*, 27: 97–105.

Seale, C. (1999) *The quality of qualitative research*. London: Sage.

Sennett, R. (2003) *Respect: the formation of character in an age of inequality*. London: Penguin.

Shakespeare, T. (1999) '"Losing the plot?": medical and activist discourses of contemporary genetics and disability', *Sociology of Health and Illness*, 21: 669–88.

Silverman, D. (1985) *Qualitative methodology and sociology*. Aldershot: Gower.

Silverman, D. (1993) *Interpreting qualitative data: methods for analysing talk, text and interaction*. London: Sage.

Silverman, D. (1998) 'The quality of qualitative health research: the open-ended interview and its alternatives', *Social Sciences in Health*, 4: 104–18.

Sim, J. and Madden, S. (2008) 'Illness experience in fibromyalgia syndrome: a meta-synthesis of qualitative studies', *Social Science and Medicine*, 67: 57–67.

Sinclair J. and Green, J. (2005) 'Understanding resolution of deliberate self harm: a qualitative interview study of patients' experiences', *British Medical Journal*, 330: 1112–6.

Smith, D. (1988) *The everyday world as problematic: a feminist sociology*. Milton Keynes: Open University Press.

Smith, R. (1997) 'Authorship: time for a paradigm shift?', *British Medical Journal*, 314: 992.

Snowdon, C., Garcia, J. and Elbourne, D. (1997) 'Making sense of randomization: responses of parents of critically ill babies to random allocation of treatment in a clinical trial', *Social Science and Medicine*, 45: 1337–55.

Stadler, J., Delany, S. and Mntambo, M. (2008) 'Women's perceptions and experiences of HIV prevention trials in Soweto, South Africa', *Social Science and Medicine*, 66: 189–200.

Stern, G. and Kruckman, L. (1983) 'Multi-disciplinary perspectives on post-partum depression: an anthropological critique', *Social Science and Medicine*, 17: 1027–41.

Stimson, G. and Webb, B. (1975) *Going to see the doctor: the consultation process in general practice*. London: Routledge & Kegan Paul.

Stone, L. and Campbell, J.G. (1984) 'The use and misuse of surveys in international development: an experiment from Nepal', *Human Organization*, 43: 27–37.

Strauss, A. (1987) *Qualitative analysis for social scientists*. Cambridge: Cambridge University Press.

Strauss, A. and Corbin, J. (1990) *Basics of qualitative research: grounded theory procedures and techniques.* Newbury Park, CA: Sage.

Temple, B. (1997) 'Watch your tongue: issues in translation and cross cultural research', *Sociology*, 31: 389–408.

ten Have, P. (1999) *Doing conversation analysis: a practical guide.* London: Sage.

Thomé, B., Esbensen, B.A., Dykes, A.-K. and Hallenberg, I.R. (2004) 'The meaning of having to live with cancer in old age', *European Journal of Cancer Care'*, 13: 399–408.

Thorogood, N. (1988) *Health and the management of daily life amongst women of Afro-Caribbean origin in Hackney.* University of London.

Thorogood, N. (1997) 'Questioning science', *British Dental Journal*, 183(5): 152–5.

Thoutenhoofd, E. (1998) 'Method in a photographic enquiry of being deaf', *Sociological Research Online*, 3(2) (www.socresonline.org.uk/socresonline/3/2/2.html).

Turner, V. (1967) *The forest of symbols: aspects of Ndembu ritual.* Ithaca, NY: Cornell University Press.

van der Geest, S. and Sarkodie, S. (1998) 'The fake patient: a research experiment in a Ghanaian hospital', *Social Science and Medicine*, 47: 1373–81.

VanderStaay, S.L. (2003) 'Believing Clayboy', *Qualitative Inquiry*, 9: 374–94.

Viney, L.L. and Bousfield, L. (1991) 'Narrative analysis: a method of psychosocial research for AIDS-affected people', *Social Science and Medicine*, 32(7): 757–65.

Vissandjée, B., Abdool, S. and Dupéré, S. (2002) 'Focus groups in rural Gujarat, India: a modified approach', *Qualitative Health Research*, 12: 826–43.

Wallerstein, N. and Bernstein, E. (1988) 'Empowerment education: Freire's ideas adapted to health education', *Health Education Quarterly*, 15(4): 379–94.

Watson, T. and de Bruin, G.P. (2007) 'Impact of cutaneous disease on the self-concept: An existential-phenomenological study of men and women with psoriasis', *Dermatology Nursing*, 19(4): 351–64.

Waxler-Morrison, N.E. (1988) 'Plural medicine in Sri Lanka: do Ayurvedic and Western medical practices differ?', *Social Science and Medicine*, 27: 531–44.

Webb, E.J., Campbell, D.T., Schwarz, R.D. and Sechrest, L. (1977) 'The use of archival sources in social research', in M. Bulmer (ed.), *Sociological research methods: an introduction.* London: Macmillan, pp. 113–30.

Wellings, K., Field, J., Johnson, A. and Wadsworth, J. (1994) *Sexual behaviour in Britain: the National Survey of Sexual Attitudes and Lifestyles.* Harmondsworth: Penguin.

Wenger, G.C. (1987) *The research relationship: practice and politics in social policy research.* London: Allen & Unwin.

Wengraf, T. (2001) *Qualitative research interviewing: biographical narrative and semi-structured interviews.* London: Sage.

West, P. (1990) 'The status and validity of accounts obtained at interview: a contrast between two studies of families with a disabled child', *Social Science and Medicine*, 30: 1229–39.

Whyte, W.F. (with K.K. Whyte) (1984) *Learning from the field: a guide from experience.* London: Sage.

Williams, C. and Heikes, E.J. (1993) 'The importance of researcher's gender in the in-depth interview: evidence from two case studies of male nurses', *Gender and Society* 7: 280–91.

Wilkinson, S. and Kitzinger, C. (2000) 'Thinking differently about thinking positive', *Social Science and Medicine*, 50: 797–811.

Winch, P. (1999) 'The role of anthropological methods in a community-based mosquito net intervention in Bagamoyo District, Tanzania', in R. Hahn (ed.), *Anthropology in public health: bridging differences in culture and society.* Oxford: Oxford University Press, pp. 44–62.

Wittig, M. (1992) *The straight mind and other essays.* Boston, MA: Beacon.

WMA General Assembly (2000) *World Medical Association Declaration of Helsinki: ethical principles for medical research involving human subjects.*

Wolcott, H. (2002) 'Writing up qualitative work ... better', *Qualitative Health Research*, 12: 91–104.

Wolff, B., Knodel, J. and Sittitrai, W. (1993) 'Focus groups and surveys as complementary research methods', in D. Morgan (ed.), *Successful focus groups: advancing the state of the art*. London: Sage, pp. 118–36.

Wright Mills, C. (1959) *The sociological imagination*. Oxford: Oxford University Press.

Yach, D. (1992) 'The use and value of qualitative methods in health research in developing countries', *Social Science and Medicine*, 35: 603–12.

Yin, R.K. (1994) *Case study research: design and methods* (2nd edn). London: Sage.

Index